Diagnosis and Treatment of Pulmonary Hypertension

Yoshihiro Fukumoto

Editor

Diagnosis and Treatment of Pulmonary Hypertension

From Bench to Bedside

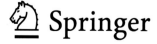 Springer

Editor
Yoshihiro Fukumoto
Department of Internal Medicine
Kurume University School of Medicine
Kurume, Japan

ISBN 978-981-287-839-7   ISBN 978-981-287-840-3   (eBook)
DOI 10.1007/978-981-287-840-3

Library of Congress Control Number: 2016961246

Printed on acid-free paper

This Springer imprint is published by Springer Nature
The registered company is Springer Nature Singapore Pte Ltd.
The registered company address is: 152 Beach Road, #22-06/08 Gateway East, Singapore 189721,
Singapore

Preface

Scientific and clinical advances continue progressively in the field of pulmonary hypertension (PH). As the accumulated evidence expands, it is important to adapt our systems to keep up with the progress. In maintaining established diagnostics and therapeutics, we have to go forward with the new advances and their potentials. PH, defined as a mean pulmonary arterial pressure (PAP) ≥ 25 mmHg at rest as assessed by right heart catheterization, is characterized by elevated pulmonary arterial pressure and increased pulmonary vascular resistance. The classification of PH has been updated, in which five major categories of the disorder are classified, including (Group 1) pulmonary arterial hypertension (PAH), (Group 2) PH due to left heart disease, (Group 3) PH due to lung diseases and/or hypoxia, (Group 4) chronic thromboembolic PH, and (Group 5) others.

Especially Group 1, PAH, is caused by small pulmonary artery obstruction due to vascular proliferation and remodeling, defined as mean PAP ≥ 25 mmHg and pulmonary capillary wedge pressure (PCWP) ≤ 15 mmHg, which is characterized by the presence of pre-capillary PH in the absence of other causes of pre-capillary PH, such as PH due to lung diseases, chronic thromboembolic pulmonary hypertension (CTEPH), or other rare diseases. The pathological changes in the pulmonary arteries in PAH include endothelial injury, proliferation and hypercontraction of vascular smooth muscle cells (VSMC), and migration of inflammatory cells. Pulmonary veno-occlusive diseases and/or pulmonary capillary hemangiomatosis (Group 1′) should be a distinct category but not completely separated from PAH as they share similar characteristics with idiopathic PAH (IPAH) but also demonstrate some differences.

Group 4, CTEPH, is caused by mechanical obstruction of pulmonary arteries due to residual pulmonary thromboembolism or in situ thrombosis, which may be initiated or aggravated by abnormalities in either the clotting cascade, endothelial cells, or platelets. Although inflammatory infiltrates are commonly detected in pulmonary endarterectomy specimens, it remains unknown whether thrombosis or platelet dysfunction is a cause or a consequence of the disorder. It has been reported that the plasma levels of factor VIII or thrombin-activatable fibrinolysis inhibitor (TAFI) is elevated in patients with CTEPH. CTEPH is regarded as a consequence of pulmonary thromboembolism (PTE) due to venous thromboembolism (VTE); however, the occurrence of CTEPH in patients with acute PTE or deep venous thrombosis is rare. Thus, it is highly possible that the pathophysiology is different between PAH and CTEPH.

PH remains a fatal disease, leading to right ventricular failure and premature death. As lifestyle modification, heavy physical activity, or isotonic exercise often causes right ventricular failure in patients with PAH/CTEPH, they should be avoided. Thus, low-level exercise is recommended in the daily life of those with PAH/CTEPH, because a low level of physical training rather improves endothelial function, exercise capacity, and quality of life. Further, high altitudes and infections should also be avoided, because a high altitude may produce hypoxic pulmonary vasoconstriction, and infections are fatal in some patients with PH.

Although significant research progress has been made in the pathogenesis of PH, the detailed mechanisms of the disorder remain to be elucidated. Also in a clinical situation, significant progress has been made for both diagnosis (e.g., new imaging techniques) and treatment (e.g., the new endothelin receptor blockers riociguat or selexipag); however, more effective and less-invasive diagnostic and/or therapeutic tools should be developed.

Although a detailed accounting of the new findings described in the book is not feasible within the narrow confines of this preface, I, as editor, would like to summarize the parts of it briefly. Part I includes the fundamentals of PH: clinical classification (Prof. Koichiro Tatsumi) and imaging for diagnosis (Drs. Nobuhiro Tahara and Yoshihiro Fukumoto). Part II focuses on pathophysiology and genetics: the role of microRNA (Dr. Aleksandra Babicheva and Prof. Jason X.-J. Yuan), sex hormone (Dr. Kaori Oshima and Prof. Masahiko Oka), Rho-kinase (Dr. Kimio Satoh and Prof. Hiroaki Shimokawa), proteinase-activated receptor 1 (Prof. Katsuya Hirano), animal models (Dr. Kohtaro Abe), human pathology (Drs. Hatsue Ishibashi-Ueda and Keiko Ohta-Ogo), and BMPR2 (Dr. Yoshihide Mitani). Part III describes the treatment of PAH: prostacyclin (Dr. Satoshi Akagi), NO-sGC-cGMP pathway (Prof. Hiroshi Watanabe and Prof. Quang-Kim Tran), endothelin receptor antagonist (Prof. Noriaki Emoto), and lung transplantation (Prof. Hiroshi Date). Part IV features the treatment of CTEPH: medical therapy (Prof. Toru Satoh), balloon pulmonary angioplasty (Drs. Hiromi Matsubara and Aiko Ogawa), and pulmonary endarterectomy (Prof. Hitoshi Ogino). The last section (Part V) focuses on right ventricular function (Drs. Kaoru Dohi and Norikazu Yamada and Prof. Masaaki Ito).

This book describes the significant progress in the understanding of PAH and CTEPH. Regarding pathophysiology of the disorders, diagnosis, and treatment, several new options have appeared in this decade, and some are under clinical trials. The usefulness of these new drugs remains to be fully examined in future studies. In this book, the experts in the field have written special articles regarding the recent progress in their own fields. I am indebted to all authors for their considerable time and effort to create high-quality articles and sincerely hope that this book can be a great help in the management of PH in terms of clinical classification, pathophysiology, genetics, diagnosis, and treatment.

Kurume, Japan   Yoshihiro Fukumoto

Contents

Part I
Fundamentals of Pulmonary Hypertension

Chapter 1
Clinical Classification

Koichiro Tatsumi

Abstract The clinical classification of pulmonary hypertension is intended to categorize in five groups of multiple clinical conditions according to similar clinical presentation, pathological findings, hemodynamic characteristics, and treatment strategy, as follows: (1) pulmonary arterial hypertension (PAH), (2) pulmonary hypertension due to left heart disease, (3) pulmonary hypertension due to lung diseases and/or hypoxia, (4) chronic thromboembolic pulmonary hypertension (CTEPH) and other pulmonary artery obstructions, and (5) pulmonary hypertension with unclear and/or multifactorial mechanisms.

Keywords Pulmonary arterial hypertension • Heritable pulmonary arterial hypertension • Nice classification • Panvasculopathy

1.1 Important Pathophysiological and Clinical Definitions of PH

The field of pathobiology and pathophysiology of pulmonary hypertension (PH) has undergone impressive growth, while the cross-link between the genetics and molecular pathogenesis has been a continued interest among various types of PH. PH is a pathophysiological disorder that may be associated with cardiovascular and respiratory diseases. Before clinical classification of PH, clinical definitions of PH should be verified. Important pathophysiological and clinical definitions of PH are described in the 2015 European Society of Cardiology (ESC) and the European Respiratory Society (ERS) guidelines for the diagnosis and treatment of pulmonary hypertension [1]:

1. Pulmonary hypertension (PH) is a hemodynamic and pathophysiological condition defined as an increase in mean pulmonary arterial pressure (mPAP)

K. Tatsumi (✉)
Department of Respirology, Graduate School of Medicine, Chiba University,
1-8-1, Inohana, Chuo-ku, Chiba 260-8670, Japan
e-mail: tatsumi@faculty.chiba-u.jp

© Springer Science+Business Media Singapore 2017
Y. Fukumoto (ed.), *Diagnosis and Treatment of Pulmonary Hypertension*,
DOI 10.1007/978-981-287-840-3_1

$\geq$25 mmHg at rest as assessed by right heart catheterization (RHC). PH can be found in multiple clinical conditions.

2. Pulmonary arterial hypertension (PAH, group 1) is a clinical condition characterized by the presence of precapillary PH and pulmonary vascular resistance (PVR) >3 Wood units, in the absence of other causes of precapillary PH such as PH due to lung diseases, chronic thromboembolic PH (CTEPH), or other rare diseases. PAH includes different forms that share a similar clinical picture and virtually identical pathological changes of the lung microcirculation.

3. There is no sufficient data to support the definition of "PH on exercise."

1.2 Definition of Pulmonary Hypertension

Clinical classification should be based on the updated theoretical and practical information on the management of patients with PH. PH is defined hemodynamically by mPAP $\geq$ 25 mmHg at rest measured by RHC [1]. Available data have shown that the normal mPAP at rest is 14 ± 3 mmHg with an upper limit of normal of approximately 20 mmHg [2, 3]. Due to the lack of reliable data that define which levels of exercise-induced changes in mPAP or PVR have prognostic implications, a disease entity "PH on exercise" cannot be defined [1, 4]. There are still insufficient data to introduce the term of "borderline PH" for patients with mPAP levels between 21 and 24 mmHg, especially because the prognostic and therapeutic implications remain unknown [2]. Patients with mPAP values between 21 and 24 mm Hg should be carefully followed, in particular when they are at risk for developing PAH such as patients with connective tissue disease (CTD) and family members of patients with idiopathic pulmonary arterial hypertension (IPAH) or heritable pulmonary arterial hypertension (HPAH). The individual cellular and molecular alterations of the pulmonary vasculature lie under each category of the clinical classification, although the definition of PH is rather simple physiological one. That is why the clinical classification of PH should be taken into account when treating patients with pulmonary hypertension.

1.3 How Can We Put All Types of Pulmonary Hypertension Together?

The answer to this question requires the consideration of two different aspects. First, the integration of multiple levels of data (hemodynamic, pathophysiological, and genetic) has the potential to deliver clinically relevant outcomes from each type of pulmonary hypertension, including the identification of pathological changes, biomarker validation, prognosis, and new therapeutic targets identification, all of which are important in the management of pulmonary hypertension. The second aspect has to do with the best way to implement all this new information in real clinical practice. The obstructive lung panvasculopathy seems to be similar in various types of pulmonary hypertension, although genetic susceptibility, acquired factors, and perivascular microenvironment pathology are different among them. The current treatment strategies have been continuously constructed in PAH, while other types of PH have no definitive information regarding the specific therapies. However, any common clinical characteristic may exist among the different types of PH. Needless to say a therapeutic system has not been well established in PH as a whole. Yet any therapeutic option is not difficult to search for and may come from other fields in clinical practice. To achieve the total understanding of PH, we need to receive multidimensional information. During the process, physicians can provide a better personalized treatment of a given patient. The personalized treatment of PH could pave the way toward the future incorporation of omics data.

1.4 From Evian to Nice

The 2nd World Symposium on pulmonary hypertension [3] held in Evian (1998) has established a clinical classification of pulmonary hypertension in order to individualize different categories of pulmonary hypertension sharing similar pathophysiological findings, similar hemodynamic characteristics, and similar management. Five groups of distinct disease entities that cause PH were identified: pulmonary arterial hypertension (group 1), pulmonary hypertension due to left heart disease (group 2), pulmonary hypertension due to chronic lung disease and/or hypoxia (group 3), chronic thromboembolic pulmonary hypertension (group 4), and pulmonary hypertension due to miscellaneous disorders that can affect the pulmonary vasculature (group 5). During the successive world meetings [5–7], a series of changes were carried out, reflecting some progresses in the understanding of the disease. However, the basic structure has since been maintained. The current clinical classification of pulmonary hypertension has been accepted in the 5th World Symposium held in 2013 in Nice, France [7, 8] and some modification by 2015 the ESC and the ERS guidelines for the diagnosis and treatment of pulmonary hypertension [1] (Table 1.1). The consensus was to maintain the general disposition of previous clinical classification.

1.5 Group 1 Modification in Nice Classification

Some modifications and updates, especially for group 1, were proposed according to new knowledge acquired in the field of PH. The agreement in the Pediatric Task Force has added some specific items related to pediatric PH in order to have a comprehensive classification common for adults and children [7] (Table 1.1). New conditions that are frequently found in children have been included in different clinical

Table 1.1 Comprehensive clinical classification of pulmonary hypertension (ESC/ERS guidelines 2015)

1. Pulmonary arterial hypertension (PAH)

    1.1 Idiopathic PAH

    1.2 Heritable PAH

        1.2.1 BMPR2 mutation

        1.2.2 Other mutations (ALK-1, ENG, SMAD9, CAV1, KCNK3)

        1.2.3 Unknown

    1.3 Drugs and toxins induced

    1.4 Associated with (APAH):

        1.4.1 Connective tissue disease

        1.4.2 Human immunodeficiency virus (HIV) infection

        1.4.3 Portal hypertension

        1.4.4 Congenital heart disease

        1.4.5 Schistosomiasis

1'. Pulmonary veno-occlusive disease (PVOD) and/or pulmonary capillary hemangiomatosis (PCH)

    1'.1 Idiopathic PVOD/PCH

    1'.2 Heritable

        1'.2.1 EIF2AK4 mutation

        1'.2.2 Other/ Unknown mutations

    1'.3 Drugs, toxins and radiation induced

    1'.4 Associated with:

        1'.4.1 Connective tissue disease

        1'.4.2 Human immunodeficiency virus (HIV) infection

1″ . Persistent pulmonary hypertension of the newborn (PPHN)

2. Pulmonary hypertension due to left heart disease

    2.1 Left ventricular systolic dysfunction

    2.2 Left ventricular diastolic dysfunction

    2.3 Valvular disease

    2.4 Congenital/acquired left heart inflow/outflow tract obstruction and congenital cardiomyopathies

    2.5 Congenital/acquired pulmonary veins stenosis

3. Pulmonary hypertension due to lung diseases and/or hypoxia

    3.1 Chronic obstructive pulmonary disease

    3.2 Interstitial lung disease

    3.3 Other pulmonary diseases with mixed restrictive and obstructive pattern

    3.4 Sleep-disordered breathing

    3.5 Alveolar hypoventilation disorders

    3.6 Chronic exposure to high altitude

    3.7 Developmental lung diseases

(continued)

Table 1.1 (continued)

4. Chronic thromboembolic pulmonary hypertension (CTEPH) and other pulmonary artery obstructions

    4.1 Chronic thromboembolic pulmonary hypertension
    4.2 Other pulmonary artery obstructions
        4.2.1 Angiosarcoma
        4.2.2 Other intravascular tumors
        4.2.3 Arteritis
        4.2.4 Congenital pulmonary arteries stenoses
        4.2.5 Parasites (hydatidosis)

5. Pulmonary hypertension with unclear and/or multifactorial mechanisms

    5.1 Hematologic disorders: chronic hemolytic anemia, myeloproliferative disorders, splenectomy
    5.2 Systemic disorders: sarcoidosis, pulmonary histiocytosis, lymphangioleiomyomatosis
    5.3 Metabolic disorders: glycogen storage disease, Gaucher disease, thyroiddisorders
    5.4 Others: tumoral thrombothic microangiopathy, fibrosing mediastinitis, chronic renal failure, segmental pulmonary hypertension

ALK-1 activin receptor-like kinase 1, *BMPR2* bone morphogenetic protein receptor 2, *CAV-1* caveolin-1, *ENG* endoglin, *KCNK3* potassium channel subfamily K member 3, *PAH* pulmonary arterial hypertension, *PH* pulmonary hypertension, *SMAD9* mothers against decapentaplegic 9

groups in order to provide a comprehensive classification appropriate to both adult and pediatric patients. Many children with PH diagnosed during neonatal through to adolescent periods are now surviving into adulthood and will thus require transition to adult care. Persistent PH of the newborn (PPHN) includes a heterogeneous group of conditions that may differ from classical PAH. As a consequence, PPHN has been subcategorized as group 1. Furthermore, some adult PH conditions develop as a consequence of lesions or substrates that have origins during childhood (such as congenital heart defects). Consistent with this philosophy, pediatric PH conditions have now been included to provide a comprehensive and unified classification system appropriate for all ages.

1.6 Pre- or Postcapillary Pulmonary Hypertension

Hemodynamically, PH is defined according to an mPAP ≥ 25 mm Hg at rest assessed using RHC. Furthermore, PH is divided according to the pulmonary artery wedge pressure (PAWP) into precapillary (PAWP ≤ 15 mmHg) and postcapillary PH (PAWP > 15 mmHg) [9]. The groups of 1 and 3~5, with the exception of group 2 left heart diseases, represent precapillary forms of PH (Fig. 1.1).

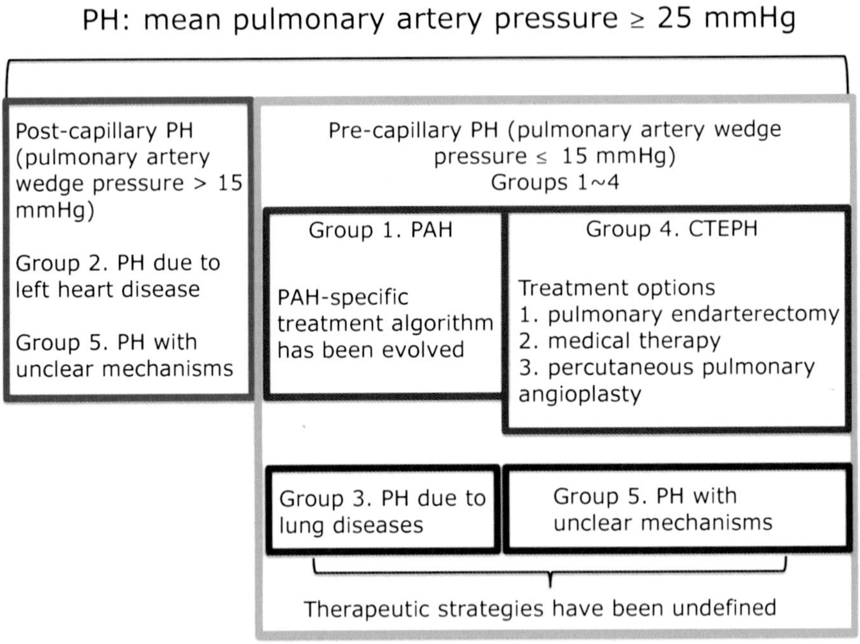

PH: mean pulmonary artery pressure ≥ 25 mmHg

Post-capillary PH (pulmonary artery wedge pressure > 15 mmHg)	Pre-capillary PH (pulmonary artery wedge pressure ≤ 15 mmHg) Groups 1~4	
Group 2. PH due to left heart disease	**Group 1. PAH**	**Group 4. CTEPH**
Group 5. PH with unclear mechanisms	PAH-specific treatment algorithm has been evolved	Treatment options 1. pulmonary endarterectomy 2. medical therapy 3. percutaneous pulmonary angioplasty
	Group 3. PH due to lung diseases	Group 5. PH with unclear mechanisms
	Therapeutic strategies have been undefined	

Fig. 1.1 Classification of pulmonary hypertension according to hemodynamic definition

1.7 Group 1: Pulmonary Arterial Hypertension (PAH)

The term PAH describes a group of PH patients characterized hemodynamically by the presence of precapillary PH, defined by a PAWP ≤15 mmHg and a pulmonary vascular resistance >3 Wood units in the absence of other causes of precapillary PH such as PH due to lung diseases, CTEPH, or other rare diseases. PAH includes different forms that share a similar clinical picture and virtually identical pathological changes of the lung microcirculation.

Recently identified gene mutations have been included in the HPAH subgroup of clinical group 1 (PAH). The new mutations are more rare as compared with the traditional bone morphogenetic protein receptor-2 (BMPR2) mutation. These abnormalities may be acquired, genetically mediated as a result of mutations in bone morphogenetic protein receptor (BMPR)-2 or activin receptor-like kinase-1 (ALK-1), or epigenetically inherited. Patients with BMPR2 or ALK-1 mutations present with higher pulmonary vascular resistance [10–12]. However, most cases of pulmonary arterial hypertension do not have known genetic triggers.

Knowledge of the pathobiology of pulmonary hypertension has been continuing to accelerate. Group 1 PAH primarily consist of an obstructive lung panvasculopathy, characterized by luminal obliteration of the distal pulmonary arteries due to vascular cell proliferation and loss of distal arterioles. Other common features include pulmonary artery endothelial dysfunction leading to vasomotor imbalance favoring vasoconstriction and therapeutic response to currently approved PAH drugs [13, 14]. This group has been the main focus of recent drug trials with PAH agents, such as endothelin receptor antagonists, phosphodiesterase type-5 inhibitors, soluble guanylate cyclase stimulators, and prostanoids.

Although pulmonary hypertension primarily affects the arteries, venous involvement such as pulmonary veno-occlusive disease (PVOD) has been increasingly recognized as an important entity. Group 1′ [pulmonary veno-occlusive disease (PVOD) and/or pulmonary capillary hemangiomatosis (PCH)] has been expanded and includes idiopathic, heritable, drug-, toxin- and radiation-induced and associated forms. Moreover, it may be that prognosis in pulmonary hypertension is determined largely by the status of the right ventricle, rather than the levels of pulmonary artery pressures.

Disordered metabolism and mitochondrial structure, inflammation, and dysregulation of growth factors lead to a proliferative, apoptosis-resistant state. Pulmonary vascular research has been evolved regarding endothelial and smooth muscle cells in intima and media pulmonary vasculature and the immediate perivascular microenvironment. The perivascular region is dominated by fibroblasts and migrating circulating cells, including inflammatory and progenitor cells [15] (Fig. 1.2).

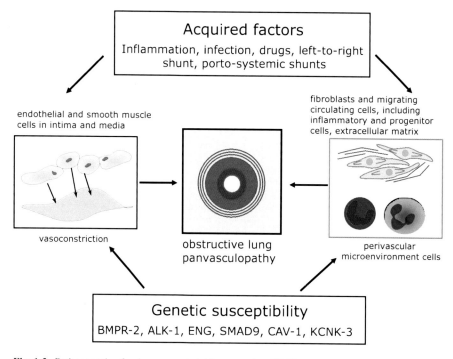

Fig. 1.2 Pathogenesis of pulmonary arterial hypertension (PAH)

1.8   Other than Group 1 PAH

No changes were made to the main classification schema in group 3 PH due to lung disease and/or hypoxia. However, the Nice meeting recommended that a subgroup of patients with severe PH due to lung disease should be differentiated from those with mild to moderate PH. This is in recognition of the fact that severe PH is actually uncommon in the setting of chronic lung diseases and those with severe PH represent a separate clinical phenotype where pulmonary vascular disease dominates the clinical picture rather than ventilatory abnormalities. The terminology of "out of proportion" PH in lung disease should be dropped, because there is no direct correlation between the extent of parenchymal disease and pulmonary hemodynamic derangement. Instead, a category of "severe PH due to lung disease," defined by a mean mPAP $\geq$ 35 mm Hg, was suggested to describe this specific phenotype [1].

A recommendation from the Nice meeting was to abandon the previous terminology of "out of proportion" PH in the context of left heart disease. This term has often been used to identify patients with left heart disease who might have a precapillary component (or pulmonary vascular disease) contributing to the increased pulmonary artery pressure (PAP). Previously, "out of proportion" left-sided PH was identified hemodynamically according to the presence of a high transpulmonary gradient (mean PAP – PAWP) > 12 mmHg.

Group 4 has been renamed as "CTEPH and other pulmonary artery (PA) obstructions," which includes CTEPH, pulmonary angiosarcoma, other intravascular tumors, arteritis, congenital pulmonary arteries stenoses, and parasites.

References

1. Galie N, Humbert M, Vachiery J-L, et al. ESC/ERS Guidelines for the diagnosis and treatment of pulmonary hypertension: the Joint Task Force for the Diagnosis and Treatment of Pulmonary Hypertension of the European Society of Cardiology (ESC) and the European Respiratory Society (ERS), endorsed by Association for European Paediatric and Congenital Cardiology (AEPC), International Society of Heart and Lung Transplantation (ISHLT). Eur Heart J. 2016;37:67–119.
2. Kovacs G, Berghold A, Scheidl S, et al. Pulmonary arterial pressure during rest and exercise in healthy subjects: a systematic review. Eur Respir J. 2009;34:888–94.
3. Fishman AP. Clinical classification of pulmonary hypertension. Clin Chest Med. 2001;22:385–91.
4. Herve P, Lau E, Sitbon O, et al. Criteria for diagnosis of exercise pulmonary hypertension. Eur Respir J. 2015;46:728–37.
5. Simonneau G, Galiè N, Rubin LJ, et al. Clinical classification of pulmonary hypertension. J Am Coll Cardiol. 2004;43 Supl:5S–12S.
6. Simonneau G, Robbins IM, Beghetti M, et al. Updated clinical classification of pulmonary hypertension. J Am Coll Cardiol. 2009;54:S43–54.
7. Simonneau G, Gatzoulis MA, Adatia I, et al. Updated clinical classification of pulmonary hypertension. J Am Coll Cardiol. 2013;62(25 Suppl):D34–41.

8. Hoeper MM, Bogaard HJ, Condliffe R, et al. Definitions and diagnosis of pulmonary hypertension. J Am Coll Cardiol. 2013;62(25 Suppl):D42–50.

9. Ivy DD, Abman SH, Barst RJ, et al. Pediatric pulmonary hypertension. J Am Coll Cardiol. 2013;62:D117–26.

10. Elliott CG, Glissmeyer EW, Havlena GT, et al. Relationship of BMPR2 mutations to vasoreactivity in pulmonary arterial hypertension. Circulation. 2006;113:2509–15.

11. Girerd B, Montani D, Coulet F, et al. Clinical outcomes of pulmonary arterial hypertension in patients carrying an ACVRL1 (ALK1) mutation. Am J Respir Crit Care Med. 2010;181:851–61.

12. Aldred MA, Comhair SA, Varella-Garcia M, et al. Somatic chromosome abnormalities in the lungs of patients with pulmonary arterial hypertension. Am J Respir Crit Care Med. 2010;182:1153–60.

13. Humbert M, Sitbon O, Simonneau G. Treatment of pulmonary arterial hypertension. N Engl J Med. 2004;351:1425–36.

14. Galie N, Corris PA, Frost A, et al. Updated treatment algorithm of pulmonary arterial hypertension. J Am Coll Cardiol. 2013;62:D60–72.

15. Tuder RM, Archer SL, Dorfmüller P, et al. Relevant issues in the pathology and pathobiology of pulmonary hypertension. J Am Coll Cardiol. 2013;62:D4–12.

Chapter 2
Diagnosis: Imaging

Nobuhiro Tahara, Tomohisa Nakamura, Hidetoshi Chibana, Eita Kumagai, Yoichi Sugiyama, Munehisa Bekki, Akihiro Honda, Atsuko Tahara, Sachiyo Igata, and Yoshihiro Fukumoto

Abstract Chronic thromboembolic pulmonary hypertension (CTEPH) is a form of pulmonary hypertension (PH) characterized by the persistence of thromboembolic obstruction in the pulmonary arteries as a result of a combination of recurrent thromboemboli, in situ thrombosis, and secondary vasculopathy in the small vessels. Without appropriate treatments, CTEPH may result in right-sided heart failure and premature death. Pulmonary endarterectomy (PEA) is able to cure CTEPH; however, approximately 40 % of the patients are inoperable due to surgically inaccessible thromboembolic materials. Recently, the balloon pulmonary angioplasty (BPA) becomes a promising treatment option for inoperable CTEPH patients with peripheral obstructive lesions or residual PH after PEA. The accurate and early diagnosis of the cause of PH determines the management and prognosis. Imaging modalities such as ventilation-perfusion lung scintigraphy, multidetector computed tomographic pulmonary angiography, and pulmonary angiography play a crucial role in the diagnosis and management for patients with CTEPH. Also, these imaging modalities enable to assess the operability in CTEPH patients. Further, recent imaging modalities are available for assessing performance or metabolism of the right ventricle. In this chapter, we describe imaging modalities for diagnosis and management of CTEPH.

Keywords Imaging • Ventilation-perfusion lung scintigraphy • Multidetector CT pulmonary angiography • Magnetic resonance imaging • Pulmonary angiography • Intravascular imaging • Molecular imaging

N. Tahara (✉) • T. Nakamura • H. Chibana • E. Kumagai • Y. Sugiyama • M. Bekki
A. Honda • A. Tahara • S. Igata • Y. Fukumoto
Department of Medicine, Division of Cardiovascular Medicine, Kurume University School of Medicine, 67 Asahi-machi, Kurume 830-0011, Japan
e-mail: ntahara@med.kurume-u.ac.jp

© Springer Science+Business Media Singapore 2017
Y. Fukumoto (ed.), *Diagnosis and Treatment of Pulmonary Hypertension,*
DOI 10.1007/978-981-287-840-3_2

Chronic thromboembolic pulmonary hypertension (CTEPH) is a form of pulmonary hypertension (PH) caused by fibrotic organization of unresolved thromboemboli in the pulmonary arteries. CTEPH is defined as a precapillary PH, confirmed by right heart catheterization with a mean pulmonary arterial pressure (PAP) $\geq$ 25 mmHg and a wedge pressure < 15 mmHg at rest, in combination with chronic thromboemboli after a long-term period (at least 3 months) of optimal therapeutic anticoagulation [1–3]. Therefore, CTEPH should be considered in any types of patient with precapillary PH.

CTEPH as a direct consequence of symptomatic pulmonary embolism (PE) is rare, leading to delayed diagnosis and treatment [4]. Hence, the natural history of CTEPH is completely unknown. Previous studies demonstrated that ranged from 0.1 to 9.1 % of patients diagnosed with acute PE develop CTEPH at 2-year follow-up [1, 3–10]. The pathogenesis of CTEPH is thought as a result of a combination of recurrent thromboemboli, in situ thrombosis, and secondary vasculopathy in the distal pulmonary bed [11, 12]. These pathogenic factors cause a progressive increase in pulmonary vascular resistance, resulting in right-sided heart failure and premature death. Therefore, patients with CTEPH have a poor prognosis without effective treatments. The 5-year survival is 30 % in CTEPH patients with a mean PAP greater than 30 mmHg [13]. Surgical pulmonary endarterectomy (PEA) is able to cure CTEPH leading to normalization of pulmonary hemodynamics and exercise capacity in the majority of patients [1–3, 10, 14], if a sufficient quantity of the organized thromboemboli is removed. Theoretically, surgical operability is given if the organized thromboemboli are not located distal to the lobar arteries. Although PEA is recommended for the treatment of CTEPH, up to 40 % of the patients are considered to be inoperable mainly due to surgically inaccessible thromboembolic materials [15–17]. The balloon pulmonary angioplasty (BPA) is a promising treatment option for inoperable CTEPH patients with peripheral obstructive lesions or residual PH after PEA [18–25]. During this decade, several Japanese centers have developed the BPA procedure and reported favorable results including significant improvements of pulmonary hemodynamics, exercise capacity, and clinical status with less concomitant complication compared to a previous report [18–21, 23–25]. The BPA procedure enables to treat peripheral weblike stenoses and intraluminal bands in subsegmental branches of the pulmonary arteries.

The imaging modality should be required for differential diagnosis in patients with suspected CTEPH. Also, it should be able to choose therapeutic options, PEA, BPA, or the combination. The accurate and early diagnosis of the cause of PH determines the management and prognosis. Identifying CTEPH is facilitated by several imaging techniques including ventilation-perfusion lung scintigraphy, multidetector computed tomographic pulmonary angiography (CTPA), pulmonary angiography, and, more recently, magnetic resonance imaging (MRI). According to the recent guidelines on PH, after a positive ventilation-perfusion scan for CTEPH, pulmonary angiography and multidetector CT can be used for detailed work-up of the pulmonary arteries [1–3, 26–28]. However, in some cases with CTEPH, the obstructive lesions cannot be detected by conventional imaging modalities. Very recently, intravascular imaging technique has been developed for the clinical assessment of the pulmonary arteries. It is useful especially to diagnose distal-type CTEPH or to demonstrate undetectable thrombi, fine webs, and thin intraluminal bands by CTPA and pulmonary angiography [29–32].

Recent and conventional imaging modalities play an important role in the diagnosis and management for patients with CTEPH. Other techniques are available for assessing performance or metabolism of the right ventricle (RV), the key determinant of patient survival. In this chapter, we describe imaging modalities for diagnosis and management of CTEPH.

2.1 Ventilation-Perfusion Lung Scintigraphy

Over 30 years, ventilation-perfusion lung scintigraphy is widely used as an imaging modality to diagnose PE. Perfusion lung scintigraphy is a modality to allow visualizing pulmonary perfusion. As localized pulmonary hypoperfusion is not highly specific for PE, the addition of ventilation scintigraphy further increases the specificity. A perfusion defect with normal ventilation (so-called ventilation-perfusion mismatched defect) usually indicates PE. The high negative predictive value of a normal ventilation-perfusion lung scintigraphy has been confirmed by a large clinical trial [33]. The positive predictive value of a high-probability scan and definitive angiogram is approximately 90 % [34]. Ventilation-perfusion lung scan is recommended to differentiate CTEPH from other types of precapillary PH [1–3, 35]. At least one unmatched ventilation-perfusion defect suggests CTEPH, while a mottled pattern perfusion scan suggests the presence of pulmonary arterial hypertension (PAH) (Fig. 2.1). Although ventilation-perfusion scan demonstrates a high sensitivity in detection of CTEPH, it can underestimate the severity of angiographic findings and pulmonary hemodynamics (Figs. 2.2 and 2.3) [36].

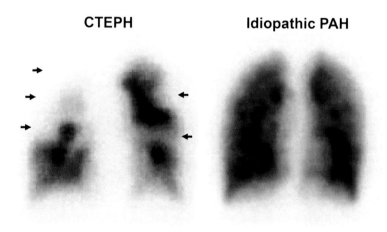

CTEPH   **Idiopathic PAH**

Fig. 2.1 Perfusion lung scintigraphy in CTEPH and IPAH. Several segmental perfusion defects suggest CTEPH (*arrows*), while a mottled pattern perfusion scan does the presence of PAH. *CTEPH* chronic thromboembolic pulmonary hypertension, *PAH* pulmonary arterial hypertension

Pulmonary angiography

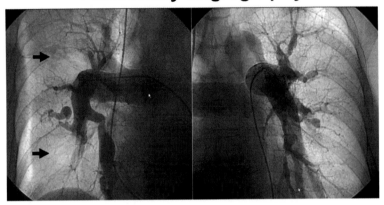

Perfusion lung scintigraphy

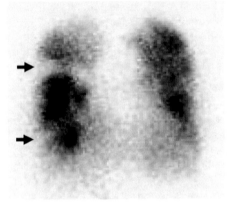

Fig. 2.2 Comparison of obstructive findings between pulmonary angiography and perfusion lung scintigraphy in a patient with CTEPH

| Pulmonary angiography | Perfusion lung scintigraphy | CT/Perfusion lung scintigraphy | 3D CTPA/Perfusion lung scintigraphy |

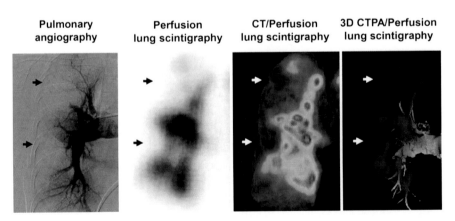

Fig. 2.3 Comparison of obstructive findings among pulmonary angiography, perfusion lung scintigraphy, merged image of multidetector CT and perfusion lung scintigraphy, and that of three-dimensional CTPA and perfusion lung scintigraphy in a patient with CTEPH. Images of perfusion lung scintigraphy and multidetector CTPA demonstrate embolic findings similar to those in pulmonary angiography (*black* and *white arrows*). *CTPA* computed tomographic pulmonary angiography

2.2   Multidetector CTPA and Dual-Energy CTPA

Multidetector CT allows detection of PE up to the segmental level with sensitivities ranging between 60 and 100 % and specificities between 81 and 98 % [37–39]. In recent years, CTPA is widely used for the evaluation of patients with suspected PE since the introduction of multidetector CT with high spatial and temporal resolution [40]. Also, there is a growing body of general agreement that CTPA is beneficial in the diagnosis of CTEPH along with a high diagnostic accuracy [41]. Three-dimensional CTPA reveals CTEPH findings consistent with those in pulmonary angiography (Fig. 2.3). Multidetector CT is also undergone to differentiate CTEPH from other pulmonary vascular diseases in patients with perfusion defects. Ventilation-perfusion scan has been largely replaced by CTPA in many centers.

Simultaneous acquisition of data sets at 80 and 140 kV can be used to visualize iodine distribution maps (regional blood volume image). Based on a three-dimensional algorithm, the technique enables iodine contrast-material extraction in tissues. These iodine maps in the pulmonary parenchyma may reflect lung perfusion. There has been much interest in the application of this technology to the assessment of acute PE [42–45]. Imaging of lung perfusion blood volume by dual-energy CTPA has been reported to be feasible for the evaluation of pulmonary perfusion and be comparable to perfusion lung scintigraphy in establishing a diagnosis of CTEPH (Fig. 2.4) [46, 47]. Dual-energy imaging technique can provide high spatial resolution images of pulmonary vascular and parenchymal anatomy in combination with thromboemboli location [48]. As such, dual-energy CTPA may

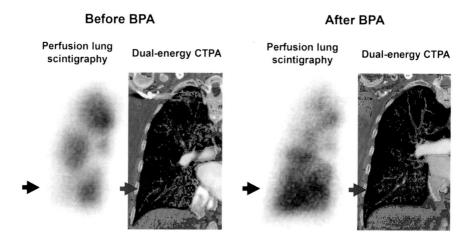

Fig. 2.4 Perfusion lung scintigraphy and dual-energy CTPA before and after BPA in a patient with inoperable CTEPH. Coronal CT images in angiographic window with merged color-coded perfusion map. BPA procedure improves lung perfusion in the right lower lobe (*black arrows*). *BPA* balloon pulmonary angioplasty

Pulmonary angiography

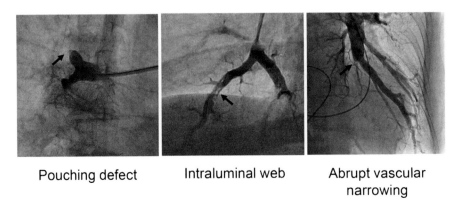

Pouching defect   Intraluminal web   Abrupt vascular
                                                        narrowing

Fig. 2.5 Angiographic findings including "pouching" defect, intraluminal web, and abrupt vascular narrowing suggest the presence of organized thromboemboli

be a promising technique in helping the patient selection for PEA or BPA. Furthermore, dual-energy CTPA has an ability to demonstrate the effect of PEA and BPA (Fig. 2.4). Dual-energy technique may further refine diagnosis and management for patient care in patients with CTEPH.

2.3 Pulmonary Angiography and Intravascular Imaging

Pulmonary angiography is the gold standard for diagnosing PE because of its ability to visualize small pulmonary arteries, which can be safely performed, combined with right heart catheterization even in patients with advanced CTEPH [49, 50]. Although perfusion defect may lead to underestimate pulmonary narrowing and obstruction in CTEPH, pulmonary angiography can detect pulmonary obstructive lesions at subsegmental levels and assess operability (Figs. 2.2 and 2.3) [1–3, 51]. Angiographic findings such as "pouching" defects, webs or bands, intimal irregularities, abrupt vascular narrowing, and complete vascular obstruction suggest the presence of organized thromboemboli in patients with CTEPH (Fig. 2.5) [52].

It is sometimes difficult for pulmonary angiography to clinically distinguish distal-type CTEPH from PAH, because both precapillary PH are characterized as having similar hemodynamic pulmonary circulation despite their different pathological vascular structures. Intravascular imaging technique has been developed for the high-resolution investigation of atherosclerosis in vivo. Based on that, there is an increasing need for intravascular imaging of the pulmonary arteries. A near-infrared light-based imaging modality with ultrahigh resolution, optical coherence tomography (OCT) or optical frequency-domain imaging (OFDI) is a useful imaging modality for differential diagnosis of CTEPH (Fig. 2.6) [29]. OCT/OFDI has demonstrated

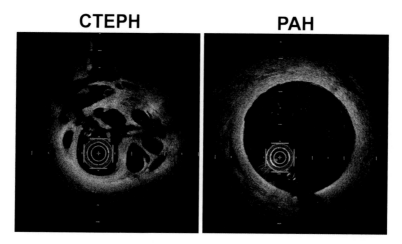

Fig. 2.6 OFDI of the pulmonary arteries from CTEPH and PAH patients. Intraluminal web in the pulmonary artery is observed in CTEPH. In contrast, the media of the pulmonary artery is thickened in PAH. *OFDI* optical frequency-domain imaging

its potential capacity to accurately detect and characterize unresolved thromboemboli in the pulmonary arteries as well as to measure the precise luminal diameter for selection of balloon size in the setting of BPA for CTEPH [29–32]. Angioscopy is an intravascular technique that projects white light through thin, flexible glass fibers loaded into catheters. Although angioscopy has not become a mainstream intravascular imaging modality, it can directly visualize the color and superficial morphology of the plaque and thrombus, which developed especially in Japan. Pulmonary angioscopy is able to observe the characterization of obstructive thromboemboli materials in the pulmonary arteries (Fig. 2.7) [32]. Intravascular modality including OCT/OFDI and angioscopy has become a potential technique for observation of vascular changes in the pulmonary arteries and may provide additional information in the assessment of patients with PH.

2.4 Magnetic Resonance Imaging

MRI is becoming increasingly useful for assessment of the pulmonary vasculature [53]. However, at present, there is no general recommendation for its use in the diagnostic examination for patients with suspected CTEPH [1–3].

RV function has a significant impact on morbidity and mortality in patients with CTEPH [54–57]. Advanced CTEPH leads to cardiac remodeling, including RV dilatation and hypertrophy, tricuspid regurgitation, and leftward ventricular septal shift, with consequent impact on cardiac function. While other modalities including echocardiography and CT cannot accurately evaluate the functional impairment of the RV [58–60], MRI is frequently utilized for assessment of RV function and remodeling with general consensus in functional and morphologic assessment of

Pulmonary angiography

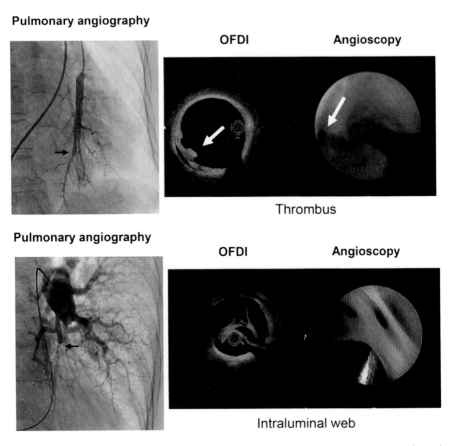

Fig. 2.7 OFDI and pulmonary angioscopy indicates thrombus (*white arrows, upper panels*) and intraluminal web (*lower panels*) lesions of the pulmonary arteries in patients with CTEPH (Reproduced and modified, with permission, from Chibana et al. (32))

patients with CTEPH [59, 61–63]. MRI demonstrated that PEA or BPA ameliorates RV dysfunction and remodeling in association with improvement of hemodynamic parameters in patients with CTEPH [23, 63].

The shortened acceleration times of blood flow in the RV outflow tract is associated with pulmonary hemodynamic parameters such as mean PAP or pulmonary vascular resistance [64–67]. Time-resolved three-dimensional phase-contrast MRI (4D flow) demonstrated that the appearance of a vortex of blood flow arises in the main pulmonary artery in patients with manifest PH, which can identify the severity of PH [68]. Very recently, it has demonstrated substantial vortex flow in the main pulmonary artery in PH and normalization of the flow form in a CTEPH patient after successful BPA (Fig. 2.8) [68–70]. The 4D-flow MRI is a promising technique for diagnostic and severity assessment for patients with PH.

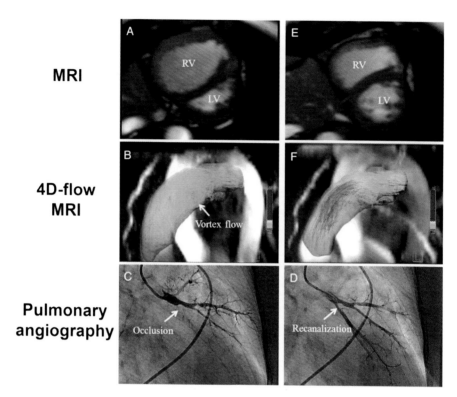

Fig. 2.8 RV remodeling and vortex flow in the main pulmonary artery are noted in a patient with distal-type CTEPH (**a, b**). Multistaged BPA procedures are successfully undergone with no serious complication (**c, d**). After the BPA procedures, RV remodeling is remarkably improved (**e**), and the vortex flow substantially diminished (**f**). *MRI* magnetic resonance imaging, *RV* right ventricle, *LV* left ventricle (Reproduced and modified, with permission, from Ota et al. (71))

2.5 Molecular Imaging

Cardiac performance is a major determinant of functional class and prognosis in PH [71–73]. Prolonged RV pressure and volume overload develops cardiac remodeling such as RV hypertrophy and dilatation, which can compensate for the increased afterload and maintain cardiac performance in patients with PH. However, RV hypertrophy and dilatation is not necessarily compensatory; some patients may lead to right-sided heart failure [73, 74]. A growing body of evidence suggests that RV performance response to afterload may depend on energy substrate metabolism [75]. The RV myocardium changes its energy substrate from fatty acid oxidation to glycolysis under augmented afterload in PH [75, 76]. Positron emission tomography (PET) imaging with 18F-fluorodeoxyglucose (FDG) has been used for the measurement of glucose uptake as an indicator of glucose metabolism in the myocardium. The RV glucose metabolism measured by FDG-PET can be expressed in association with the increased workload (Fig. 2.9) [76–82]. In addition, enhanced FDG

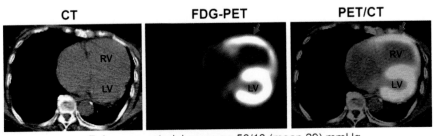

Pulmonary arterial pressure 56/13 (mean 29) mmHg

Cardiac index 1.75 L/min/m²

Pulmonary vascular resistance 11.4 Wood units

Fig. 2.9 CT, FDG-PET, and PET/CT images in a patient with CTEPH with pulmonary hemodynamic parameters. Note the intense FDG uptake comparable to the left ventricle in the right ventricle (*red arrows*). *FDG* 18F-fluorodeoxyglucose, *PET* positron emission tomography

uptake in the RV free wall may be an independent factor for prognosis in patients with PAH and CTEPH [83, 84]. FDG-PET imaging is a promising modality having an ability to demonstrate PH severity and clinical outcome.

References

1. Tanabe N, Sugiura T, Tatsumi K. Recent progress in the diagnosis and management of chronic thromboembolic pulmonary hypertension. Respir Invest. 2013;51:134–46.
2. Kim NH, Delcroix M, Jenkins DP, Channick R, Dartevelle P, Jansa P, Lang I, Madani MM, Ogino H, Pengo V, Mayer E. Chronic thromboembolic pulmonary hypertension. J Am Coll Cardiol. 2013;62(25 Suppl):D92–9.
3. Galiè N, Humbert M, Vachiery JL, Gibbs S, Lang I, Torbicki A, Simonneau G, Peacock A, Vonk Noordegraaf A, Beghetti M, Ghofrani A, Gomez Sanchez MA, Hansmann G, Klepetko W, Lancellotti P, Matucci M, McDonagh T, Pierard LA, Trindade PT, Zompatori M, Hoeper M, Aboyans V, Vaz Carneiro A, Achenbach S, Agewall S, Allanore Y, Asteggiano R, Paolo Badano L, Albert Barberà J, Bouvaist H, Bueno H, Byrne RA, Carerj S, Castro G, Erol Ç, Falk V, Funck-Brentano C, Gorenflo M, Granton J, Iung B, Kiely DG, Kirchhof P, Kjellstrom B, Landmesser U, Lekakis J, Lionis C, Lip GY, Orfanos SE, Park MH, Piepoli MF, Ponikowski P, Revel MP, Rigau D, Rosenkranz S, Völler H, Luis Zamorano J. 2015 ESC/ERS Guidelines for the diagnosis and treatment of pulmonary hypertension: The Joint Task Force for the Diagnosis and Treatment of Pulmonary Hypertension of the European Society of Cardiology (ESC) and the European Respiratory Society (ERS): Endorsed by: Association for European Paediatric and Congenital Cardiology (AEPC), International Society for Heart and Lung Transplantation (ISHLT). Eur Heart J. 2016;37(1):67–119.
4. Fedullo PF, Auger WR, Kerr KM, Rubin LJ. Chronic thromboembolic pulmonary hypertension. N Engl J Med. 2001;345(20):1465–72.
5. Pengo V, Lensing AW, Prins MH, Marchiori A, Davidson BL, Tiozzo F, Albanese P, Biasiolo A, Pegoraro C, Iliceto S, Prandoni P, Thromboembolic Pulmonary Hypertension Study Group. Incidence of chronic thromboembolic pulmonary hypertension after pulmonary embolism. N Engl J Med. 2004;350(22):2257–64.

6. Becattini C, Agnelli G, Pesavento R, Silingardi M, Poggio R, Taliani MR, Ageno W. Incidence of chronic thromboembolic pulmonary hypertension after a first episode of pulmonary embolism. Chest. 2006;130(1):172–5.

7. Dentali F, Donadini M, Gianni M, Bertolini A, Squizzato A, Venco A, Ageno W. Incidence of chronic pulmonary hypertension in patients with previous pulmonary embolism. Thromb Res. 2009;124(3):256–8.

8. Klok FA, van Kralingen KW, van Dijk AP, Heyning FH, Vliegen HW, Huisman MV. Prospective cardiopulmonary screening program to detect chronic thromboembolic pulmonary hypertension in patients after acute pulmonary embolism. Haematologica. 2010;95(6):970–5.

9. Lang IM, Pesavento R, Bonderman D, Yuan JX. Risk factors and basic mechanisms of chronic thromboembolic pulmonary hypertension: a current understanding. Eur Respir J. 2013;41(2):462–8.

10. Hoeper MM, McLaughlin VV, Dalaan AM, Satoh T, Galiè N. Treatment of pulmonary hypertension. Lancet Respir Med. 2014;2(7):573–82.

11. Castañer E, Gallardo X, Ballesteros E, Andreu M, Pallardó Y, Mata JM, Riera L. CT diagnosis of chronic pulmonary thromboembolism. Radiographics. 2009;29(1):31–50.

12. Galiè N, Kim NH. Pulmonary microvascular disease in chronic thromboembolic pulmonary hypertension. Proc Am Thorac Soc. 2006;3(7):571–6.

13. Riedel M, Stanek V, Widimsky J, Prerovsky I. Longterm follow-up of patients with pulmonary thromboembolism. Late prognosis and evolution of hemodynamic and respiratory data. Chest. 1982;81(2):151–8.

14. Mayer E, Jenkins D, Lindner J, D'Armini A, Kloek J, Meyns B, Ilkjaer LB, Klepetko W, Delcroix M, Lang I, Pepke-Zaba J, Simonneau G, Dartevelle P. Surgical management and outcome of patients with chronic thromboembolic pulmonary hypertension: results from an international prospective registry. J Thorac Cardiovasc Surg. 2011;141(3):702–10.

15. Mayer E. Surgical and post-operative treatment of chronic thromboembolic pulmonary hypertension. Eur Respir Rev. 2010;19(115):64–7.

16. Pepke-Zaba J, Delcroix M, Lang I, Mayer E, Jansa P, Ambroz D, Treacy C, D'Armini AM, Morsolini M, Snijder R, Bresser P, Torbicki A, Kristensen B, Lewczuk J, Simkova I, Barberà JA, de Perrot M, Hoeper MM, Gaine S, Speich R, Gomez-Sanchez MA, Kovacs G, Hamid AM, Jaïs X, Simonneau G. Chronic thromboembolic pulmonary hypertension (CTEPH): results from an international prospective registry. Circulation. 2011;124(18):1973–81.

17. Jenkins D, Mayer E, Screaton N, Madani M. State-of-the-art chronic thromboembolic pulmonary hypertension diagnosis and management. Eur Respir Rev. 2012;21(123):32–9.

18. Feinstein JA, Goldhaber SZ, Lock JE, Ferndandes SM, Landzberg MJ. Balloon pulmonary angioplasty for treatment of chronic thromboembolic pulmonary hypertension. Circulation. 2001;103(1):10–3.

19. Sugimura K, Fukumoto Y, Satoh K, Nochioka K, Miura Y, Aoki T, Tatebe S, Miyamichi-Yamamoto S, Shimokawa H. Percutaneous transluminal pulmonary angioplasty markedly improves pulmonary hemodynamics and long-term prognosis in patients with chronic thromboembolic pulmonary hypertension. Circ J. 2012;76(2):485–8.

20. Mizoguchi H, Ogawa A, Munemasa M, Mikouchi H, Ito H, Matsubara H. Refined balloon pulmonary angioplasty for inoperable patients with chronic thromboembolic pulmonary hypertension. Circ Cardiovasc Interv. 2012;5(6):748–55.

21. Kataoka M, Inami T, Hayashida K, Shimura N, Ishiguro H, Abe T, Tamura Y, Ando M, Fukuda K, Yoshino H, Satoh T. Percutaneous transluminal pulmonary angioplasty for the treatment of chronic thromboembolic pulmonary hypertension. Circ Cardiovasc Interv. 2012;5(6):756–62.

22. Andreassen AK, Ragnarsson A, Gude E, Geiran O, Andersen R. Balloon pulmonary angioplasty in patients with inoperable chronic thromboembolic pulmonary hypertension. Heart. 2013;99(19):1415–20.

23. Fukui S, Ogo T, Morita Y, Tsuji A, Tateishi E, Ozaki K, Sanda Y, Fukuda T, Yasuda S, Ogawa H, Nakanishi N. Right ventricular reverse remodelling after balloon pulmonary angioplasty. Eur Respir J. 2014;43(5):1394–402.

24. Yanagisawa R, Kataoka M, Inami T, Shimura N, Ishiguro H, Fukuda K, Yoshino H, Satoh T. Safety and efficacy of percutaneous transluminal pulmonary angioplasty in elderly patients. Int J Cardiol. 2014;175(2):285–9.

25. Inami T, Kataoka M, Ando M, Fukuda K, Yoshino H, Satoh T. A new era of therapeutic strategies for chronic thromboembolic pulmonary hypertension by two different interventional therapies; pulmonary endarterectomy and percutaneous transluminal pulmonary angioplasty. PLoS One. 2014;9(4):e94587.

26. Jaff MR, McMurtry MS, Archer SL, Cushman M, Goldenberg N, Goldhaber SZ, Jenkins JS, Kline JA, Michaels AD, Thistlethwaite P, Vedantham S, White RJ, Zierler BK. American Heart Association Council on Cardiopulmonary, Critical Care, Perioperative and Resuscitation; American Heart Association Council on Peripheral Vascular Disease; American Heart Association Council on Arteriosclerosis, Thrombosis and Vascular Biology. Management of massive and submassive pulmonary embolism, iliofemoral deep vein thrombosis, and chronic thromboembolic pulmonary hypertension: a scientific statement from the American Heart Association. Circulation. 2011;123(16):1788–1830.

27. Galiè N, Hoeper MM, Humbert M, Torbicki A, Vachiery JL, Barbera JA, Beghetti M, Corris P, Gaine S, Gibbs JS, Gomez-Sanchez MA, Jondeau G, Klepetko W, Opitz C, Peacock A, Rubin L, Zellweger M, Simonneau G; ESC Committee for Practice Guidelines (CPG). Guidelines for the diagnosis and treatment of pulmonary hypertension: the Task Force for the Diagnosis and Treatment of Pulmonary Hypertension of the European Society of Cardiology (ESC) and the European Respiratory Society (ERS), endorsed by the International Society of Heart and Lung Transplantation (ISHLT). Eur Heart J. 2009;30(20):2493–537.

28. Brown K, Gutierrez AJ, Mohammed TL, Kirsch J, Chung JH, Dyer DS, Ginsburg ME, Heitkamp DE, Kanne JP, Kazerooni EA, Ketai LH, Parker JA, Ravenel JG, Saleh AG, Shah RD, Steiner RM, RD S, Expert Panel on Thoracic Imaging. ACR Appropriateness Criteria® pulmonary hypertension. J Thorac Imaging. 2013;28(4):W57–60.

29. Tatebe S, Fukumoto Y, Sugimura K, Nakano M, Miyamichi S, Satoh K, Oikawa M, Shimokawa H. Optical coherence tomography as a novel diagnostic tool for distal type chronic thromboembolic pulmonary hypertension. Circ J. 2010;74(8):1742–4.

30. Tatebe S, Fukumoto Y, Sugimura K, Miura Y, Nochioka K, Aoki T, Miura M, Yamamoto S, Yaoita N, Satoh K, Shimokawa H. Optical coherence tomography is superior to intravascular ultrasound for diagnosis of distal-type chronic thromboembolic pulmonary hypertension. Circ J. 2013;77(4):1081–3.

31. Sugimura K, Fukumoto Y, Miura Y, Nochioka K, Miura M, Tatebe S, Aoki T, Satoh K, Yamamoto S, Yaoita N, Shimokawa H. Three-dimensional-optical coherence tomography imaging of chronic thromboembolic pulmonary hypertension. Eur Heart J. 2013;34(28):2121.

32. Chibana H, Tahara N, Itaya N, Sasaki M, Sasaki M, Nakayoshi T, Ohtsuka M, Yokoyama S, Sasaki KI, Ueno T, Fukumoto Y. Optical frequency-domain imaging and pulmonary angioscopy in chronic thromboembolic pulmonary hypertension. Eur Heart J. 2016 pii: ehv736.

33. Anderson DR, Kahn SR, Rodger MA, Kovacs MJ, Morris T, Hirsch A, Lang E, Stiell I, Kovacs G, Dreyer J, Dennie C, Cartier Y, Barnes D, Burton E, Pleasance S, Skedgel C, O'Rouke K, Wells PS. Computed tomographic pulmonary angiography vs ventilation-perfusion lung scanning in patients with suspected pulmonary embolism: a randomized controlled trial. JAMA. 2007;298(23):2743–53.

34. PIOPED Investigators. Value of the ventilation/perfusion scan in acute pulmonary embolism. Results of the prospective investigation of pulmonary embolism diagnosis (PIOPED). JAMA. 1990;263(20):2753–9.

35. Hoeper MM, Mayer E, Simonneau G, Rubin LJ. Chronic thromboembolic pulmonary hypertension. Circulation. 2006;113(16):2011–20.

36. Ryan KL, Fedullo PF, Davis GB, Vasquez TE, Moser KM. Perfusion scan findings understate the severity of angiographic and hemodynamic compromise in chronic thromboembolic pulmonary hypertension. Chest. 1988;93(6):1180–5.

37. Ghaye B, Szapiro D, Mastora I, Delannoy V, Duhamel A, Remy J, Remy-Jardin M. Peripheral pulmonary arteries: how far in the lung does multi-detector row spiral CT allow analysis? Radiology. 2001;219(3):629–36.
38. Coche E, Verschuren F, Keyeux A, Goffette P, Goncette L, Hainaut P, Hammer F, Lavenne E, Zech F, Meert P, Reynaert MS. Diagnosis of acute pulmonary embolism in outpatients: comparison of thin-collimation multi-detector row spiral CT and planar ventilation-perfusion scintigraphy. Radiology. 2003;229(3):757–65.
39. Stein PD, Fowler SE, Goodman LR, Gottschalk A, Hales CA, Hull RD, Leeper Jr KV, Popovich Jr J, Quinn DA, Sos TA, Sostman HD, Tapson VF, Wakefield TW, Weg JG, PK W, PIOPED II Investigators. Multidetector computed tomography for acute pulmonary embolism. N Engl J Med. 2006;354(22):2317–27.
40. Bettmann MA, Baginski SG, White RD, Woodard PK, Abbara S, Atalay MK, Dorbala S, Haramati LB, Hendel RC, Martin 3rd ET, Ryan T, Steiner RM. ACR Appropriateness Criteria® acute chest pain–suspected pulmonary embolism. J Thorac Imaging. 2012;27(2):W28–31.
41. Reichelt A, Hoeper MM, Galanski M, Keberle M. Chronic thromboembolic pulmonary hypertension: evaluation with 64-detector row CT versus digital substraction angiography. Eur J Radiol. 2009;71(1):49–54.
42. Pontana F, Faivre JB, Remy-Jardin M, Flohr T, Schmidt B, Tacelli N, Pansini V, Remy J. Lung perfusion with dual-energy multidetector-row CT (MDCT): feasibility for the evaluation of acute pulmonary embolism in 117 consecutive patients. Acad Radiol. 2008;15(12):1494–504.
43. Thieme SF, Becker CR, Hacker M, Nikolaou K, Reiser MF, Johnson TR. Dual energy CT for the assessment of lung perfusion–correlation to scintigraphy. Eur J Radiol. 2008;68(3):369–74.
44. Fink C, Johnson TR, Michaely HJ, Morhard D, Becker C, Reiser M, Nikolaou K. Dual-energy CT angiography of the lung in patients with suspected pulmonary embolism: initial results. Rofo. 2008;180(10):879–83.
45. Thieme SF, Johnson TR, Lee C, McWilliams J, Becker CR, Reiser MF, Nikolaou K. Dual-energy CT for the assessment of contrast material distribution in the pulmonary parenchyma. AJR Am J Roentgenol. 2009;193(1):144–9.
46. Nakazawa T, Watanabe Y, Hori Y, Kiso K, Higashi M, Itoh T, Naito H. Lung perfused blood volume images with dual-energy computed tomography for chronic thromboembolic pulmonary hypertension: correlation to scintigraphy with single-photon emission computed tomography. J Comput Assist Tomogr. 2011;35(5):590–5.
47. Hoey ET, Mirsadraee S, Pepke-Zaba J, Jenkins DP, Gopalan D, Screaton NJ. Dual-energy CT angiography for assessment of regional pulmonary perfusion in patients with chronic thromboembolic pulmonary hypertension: initial experience. AJR Am J Roentgenol. 2011;196(3):524–32.
48. Remy-Jardin M, Faivre JB, Pontana F, Hachulla AL, Tacelli N, Santangelo T, Remy J. Thoracic applications of dual energy. Radiol Clin N Am. 2010;48(1):193–205.
49. Stein PD, Athanasoulis C, Alavi A, Greenspan RH, Hales CA, Saltzman HA, Vreim CE, Terrin ML, Weg JG. Complications and validity of pulmonary angiography in acute pulmonary embolism. Circulation. 1992;85(2):462–8.
50. Pitton MB, Düber C, Mayer E, Thelen M. Hemodynamic effects of nonionic contrast bolus injection and oxygen inhalation during pulmonary angiography in patients with chronic major-vessel thromboembolic pulmonary hypertension. Circulation. 1996;94(10):2485–91.
51. JCS Joint Working Group. Guidelines for the diagnosis, treatment and prevention of pulmonary thromboembolism and deep vein thrombosis (JCS 2009). Circ J. 2011;75(5):1258–81.
52. Auger WR, Fedullo PF, Moser KM, Buchbinder M, Peterson KL. Chronic major-vessel thromboembolic pulmonary artery obstruction: appearance at angiography. Radiology. 1992;182(2):393–8.
53. Gan CT, Lankhaar JW, Westerhof N, Marcus JT, Becker A, Twisk JW, Boonstra A, Postmus PE, Vonk-Noordegraaf A. Noninvasively assessed pulmonary artery stiffness predicts mortality in pulmonary arterial hypertension. Chest. 2007;132(6):1906–12.

54. Moser KM, Auger WR, Fedullo PF. Chronic major-vessel thromboembolic pulmonary hypertension. Circulation. 1990;81(6):1735–43.
55. Jamieson SW, Kapelanski DP, Sakakibara N, Manecke GR, Thistlethwaite PA, Kerr KM, Channick RN, Fedullo PF, Auger WR. Pulmonary endarterectomy: experience and lessons learned in 1,500 cases. Ann Thorac Surg. 2003;76(5):1457–62. discussion 1462-4
56. Fedullo PF, Auger WR, Kerr KM, Kim NH. Chronic thromboembolic pulmonary hypertension. Semin Respir Crit Care Med. 2003;24(3):273–86.
57. Dartevelle P, Fadel E, Mussot S, Chapelier A, Hervé P, de Perrot M, Cerrina J, Ladurie FL, Lehouerou D, Humbert M, Sitbon O, Simonneau G. Chronic thromboembolic pulmonary hypertension. Eur Respir J. 2004;23(4):637–48.
58. Grothues F, Moon JC, Bellenger NG, Smith GS, Klein HU, Pennell DJ. Interstudy reproducibility of right ventricular volumes, function, and mass with cardiovascular magnetic resonance. Am Heart J. 2004;147(2):218–23.
59. Kreitner KF, Ley S, Kauczor HU, Mayer E, Kramm T, Pitton MB, Krummenauer F, Thelen M. Chronic thromboembolic pulmonary hypertension: pre- and postoperative assessment with breath-hold MR imaging techniques. Radiology. 2004;232(2):535–43.
60. Vonk-Noordegraaf A, Souza R. Cardiac magnetic resonance imaging: what can it add to our knowledge of the right ventricle in pulmonary arterial hypertension? Am J Cardiol. 2012;110(6 Suppl):25S–31S.
61. Coulden R. State-of-the-art imaging techniques in chronic thromboembolic pulmonary hypertension. Proc Am Thorac Soc. 2006;3(7):577–83.
62. Kreitner KF, Kunz RP, Ley S, Oberholzer K, Neeb D, Gast KK, Heussel CP, Eberle B, Mayer E, Kauczor HU, Düber C. Chronic thromboembolic pulmonary hypertension – assessment by magnetic resonance imaging. Eur Radiol. 2007;17(1):11–21.
63. Reesink HJ, Marcus JT, Tulevski II, Jamieson S, Kloek JJ, Vonk Noordegraaf A, Bresser P. Reverse right ventricular remodeling after pulmonary endarterectomy in patients with chronic thromboembolic pulmonary hypertension: utility of magnetic resonance imaging to demonstrate restoration of the right ventricle. J Thorac Cardiovasc Surg. 2007;133(1):58–64.
64. Tardivon AA, Mousseaux E, Brenot F, Bittoun J, Jolivet O, Bourroul E, Duroux P. Quantification of hemodynamics in primary pulmonary hypertension with magnetic resonance imaging. Am J Respir Crit Care Med. 1994;150(4):1075–80.
65. Laffon E, Vallet C, Bernard V, Montaudon M, Ducassou D, Laurent F, Marthan R. A computed method for noninvasive MRI assessment of pulmonary arterial hypertension. J Appl Physiol (1985). 2004;96(2):463–8.
66. Kondo C, Caputo GR, Masui T, Foster E, O'Sullivan M, Stulbarg MS, Golden J, Catterjee K, Higgins CB. Pulmonary hypertension: pulmonary flow quantification and flow profile analysis with velocity-encoded cine MR imaging. Radiology. 1992;183(3):751–8.
67. Mousseaux E, Tasu JP, Jolivet O, Simonneau G, Bittoun J, Gaux JC. Pulmonary arterial resistance: noninvasive measurement with indexes of pulmonary flow estimated at velocity-encoded MR imaging–preliminary experience. Radiology. 1999;212:896–902.
68. Reiter G, Reiter U, Kovacs G, Kainz B, Schmidt K, Maier R, Olschewski H, Rienmueller R. Magnetic resonance-derived 3-dimensional blood flow patterns in the main pulmonary artery as a marker of pulmonary hypertension and a measure of elevated mean pulmonary arterial pressure. Circ Cardiovasc Imaging. 2008;1(1):23–30.
69. Odagiri K, Inui N, Miyakawa S, Hakamata A, Wei J, Takehara Y, Sakahara H, Sugiyama M, Alley MT, Tran QK, Watanabe H. Abnormal hemodynamics in the pulmonary artery seen on time-resolved 3-dimensional phase-contrast magnetic resonance imaging (4D-flow) in a young patient with idiopathic pulmonary arterial hypertension. Circ J. 2014;78(7):1770–2.
70. Ota H, Sugimura K, Miura M, Shimokawa H. Four-dimensional flow magnetic resonance imaging visualizes drastic change in vortex flow in the main pulmonary artery after percutaneous transluminal pulmonary angioplasty in a patient with chronic thromboembolic pulmonary hypertension. Eur Heart J. 2015;36(25):1630.

71. Miura Y, Fukumoto Y, Sugimura K, Oikawa M, Nakano M, Tatebe S, Miyamichi S, Satoh K, Shimokawa H. Identification of new prognostic factors of pulmonary hypertension. Circ J. 2010;74(9):1965–71.

72. Nickel N, Golpon H, Greer M, Knudsen L, Olsson K, Westerkamp V, Welte T, Hoeper MM. The prognostic impact of follow-up assessments in patients with idiopathic pulmonary arterial hypertension. Eur Respir J. 2012;39(3):589–96.

73. Ryan JJ, Archer SL. The right ventricle in pulmonary arterial hypertension: disorders of metabolism, angiogenesis and adrenergic signaling in right ventricular failure. Circ Res. 2014;115(1):176–88.

74. Guarracino F, Cariello C, Danella A, Doroni L, Lapolla F, Vullo C, Pasquini C, Stefani M. Right ventricular failure: physiology and assessment. Minerva Anestesiol. 2005;71(6):307–12.

75. Neubauer S. The failing heart–an engine out of fuel. N Engl J Med. 2007;356(11):1140–51.

76. Ahmadi A, Ohira H, Mielniczuk LM. FDG PET imaging for identifying pulmonary hypertension and right heart failure. Curr Cardiol Rep. 2015;17(1):555.

77. Oikawa M, Kagaya Y, Otani H, Sakuma M, Demachi J, Suzuki J, Takahashi T, Nawata J, Ido T, Watanabe J, Shirato K. Increased [18F]fluorodeoxyglucose accumulation in right ventricular free wall in patients with pulmonary hypertension and the effect of epoprostenol. J Am Coll Cardiol. 2005;45(11):1849–55.

78. Basu S, Alavi A. Avid FDG uptake in the right ventricle coupled with enhanced intercostal muscle hypermetabolism in pneumoconiosis. Clin Nucl Med. 2007;32(5):407–8.

79. Can MM, Kaymaz C, Tanboga IH, Tokgoz HC, Canpolat N, Turkyilmaz E, Sonmez K, Ozdemir N. Increased right ventricular glucose metabolism in patients with pulmonary arterial hypertension. Clin Nucl Med. 2011;36(9):743–8.

80. Hagan G, Southwood M, Treacy C, Ross RM, Soon E, Coulson J, Sheares K, Screaton N, Pepke-Zaba J, Morrell NW, Rudd JH. (18)FDG PET imaging can quantify increased cellular metabolism in pulmonary arterial hypertension: a proof-of-principle study. Pulm Circ. 2011;1(4):448–55.

81. Yang T, Wang L, Xiong CM, He JG, Zhang Y, Gu Q, Zhao ZH, Ni XH, Fang W, Liu ZH. The ratio of (18)F-FDG activity uptake between the right and left ventricle in patients with pulmonary hypertension correlates with the right ventricular function. Clin Nucl Med. 2014;39(5):426–30.

82. Ohira H, deKemp R, Pena E, Davies RA, Stewart DJ, Chandy G, Contreras-Dominguez V, Dennie C, Mc Ardle B, Mc Klein R, Renaud JM, DaSilva JN, Pugliese C, Dunne R, Beanlands R, Mielniczuk LM. Shifts in myocardial fatty acid and glucose metabolism in pulmonary arterial hypertension: a potential mechanism for a maladaptive right ventricular response. Eur Heart J Cardiovasc Imaging. 2015. pii: jev136. [Epub ahead of print].

83. Tatebe S, Fukumoto Y, Oikawa-Wakayama M, Sugimura K, Satoh K, Miura Y, Aoki T, Nochioka K, Miura M, Yamamoto S, Tashiro M, Kagaya Y, Shimokawa H. Enhanced [18F]fluorodeoxyglucose accumulation in the right ventricular free wall predicts long-term prognosis of patients with pulmonary hypertension: a preliminary observational study. Eur Heart J Cardiovasc Imaging. 2014;15(6):666–72.

84. Li W, Wang L, Xiong CM, Yang T, Zhang Y, Gu Q, Yang Y, Ni XH, Liu ZH, Fang W, He JG. The prognostic value of 18F-FDG uptake ratio between the right and left ventricles in idiopathic pulmonary arterial hypertension. Clin Nucl Med. 2015;40(11):859–63.

Part II
Pathophysiology and Genetics

Chapter 3
Pathogenic and Therapeutic Role of MicroRNA in Pulmonary Arterial Hypertension

Aleksandra Babicheva, Kimberly M. McDermott, Samuel C. Williams, Allison M. Yee, Swetaleena Dash, Marisela Rodriquez, Nadia Ingabire, Ayako Makino, and Jason X.-J. Yuan

Abstract MicroRNAs (miRNAs) are small noncoding RNAs that play an integral role in regulating gene expression. Increasing evidence supports the important role of miRNAs in the development and progression of pulmonary arterial hypertension (PAH). The function of miRNAs can also be efficiently and specifically regulated using a number of therapeutic strategies, supporting their potential as targets for the treatment of PAH. In this chapter we briefly describe the biogenesis of miRNAs, summarize our current knowledge of the role of various miRNAs in the pathogenic mechanisms of PAH, introduce strategies of targeting miRNAs to treat the disease, review the preclinical results and potential for using miRNAs for treatment of PAH in in vivo models, and finally discuss the current challenges facing the field to deliver miRNA-targeting therapeutics specifically and efficiently to patients.

Keywords miRNA • Pulmonary hypertension • AntagomiR • miRNA mimic

A. Babicheva • K.M. McDermott • S.C. Williams • A.M. Yee • S. Dash • M. Rodriquez
N. Ingabire
Division of Translational and Regenerative Medicine, Department of Medicine, The
University of Arizona College of Medicine, Tucson, AZ 85721, USA

A. Makino
Department of Physiology, The University of Arizona College of Medicine,
Tucson, AZ 85721, USA

J.X.-J. Yuan (✉)
Division of Translational and Regenerative Medicine, Department of Medicine, The
University of Arizona College of Medicine, Tucson, AZ 85721, USA

Department of Physiology, The University of Arizona College of Medicine,
Tucson, AZ 85721, USA
e-mail: jasonyuan@email.arizona.edu

© Springer Science+Business Media Singapore 2017
Y. Fukumoto (ed.), *Diagnosis and Treatment of Pulmonary Hypertension*,
DOI 10.1007/978-981-287-840-3_3

3.1   Introduction

Pulmonary arterial hypertension (PAH) is a progressive and fatal disease that predominantly affects women. PAH is distinguished from other forms of pulmonary
hypertension and itself includes four subcategories: idiopathic (IPAH), heritable
(HPAH), associated (APAH), and drug-/toxin-induced PAH [1]. Pulmonary hypertension is defined by a mean pulmonary arterial pressure (mPAP) of mPAP$\geq$25 mmHg at
rest or mPAP$\geq$30 mmHg during exercise, which is determined by right heart catheterization [2, 3]. The increased PAP in patients with PAH is due primarily to increased
pulmonary vascular resistance (PVR), and the increased PVR is regarded to be multifactorial and involves both genetic and environmental stimuli [4]. Regardless of the
initial cause of the disease, the elevated PVR in patients with PAH is caused by the
combined effects of four pathologic features: (1) sustained pulmonary vasoconstriction (due to smooth muscle contraction), (2) concentric pulmonary vascular wall
thickening (due to increased cell proliferation, migration, and inhibited cell apoptosis), (3) in situ thrombosis (which leads to embolic obliteration of pulmonary arterioles), and (4) increased pulmonary arterial wall stiffness and/or extracellular matrix
remodeling (which restricts the recruitment and extension of small pulmonary arteries, precapillary arterioles, and capillaries). Cellular mechanisms that contribute
to increased PVR and the pathologic features defined above include increased
proliferation, resistance to apoptosis, vascular remodeling, vasoconstriction, increased
migration, increased wall stiffness, changes in metabolism, and inflammation.

   The consequences of increased PVR are dire for patients because it leads to
increased afterload for right ventricle and ultimately to right heart failure. Currently,
treatment for PAH is limited resulting in high mortality and low survival rate after
diagnosis [5]. In this chapter, we review the biogenesis of microRNAs (miRNAs),
the role of miRNAs in the pathogenic mechanisms involved in pulmonary vascular
remodeling and sustained pulmonary vasoconstriction, and the development and
progression of PAH and discuss current strategies and challenges for targeting miR-
NAs for treatment of PAH.

3.2   The Biogenesis of miRNAs

The discovery of small noncoding RNA (ncRNA) has revolutionized our understanding of gene regulation. Among ncRNAs, miRNAs are single-stranded RNA
located in intergenic or intronic regions as individual or clustered genes. They are
endogenously expressed in animals, plants, and viruses and have an ability to bind
to the 3′-untranslated regions (3′-UTR) of the targeted mRNAs. This interaction
prevents protein production by suppressing protein synthesis and/or by initiating
mRNA degradation [6, 7]. Here, we briefly discuss the canonical mechanism by
which miRNAs are processed to their final functional form. The generation of miR-
NAs starts in the nucleus where RNA polymerase II and III transcribe a long

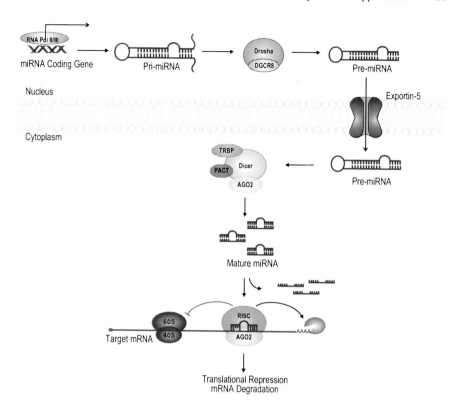

Fig. 3.1 Canonical miRNA biogenesis and function. MicroRNAs (*miRNAs*) are transcribed by RNA polymerase II or III resulting in production of primary miRNA (*pri-miRNA*) hairpins. Pri-miRNAs are then processed by the Drosha–DGCR8 complex to generate precursor miRNAs (*pre-miRNAs*). Pre-miRNAs are transported into the cytoplasm by exportin 5 where they are processed into the final mature double-stranded miRNA by the Dicer–TRBP complex. The passenger strand is released and the guide strand is loaded into Argonaute 2 (*AGO2*)-containing RNA-induced silencing complexes (*RISCs*). The guide strand of the miRNA binds by base-pairing to the target mRNA to suppress downstream target gene expression by promoting degradation of the target mRNA or suppression of translation

primary miRNA transcript (pri-miRNA) (Fig. 3.1). A ribonuclease III is called Drosha and the double-stranded DNA-binding protein, DGCR8 (also referred to as the Microprocessor complex), and they cleave the pri-miRNA into a precursor miRNA (pre-miRNA, 70–100 nucleotides in length). The pre-miRNA is then exported from the nucleus to the cytoplasm by the nuclear export factor exportin-5 where they undergo further processing [8].

Once the pre-miRNA reaches the cytoplasm, it is recognized by the ribonuclease III Dicer and its cofactors (PACT and TRBP) that further process it into the 18–25 nucleotide miRNA duplex. This duplex consists of a miRNA guide strand and passenger strand. The miRNA guide strand is incorporated into the RNA-induced silencing complex (RISC), whereas the passenger strand is mostly degraded. The miRNA/RISC complex then binds to the target mRNA transcript. The mRNA target specificities of miRNAs are primarily encoded within a 6–8 nt "seed region" near the 5′ end of the miRNA. miRNAs can be classified into families based on similar function, and often these miRNA family members share high sequence conservation in the seed region. The number and position of pairing mismatches between the miRNA and the target mRNA contributes to the efficiency of posttranscriptional repression. miRNA binding to the 3′-UTR of a target mRNA transcript can result in repression of translation or degradation of the target mRNA by cleavage or deadenylation of the mRNA [9, 10]. Furthermore, it has been recently demonstrated that miRNAs can also bind to the 5′-untranslated region (5′-UTR) of genes to repress or activate transcription of certain genes. Inhibition of translation can be mediated by binding miRNAs to the 5′-UTR, similar to that observed for binding to the 3′-UTR. However, data suggests that the association of miRNAs with the 5′-UTR generally induces an activation of translation rather than a repression. For example, miRNAs can stabilize RNA and slow their decay to increase gene expression [11–13].

It has been shown that misprocessing of miRNAs is implicated in the development of disease. A study by Albinsson et al. demonstrated that Dicer knockout mice exhibited thin-walled blood vessels due to decreased smooth muscle proliferation as well as reduced contractility of smooth muscle cells (SMC) in early embryogenesis (days 15–16) [14]. In contrast, Caruso et al. showed decreased expression of both Dicer and Drosha in animal models of pulmonary hypertension (PH) with increased proliferation of SMCs [15]. Also, hypoxia has been shown to play a critical role in the downregulation of Drosha and Dicer in cancer cells, leading to dysregulation of miRNA biogenesis [16]. Indeed, Dicer protein level is decreased in human umbilical vein endothelial cells exposed to hypoxia after 48 h [17]. These results suggest that PH-related deregulation of miRNA biogenesis is involved in the progression of disease. Future studies are needed to resolve these conflicting results and to determine the expression and function of Dicer and Drosha in human patients with PAH. Regardless, these findings highlight the importance of distinguishing between the global dysregulation of miRNAs and that of specific miRNAs in understanding their mechanistic contribution to the pathogenesis of PAH.

3.3 Specific miRNAs Involved in the Pathogenesis of PAH

Currently over 2500 human miRNAs have been identified in the miRBase 20.0 database. A single miRNA can regulate multiple target mRNAs, and it has been estimated that these molecules regulate approximately 60 % of human genes [18–20]. For most miRNAs, there is still little known about their effects on genes regulation. Progress has been made in understanding how a handful of miRNAs regulate gene expression in PH. In this section, we will discuss the molecular mechanisms by which miRNAs contribute to the pathogenesis of PH. The miRNAs we will discuss include the following: 21a, 210, and 143/145 cluster, 124 and 130/301 cluster, and 204, 424/503, and 17/92 cluster.

3.3.1   miR-21a and the BMP Pathway

miR-21a has been shown to have increased expression in human pulmonary arterial endothelial cell (HPAEC) and smooth muscle cell (HPASMC) exposed to hypoxia for 24–72 h [21, 22]. In contrast, decreased expression of miR-21a has been observed in human lung tissue, HPAEC, and HPASMC from patients with IPAH (Table 3.1) [15, 23]. Bone morphogenetic protein receptor 2 (BMPR2) is a member of the transforming growth factor-β (TGF-β) family, which encodes a tyrosine kinase receptor on the plasma membrane activated by BMP ligands. Mutations in BMPR2 have been linked to the pathogenesis of PAH, and decreased BMPR2 protein level is observed in patients with IPAH and rat models of PH induced by hypoxia or monocrotaline (MCT) [24–26]. Several lines of evidence suggest that BMP can increase expression of miR-21a (Fig. 3.2) [21, 27]. Experimental knock-down of either BMPR2 or SMAD5 (a downstream regulator of BMP signaling) using siRNAs resulted in downregulation of miR-21a when cells were treated with BMP ligand [21, 28]. Moreover, miR-21 expression is decreased in both PAEC and PASMC isolated from explant lungs of patients with HPAH and IPAH associated with BMPR2 mutations [23].

It has also been demonstrated that exogenous overexpression of miR-21a decreased BMPR2 protein levels in HPAEC (Table 3.1), suggesting a negative feed-back loop between BMPR2 and miR-21a (Fig. 3.2) [21]. Although this evidence implies that miR-21a contributes to the progression of PH through BMPR2, it is still unknown which one is the trigger to development of PH. Therefore, it is critical to examine the time course of miR-21a and BMPR2 expression levels during the development of PH. In independence of the BMPR2-miR-21a cascade, there are two alternative pathways that may regulate miR-21a expression levels: Akt2/mTOR and hypoxia-inducible factor 1α (HIF-1α) signaling pathways (Fig. 3.2) [29].

Increased expression of miR-21 was observed in lung tissue from mice 1–3 weeks following exposure to hypoxia and therefore may play a significant role at early stages to provoke PH through targeting of multiple genes (Fig. 3.2) [22, 30, 31]. It directly targets the pro-apoptotic protein programmed cell death protein 4 (PDCD4) and peroxisome proliferator-activated receptor-γ (PPARγ). Overexpression of miR-21a decreased expression of PDCD4 and PPARγ and resulted in resistance to apoptosis and increased proliferation (Table 3.1) [32, 33]. Phosphatase and tensin homolog (PTEN) is also a validated target of miR-21a. Overexpression with miR-21a suppressed PTEN and consequently stimulated HPASMC proliferation. Finally, miR-21a repressed Sprouty 2 (SPRY2) expression, which induced molecular changes consistent with enhanced cell proliferation and migration [28]. PDCD4, PTEN, and SPRY2 quantification in PH remains to be established, whereas decreased PPARγ gene expression was observed in human lung tissue with primary and secondary PH [34]. In contrast, PPARγ staining was higher in the medial layer of pulmonary arteries from patients with IPAH [35]. These data also serve as evidence to support that miR-21a has a biphasic regulation during the development of PH.

Table 3.1 miRNA-based regulation of PH-associated signaling pathways

miRNA	Regulation	Species/tissues/cells	Target gene(s)	PH-related function	Ref
miR-17-92 cluster	↓	Human IPF lung fibroblasts	DNMT*-1↑	Idiophatic pulmonary fibrosis↑	[98]
	↓	Human PAH PASMC	PDLIM5*↑	Vascular remodeling ↓	[71]
			TGF-β3↓/SMAD3↓		
miR-17	↑	Human PAEC	BMPR2↓	Proliferation ↑	[72]
	↑	Human PASMC	p21 ↓	Proliferation ↑	[74]
miR-20a	↑	Mouse lung tissue	BMPR2↓	Vascular remodeling ↑	[75]
		Human PASMC			
miR-21	↑	Rat CASMC	PTEN↓/Akt ↑/ Bcl-2 ↑	Proliferation ↑/apoptosis↓	[99]
	↑	Human PASMC	PTEN ↓	Proliferation ↑	[22]
		Mouser lung tissue			
	↑	Rat AoSMC	PDCD-4* ↓/AP-1↑	Apoptosis ↓	[32]
	↑	Human PAEC	PDCD-4↓	Apoptosis ↓	[33]
	↑	Human PASMC	PDCD-4 ↓	Proliferation ↑	[28]
			SPRY2 ↓	Migration↑	
			PPARγ*↓	Proliferation ↑	
	↑	Human PAEC	BMPR2*↓	Proliferation ↑	[21]
			RhoB↓	Apoptosis ↓	
				Angiogenesis ↓	
				Vascular relaxation↓	
	↑	Human PAEC, PASMC	DDAH1/2↓	Proliferation ↑	[30]
		Mouse lung tissue			
		Human PAH lung tissue			
	↑	Human AoSMC	AP-1*↑/α-SMA ↑	Proliferation ↑/migration↑	[100]
	↓	IPAH lung tissue	–	–	[15]
		Human PAH PASMC			
		Human PAH PAEC			
miR-27a	↑	Mouse lung tissue	PPARγ*↓/ET-1↑	Proliferation ↑	[101]
		Human PAEC			
miR-27b	↑	Human PAEC	PPARγ*↓/NO↓	Vascular remodeling ↑	[102]
		Rat lung tissue		Vascular relaxation↓	
miR-124	↓	Mouse lung tissue	NFAT↑/CAMTA1↑/	Proliferation ↑	[56]
		Human PASMC	PTBP1 ↑	Vascular remodeling ↑	

(continued)

Table 3.1 (continued)

miRNA	Regulation	Species/tissues/cells	Target gene(s)	PH-related function	Ref
	↓	Human PAF	HIF-2a↑/p21↓	Proliferation ↑	[57]
		Bovine PAF	PTBP1*↑/Notch1↑	Migration↑	
			MCP1*↑	Inflammation↑	
miR-130/301	↑	Human PASMC	PPARγ↓/ET-1↑	Vascular relaxation↓	[61]
		Human PAEC	/eNOS↓		
	↑	Human PASMC	PPARγ*↓/STAT3↑	Proliferation ↑	[60]
		Human PAEC	/miR-204↓	Proliferation ↑	
			PPARγ*↓/apelin↓	Apoptosis ↓	
			/miR-424/503↓		
	↑	Human PASMC, PAEC	p21* ↓	Proliferation ↑	[76]
miR-143/145	↑	Human PASMC	KLF4↓	Vascular remodeling↓	[49]
	↓	Rat AoSMC	α-SMA↓/KLF4*↑/	Vascular remodeling↑	[50]
			myocardin*↑Elk-1*↑	Proliferation ↑	
miR-145	↑	Mouse lung tissue	–	Vascular remodeling↑	[46]
	↑	Human PAH lung tissue	KLF4↑	Vascular relaxation↓	[46, 47]
	↓	Rat AoSMC, AoEC	α-SMA↓/calponin↓/	Vascular remodeling↑	[51]
			SM-MHC↓/ KLF5*↑		
			/myocardin↓		
	↓	Mouse AoSMC	α-SMA↓	Vascular remodeling↑	[103]
miR-143	↑	Human PASMC, PAEC	–	Apoptosis ↓	[104]
		Human PAH PASMC		Migration↑	
	↓	Rat AoSMC	FRA-1↑/PTEN↓	Proliferation↑	[105]
miR-204	↓	Human PASMC	SHP2↑/NFAT↑/	Proliferation ↑	[64, 65]
			HIF-1α↑	Apoptosis ↓	
	↓	Mouse AoSMC	Runx2*↑	Calcification↑	[66]
miR-210	↑	Human PASMC	E2F3*↓	Apoptosis ↓	[40]
		Mouse lung tissue			
	↑	Human PASMC	MKP-1↓	Proliferation ↑	[45]
	↑	Human PASMC, PAEC	ISCU1/2*↓	Fe-S deficiency↑	[42]
		Mouse PASMC, PAEC		Mitochondrial metabolism↓	[41]
				Proliferation ↑	

(continued)

Table 3.1 (continued)

miRNA	Regulation	Species/tissues/cells	Target gene(s)	PH-related function	Ref
miR-424/503	↓	Human PAEC	FGF2*↑	Proliferation ↑	[60, 70]
miR-424	↑	Human MVEC	CUL2*↓/HIF-1α↑ /HIF-2α↑	Angiogenesis↑	[106]

Asterisk (*) denotes mRNAs that have been shown to be direct targets of the associated miRNA

RhoB has been identified as another target of miR-21a [21]. Knockdown of miR-21a restored RhoB expression and Rho-kinase activity in mice. However, despite the increased miR-21a expression observed in hypoxia-treated HPAEC [21], RhoB has been shown to have twofold elevated level in HPAEC and HPASMC under hypoxia [36], as well as in chronic hypoxia-induced mouse lung tissue [37]. Moreover, RhoB activation is likely an early event in PH because it stabilizes HIF-1α during hypoxia in vivo and in vitro. Also, RhoB activation mediates proliferative and migratory responses of both cell types in response to hypoxia [36].

3.3.2 miR-210 and the HIF-1α Pathway

miR-210 expression has been shown to be increased in response to hypoxia in a variety of cell types and therefore has been termed a "hypoxamiR" [38, 39]. Increased expression of miR-210 was observed in the small pulmonary arterioles in human PAH lung tissues resulting from activation of HIF-1α (Fig. 3.2) [40, 41]. Direct targets of miR-210 include iron–sulfur cluster assembly proteins 1/2 (ISCU1/2), which altered mitochondrial metabolic integrity through Fe-S deficiencies involved in hypoxia-dependent PH in mice (Table 3.1) [41, 42]. Thus, these coordinated changes allow HIF-1α to have control over energy production and cellular survival during hypoxic stress. Guo et al. demonstrated that hypoxia-induced expression of miR-210 also plays an anti-apoptotic role in HPASMC by directly targeting the cell-cycle regulator E2F3 [40]. Thus, miR-210 may have anti-apoptotic effects that protect HPASMCs from cell death during hypoxia [43, 44]. In addition, mitogen-activated protein kinase phosphatase 1 (MKP-1) has been shown to be a target of miR-210 [45]. MKP-1 is an inhibitor of extracellular-signal-regulated kinases (ERK), a key activator of the mitotic Ras pathway. Indeed, Jin et al. revealed that inhibition of miR-210 led to increased MKP-1 expression and decreased proliferation in HPASMC [45]. Overexpression of miR-210 resulted in decreased expression of MKP-1, but alone did not affect cell proliferation in HPASMC. Expression of MKP-1 have not been quantified in PAH patients.

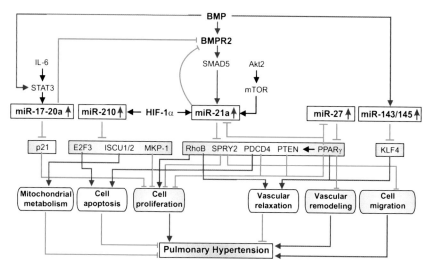

Fig. 3.2 Schematic representation of miRNAs associated with the BMP pathway in PH. At early stage (24–72 h) of PH, BMPR2 activation increases miR-21a expression. In turn, miR-21a negatively regulates BMPR2 which results in decrease in BMPR2 protein expression at later stage of PH (negative feedback loop). At early stages, increased miR-21a targets RhoB, SPRY2, PDCD4, PTEN, and PPARγ to induce/inhibit PH-related cell functions. miR-27 also targets PPARγ to contribute to vascular remodeling. PPARγ activation can induce PTEN as well as suppress both miR-21a and miR-27. miR-21a and miR-27 both can be activated by HIF-1α. miR-210 targets E2F3, ISCU1/2, and MKP-1 to induce/inhibit PH-related cell functions. BMP can also induce STAT3 and miR-143/145 cluster. miR-17-20a can be activated by IL-6 in a STAT3-dependent manner. miR-17-20a contributes to impaired BMPR2 expression and to increased proliferation by inhibiting p21. Elevated level of miR-143/145 also results in decreased vasodilatation by suppressing KLF4. Genes grouped together in yellow boxes indicate targets of the associated miRNA. The *blue arrows* indicate decreased expression, and the *red arrows* indicate increased expression of miRNAs observed in PH. The *red lines* denote activation and the *blue lines* denote inhibition of associated genes/phenotypes

3.3.3 MiR143/145 and the KLF4 Pathway

Increased expression of miR-145 has been observed in human PAH-PASMCs, lung tissue from BMPR2-deficient mouse, and HPASMC from patients with BMPR2 mutations [46]. These results are consistent with data demonstrating decreased expression of Krüppel-like factor 4 (KLF4) in lung tissue from PAH patients (Table 3.1) [46, 47]. KLF4 is a group of transcription factors expressed in the vascular endothelium that exert anti-inflammatory and anticoagulant effects as well as increased endothelial nitric oxide synthase (eNOS) expression leading to increased eNOS activity [48]. BMP4 and TGF-β can induce contractile gene expression in HPASMC, and this was shown to be dependent on the increased expression of the miR-143-145 cluster (Fig. 3.2) [49]. Moreover, BMP4 and TGF-β inhibited expression of KLF4 via miR-143/145. The authors suggest a dominant role of miR-145 in the TGF-β or BMP4-mediated control of KLF4. miR-145 knockout mice exhibited increased KLF4 compared to wild-type mice [46]. Furthermore, miR-145 knockout mice, as well as antagomiR-145-treated mice, did not develop PH in hypoxic conditions, suggesting that miR-145 is essential for the PH progression. Functionally, increased expression of KLF4 and KLF5 resulted in decreased expression of smooth muscle cell markers including α-SMA, calponin, and SM-MHC [50, 51]. Inhibition of KLF4 led to decreased eNOS expression and therefore decreased eNOS activity [52]. Together these results suggest that inhibition of KLF4 contributes to vasoconstriction in PH.

3.3.4   miR-124/NFAT Pathway

The nuclear factor of activated T cells (NFAT) is a family of transcription factors that were first described to be important in immune response. NFAT consists of five members including four calcium-responsive isoforms (NFAT1-NFAT4). In the nucleus NFAT1–NFAT4 activate transcription of downstream target genes that play an important role in cellular functions associated with PH including proliferation and vascular remodeling. Recent studies revealed that NFAT family member expression was increased in PAH-HPASMC and HPASMC exposed to hypoxia resulting in increased cell proliferation and resistance to apoptosis [53]. In addition, increased expression and activity of NFAT was observed in PAH patients and animal models with chronic hypoxia-induced PH [54, 55].

Kang et al. reported that miR-124 directly targeted the 3′-UTR of NFATc1 and attenuated proliferation of PAH-PASMCs (Table 3.1) [56]. In HPASMC and mouse lung tissue, hypoxia induced a decrease in miR-124 expression, consistent with NFAT activation during this process. Functionally, miR-124 exhibits not only anti-proliferative but also pro-differentiation effects in PASMC due to suppression of the NFAT pathway [56]. In addition, miR-124 has been implicated in the remodeling of pulmonary artery fibroblasts (PAF) in IPAH patient samples. Decreased level of miR-124 correlated with hyper-proliferation of IPAH-PAF and the overexpression of miR-124 was shown to inhibit proliferation [57]. Another study indicates that miR-124 inhibited NFAT signaling by suppressing CAMTA1 (calmodulin-binding transcription activator 1) and PTBP1 (polypyrimidine tract-binding protein 1), which are required for NFAT dephosphorylation and translocation to the nucleus (Fig. 3.3) [56].

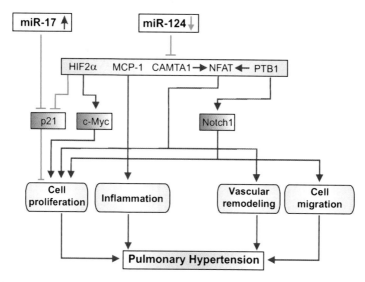

Fig. 3.3 Schematic representation of the pathways regulated by miR-124 in PH. Decreased expression of miR-124 leads to increased expression of HIF-2α, MCP-1, CAMTA1, NFAT, and PTB1 to induce/inhibit PH-related cell functions. CAMTA1 and PTB1 both contribute to NFAT activation. PTB1 mediates Notch1 signaling. HIF-2α induces proliferation by inhibiting p21 and stimulating c-Myc. Increased miR-17 also contributes to increased proliferation by inhibition of p21. Genes grouped together in *yellow boxes* indicate targets of the associated miRNA. The *blue arrows* indicate decreased expression, and the *red arrows* indicate increased expression of miR-NAs observed in PH. The *red lines* denote activation and the *blue lines* denote inhibition of associated genes/phenotypes

3.3.5   miR-124 and Other PH-Associated Pathways

miR-124 has additional targets distinct from the NFAT pathway. For example, miR-124 was also shown to inhibit expression of PTBP1, which regulates fibroblast proliferation and migration through multiple cell cycle-related genes including NOTCH1, PTEN, and FOXO3 [57]. Along with decreased level of miR-124, elevated HIF-2α expression was observed in IPAH-PAF, which has been identified as a protein that is essential for the hyper-proliferative and pro-migratory phenotype of adventitial fibroblasts in PH. miR-124 mimic was also shown to decrease level of HIF-2α in IPAH-PAF. HIF-2α is involved in cell cycle progression by inhibiting p21 expression and enhancing activation of c-Myc (Fig. 3.3) [57, 58]. Inflammation is now recognized as an important contributor to the pathogenesis of PH. Compared to control subjects, patients with PAH exhibited higher level of monocyte chemoattractant protein (MCP-1, chemokines) in plasma and the lung [59]. Decreased expression of miR-124 was also accompanied by increased expression of the monocyte chemoattractant protein (MCP-1) in IPAH-PAF (Table 3.1) [57].

3.3.6 miR-130/301, PPARγ, and miR-204 Pathway

miR-130/301 family was characterized as a master regulator of a hierarchy of pathogenic pathways relevant to PH. PH-associated PASMCs and PAECs in both murine
and human were shown to have increased expression of miR-130/301. Increased
expression of miR-130/301 activated the signal transducer and activator of transcription 3 (STAT3) signaling pathway in HPASMC by targeting inhibition of
PPARγ and ultimately leading to increased proliferation (Table 3.1) [60].
Furthermore, inhibition of PPARγ by miR130/301 leads to increase in endothelin-1
(ET-1) expression (a vasoconstriction factor) in HPASMC [61].

STAT3 is negatively regulated by PPARγ; thus, the PH-associated inhibition
of PPARγ is thought to lead to STAT3 activation and increased proliferation seen
in IPAH patients [62, 63]. STAT3 activation in HPASMC inhibited expression of
miR-204, which resulted in increased activation of the Src activator (SHP2), and
this reinforced STAT3 activation via a positive feedback loop that requires Src
(Fig. 3.4) [64, 65]. Additionally, miR-204 has been identified as a negative regulator of mouse aorta calcification that inhibited expression of a key transcription
factor for osteogenesis – Runx2 [66]. Thus miR-204 likely contributes in arterial
wall stiffness as well, which is one of the major causes for elevated PVR in
patients with PAH [67].

3.3.7 miR-130/301, Apelin, and miR-424/503

In HPAEC increased expression of miR-130/301 activated apelin signaling pathway by targeting inhibition of PPARγ and ultimately leading to increased proliferation (Table 3.1) [60]. Apelin is an important peptide in PH due to its role in the
regulation of proliferation of endothelial cells [68]. Apelin is normally activated
by PPARγ; thus, decreased expression of PPARγ seen in PA sections from humans
with PAH [35] is consistent with the observed decreased expression of apelin seen
in serum from PAH patients [69]. Lower expression of apelin resulted in decreased
miR-424 and miR-503 expression in PAH-HPAEC and animal PH models [70].
However, no significant changes in both miRNA levels were observed in PAH-
HPASMC. Nevertheless, overexpression of miR-424 and miR-503 in HPAECs
significantly reduced the proliferative response of the HPASMCs in a paracrine
manner. This information provides convincing evidence that both apelin and
miR-424/503 are integral to PH pathogenesis and potential targets for therapeutic
intervention.

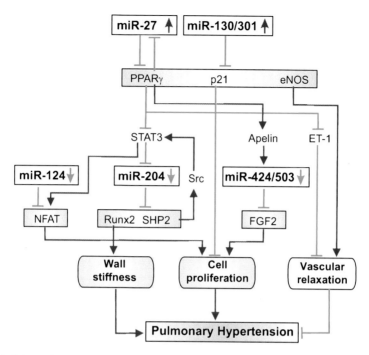

Fig. 3.4 Schematic representation of the pathways regulated by miR-130/301 in PH. miR-130/301 inhibits PPARγ, p21, and eNOS to induce/inhibit PH-related cell functions. PPARγ can be suppressed by miR-27 as well. Decreased level of PPARγ results in STAT3 and ET-1 activation. STAT3 inhibits miR-204 to increase Runx2 and SHP2 expression. Runx2 contributes to increased wall stiffness, whereas SHP2 maintains STAT3 activation through induction of Scr. NFAT also mediates proliferative effects of STAT3. Lower level of PPARγ leads to decreased miR-424/503 expression in an apelin-dependent manner and is involved in decreased vasodilatation and increased proliferation. Genes grouped together in *yellow boxes* indicate targets of the associated miRNA. The *blue arrows* indicate decreased expression, and the *red arrows* indicate increased expression of miRNAs observed in PH. The *red lines* denote activation and the *blue lines* denote inhibition of associated genes/phenotypes

3.3.8   miR-17-92 and the Cell Cycle

miR-17-92 cluster produces a single polycistronic transcript which yields six mature miRNAs: 17, 18a, 19a, 19b, 20a, and 92a. miR-17-92 was shown to directly target the 3′-UTR of PDZ and LIM domain protein 5 (PDLIM5), which is essential for miR-17-92-mediated TGF-β3/SMAD signaling and consequently SMC phenotypes (Table 3.1) [71]. This study identified PDLIM5 as a negative regulator of TGFβ/SMAD signaling and revealed that loss of PDLIM5 provoked hypoxia-induced pulmonary vascular remodeling and overexpression of PDLIM5 suppressed PH.

Gene expression of miR-17-92 was shown to be elevated by interleukin-6 (IL-6) in a STAT3-dependent manner (Fig. 3.2) [72]. Consistent with this, patients with IPAH were found to have higher serum levels of IL-6 as compared with healthy controls. Moreover, transgenic mice overexpressing IL-6 developed spontaneous pulmonary hypertension [73]. This is also consistent with the observed increased expression of miR-17 at early stages of hypoxia- and MCT-induced PH in mouse and rat models [74]. In contrast, Chen et al. revealed decreased expression of miR-17-92 in HPASMCs from IPAH patients [71]. However, in normal human and mouse PASMCs, the level of miR-17-92 was increased after exposure to hypoxia for the initial 6 h but decreased after 24 h of exposure to hypoxia. Thus, miR-17-92 appears to contribute to PH via biphasic regulation: (1) at early stages of remodeling of blood vessels, enhanced miR-17-92 expression may inhibit p21 and provoke PH; (2) in the late progressive stages, decreased expression of miR-17-92 may increase expression of PDLIM5 and therefore stimulate vascular remodeling.

3.3.9   PH-Associated miRNA Cross Talk and Redundancy

As illustrated in Figs. 3.2, 3.3, and 3.4, multiple miRNAs often affect the same pathway. This cross talk between pathways and redundancy in the regulation of pathways reinforces their importance in the pathobiology of PH. For example, BMPR2 can be inhibited by both miR-17-20a and miR-21a (Fig. 3.2) [21, 75]. PPARγ activity is also inhibited by multiple miRNAs including miR-130/301, miR-21a, and miR-27 (Figs. 3.2 and 3.4). miR-130/301 family appears to be involved in the development of increased proliferation in PH through targets other than PPARγ (Fig. 3.4). Brock et al. demonstrated that p21 is a direct target of miR-130 using reporter gene analysis [76]. In normoxic HPAECs, forced expression of miR-130a also resulted in decreased expression of eNOS and correlated with decreased vascular relaxation [61].

3.4   General Advances in miRNA Therapeutics

With a growing number of miRNAs being identified as regulators of disease, several approaches to miRNA therapy have been developed. The use of miRNA therapy in patients is becoming more realistic, and studies are showing promising results for a diverse range of diseases. There are two basic therapeutic strategies for miRNAs: replacement or inhibition and many miRNA therapies are in preclinical and clinical trials. The most advanced compounds currently in clinical trial are anti-miR-122 for the hepatitis C virus therapy followed by miR-34a for cancer treatment and anti-miR-33a/b for atherosclerosis [77–81]. In addition to these therapeutic approaches, miRNA treatment delivery methods have also evolved. Vectors have been designed and packaged in nanoparticles, liposomal molecules, or viruses to deliver miRNA treatments to disease-related cells.

Many miRNAs have been found to have decreased expression in different types of cancers and disease processes [82]. Therefore, miRNA replacement therapy works to replace the inhibited miRNAs through miRNA mimics [83, 84]. miRNA mimics are composed of oligonucleotides with the same sequence as the mature miRNA and can be either double-stranded DNA or single-stranded RNA [84]. However, studies indicate that double-stranded oligonucleotides have a higher potency (100–1000-fold) than single-stranded oligonucleotides [84, 85].

For diseases that have increased expression of miRNA, miRNA sponges offer a solution to inhibit a whole family of miRNAs allowing for a broader range of control over miRNA expression. miRNA sponges create a loss of function due to competitive inhibition of the miRNA of interest [86, 87]. Ebert et al. demonstrated that miRNA sponges expressed at high levels inhibited a family of miRNA through complementary binding to a common seed region [87]. The inhibiting effects of miRNA sponges appear to be long lasting making them an attractive method for clinical treatment [86, 88].

Another miRNA inhibition therapy is antisense oligonucleotides (also referred to as antagomiRs) with locked nucleic acid (LNA) modifications. LNA-based antisense oligonucleotides bind to and inhibit miRNAs directly, acting as anti-miRNAs. One of the benefits of LNA-based anti-miRNAs is that they work in a similar manner as small interfering RNAs (siRNAs), which have been shown to work as therapeutic agents and several are currently in clinical trials. A limitation of LNA-based anti-miRNAs is that oligonucleotides are rapidly degraded by serum nucleases and therefore need to be chemically modified to stay in serum for longer periods of time [89]. Additionally, they can only target one miRNA at a time as shown by Montgomery et al. in a preclinical trial [88].

3.5   Potential for miRNA Target Therapies in PAH

While there are currently no clinical trials targeting miRNAs for the treatment of PAH, preclinical studies highlighted below open new avenues for the treatment of PAH using miRNA-based therapeutics.

3.5.1   PAH miRNA Replacement Therapy

Several examples using miRNA mimics suggest that replacement therapy may be a useful treatment strategy. Overexpression of miR-124 was shown to inhibit proliferation in PAF from patients with IPAH [57]. Treatment with a synthetic miR-204 mimic in MCT-induced PH rats showed a significant decrease in PAP, decreased pulmonary artery remodeling, attenuated PASMC proliferation, and increased PASMC apoptosis [64]. Since miR-204 has been identified as a negative regulator of mouse aorta calcification that functions through repressing a key transcription factor for osteogenesis, Runx2 (Fig. 3.4) [66], miR-204 likely contributes to arterial wall stiffness as well, which is one of the major causes for elevated PVR in patients with

PAH [67]. Kim et al. showed that overexpressing miR-424 and miR-503 provided a protective effect that ameliorates PH by markedly reducing right ventricular systolic pressure (RVSP) and right heart hypertrophy [70]. This is consistent with reported reversal of PH in mice with daily i.p. injections of 200 µg/kg apelin for 2 weeks compared to vehicle [90]. This information provides convincing evidence that miR-424/503 are also potential targets for therapeutic intervention.

3.5.2 PAH miRNA Inhibition Therapy

Preclinical data suggests that inhibition of critical miRNAs with antagomiRs also has promise. Treatment of HPASMC with antagomiR-21a restored PTEN expression and inhibited hypoxia-induced proliferation, further supporting the important role of miR-21a in PH pathogenesis [28]. Jin et al. inhibited miR-210 and observed re-expression of MKP-1 and consequently prevented hypoxia-induced cell proliferation. AntagomiR-145 has been shown to have a protective effect against hypoxia-induced PH in mice by significantly reducing RVSP and pulmonary vascular remodeling [46]. An antagomiR-17 improved hemodynamic and structural changes presumably by inducing a well-known inhibitor of SMC proliferation, p21 [74]. Inhibition of miR-17-92 also resulted in increased PDLIM5 and prevented lung and heart vascular remodeling in PH [71].

3.5.3 PAH miRNA Diagnostics

Accumulating evidence suggested that circulating miRNAs could be developed as biomarkers for early diagnosis of the onset of PAH. Decreased level of miR-21 was reported in lung tissue as well as in serum from patients with IPAH [15]. Courboulin et al. reported that decreased expression of miR-204 in white blood cells correlated with PAH severity and might serve as a circulatory biomarker of PAH [64]. Also, increasing higher plasma levels of miR-130/301 family members were observed in patients with increasing hemodynamic severity of PH [60]. Another study used high-density microarrays to identify circulating miRNAs in 12 well-characterized IPAH patients [91]. These results support that miR-130, miR-204, miR-145, and miR-27a can potentially be used as biomarkers for earlier and more accurate diagnosis of IPAH.

3.6 Target miRNAs for Treatment

These data collectively suggest that targeting miRNAs for treatment of PAH could be a powerful technology, but it is clear that there are several challenges that still need to be overcome.

As mentioned earlier, over 2500 mature human miRNAs are registered in miR-Base. Many of these belong to miRNA families with similar seed regions. Under physiological conditions, anti-miRNAs target all miRNAs within the same family with identical seed regions. This lack of target specificity may lead to harmful off-target effects of the anti-miRNA. Reports of successful targeting of the 3′ sequence of miRNAs or targeting the translation of pre-miRNAs suggests that these alternative strategies for inhibiting miRNAs may improve target specificity [92–95].

Molecules used to target miRNAs, both the miRNA target technology and the delivery system, may be detected by the innate and adaptive arms of the immune system constituting serious toxicological concerns. Chemical modification of oligonucleotides helps to increase their RNA-binding affinity and resistance to cellular nucleases. However, these chemical modifications can induce sequence-independent toxicity in vivo [96]. Kerkmann et al. modified the sense strand nucleotides with poly(A) and minimized these immunostimulatory effects demonstrating that it is possible to derive safe oligonucleotide treatments [95].

Strategies will also need to be carefully considered in order to achieve the desired delivery of miRNA-targeted treatments to the disease site (distal pulmonary arterioles) to improve therapeutic efficacy and decrease systemic and local side effects. Not only is it important to deliver appropriate levels of the miRNA targeted treatment to the affected cells, but it is also critical that normal surrounding tissues be avoided to prevent on-target side effects in normal cells. A potential therapeutic target for PAH is the miR-17-92 cluster that is increased at early stages of PH and contributes to increased proliferation, vascular remodeling, RVSP, and right heart hypertrophy. However, miR-17-92 is expressed in many normal tissues, and targeted deletion of miR-17–92 in mice causes death of neonates owing to lung hypoplasia and a ventricular septal defect [97]. Therefore, it is critical to develop targeted delivery approaches specifically to diseased cells. Identification of a cell surface antigen expressed uniquely on the diseased cells would allow use of antibodies or ligand binding domains to target the miRNA therapeutic to the appropriate cell type.

3.7 Summary and Future Research Directions

Multiple molecular mechanisms are involved in the development and progression of sustained pulmonary vasoconstriction, concentric pulmonary vascular remodeling, in situ thrombosis, and increased pulmonary vascular wall stiffness. As a posttranscriptional regulator, miRNAs are involved in the downregulation of multiple genes that cause vasodilation of pulmonary arteries and arterioles and regression of thickened pulmonary vascular wall and eventually contribute to the development and progression of PAH. miRNAs are also indirectly involved in the upregulation of many genes that contribute to cell proliferation and growth, dedifferentiation, and migration, which subsequently result in concentric pulmonary vascular wall thickening leading to the increased PVR and pulmonary hypertension. It is thus important to understand the precise sequence of events by which certain miRNAs regulate key genes (e.g., *BMPR2*, *TRPC6*, *KCNA5*, *CASR*, *CAV1*) that are involved in the development and progression of PAH. It is also critical to identify specific miRNAs that are major modulators of the pathogenic genes or signaling pathways involved in PAH.

Acknowledgment This work was supported by the grants obtained from the National Heart, Lung, and Blood Institute of the National Institutes of Health (HL115014, HL066012, and HL098053). The authors would like to thank Nikita Babichev for assistance with graphic layout of the figures.

References

1. Hoeper MM, Simon RGJ. The changing landscape of pulmonary arterial hypertension and implications for patient care. Eur Respir Rev. 2014;23(134):450–7. doi:10.1183/09059180.00007814.
2. Kovacs G, Berghold A, Scheidl S, Olschewski H. Pulmonary arterial pressure during rest and exercise in healthy subjects: a systematic review. Eur Respir J. 2009;34(4):888–94. doi:10.1183/09031936.00145608.
3. Thum T, Batkai S. MicroRNAs in right ventricular (dys)function (2013 Grover Conference series). Pulm Circ. 2014;4(2):185–90. doi:10.1086/675981 PC2013103 [pii]
4. Kim GH, Ryan JJ, Marsboom G, Archer SL. Epigenetic mechanisms of pulmonary hypertension. Pulm Circ. 2011;1(3):347–56. doi:10.4103/2045-8932.87300 PC-1-347 [pii]
5. Frumkin LR. The pharmacological treatment of pulmonary arterial hypertension. Pharmacol Rev. 2012;64(3):583–620. doi:10.1124/pr.111.005587.
6. Joshi SR, McLendon JM, Comer BS, Gerthoffer WT. MicroRNAs-control of essential genes: implications for pulmonary vascular disease. Pulm Circ. 2011;1(3):357–64. doi:10.4103/2045-8932.87301 PC-1-357 [pii]
7. White K, Loscalzo J, Chan SY. Holding our breath: the emerging and anticipated roles of microRNA in pulmonary hypertension. Pulm Circ. 2012;2(3):278–90. doi:10.4103/2045-8932.101395.
8. Winter J, Jung S, Keller S, Gregory RI, Diederichs S. Many roads to maturity: microRNA biogenesis pathways and their regulation. Nat Cell Biol. 2009;11(3):228–34. doi:10.1038/ncb0309-228.
9. Geraci MW. Integrating molecular genetics and systems approaches to pulmonary vascular diseases. Pulm Circ. 2013;3(1):171–5. doi:10.4103/2045-8932.109959 PC-3-171 [pii]
10. Sessa R, Hata A. Role of microRNAs in lung development and pulmonary diseases. Pulm Circ. 2013;3(2):315–28. doi:10.4103/2045-8932.114758 PC-3-315 [pii]
11. Da Sacco L, Masotti A. Recent insights and novel bioinformatics tools to understand the role of microRNAs binding to 5′ untranslated region. Int J Mol Sci. 2012;14(1):480–95. doi:10.3390/ijms14010480 ijms14010480 [pii]
12. Towler BP, Jones CI, Newbury SF. Mechanisms of regulation of mature miRNAs. Biochem Soc Trans. 2015;43(6):1208–14. doi:10.1042/BST20150157. BST20150157 [pii]
13. Barrett LW, Fletcher S, Wilton SD. Regulation of eukaryotic gene expression by the untranslated gene regions and other non-coding elements. Cell Mol Life Sci. 2012;69(21):3613–34. doi:10.1007/s00018-012-0990-9.
14. Albinsson S, Suarez Y, Skoura A, Offermanns S, Miano JM, Sessa WC. MicroRNAs are necessary for vascular smooth muscle growth, differentiation, and function. Arterioscler Thromb Vasc Biol. 2010;30(6):1118–26. doi:10.1161/ATVBAHA.109.200873.
15. Caruso P, MacLean MR, Khanin R, McClure J, Soon E, Southgate M, et al. Dynamic changes in lung microRNA profiles during the development of pulmonary hypertension due to chronic hypoxia and monocrotaline. Arterioscler Thromb Vasc Biol. 2010;30(4):716–23. doi:10.1161/ATVBAHA.109.202028.

16. Rupaimoole R, Wu SY, Pradeep S, Ivan C, Pecot CV, Gharpure KM, et al. Hypoxia-mediated downregulation of miRNA biogenesis promotes tumour progression. Nat Commun. 2014;5:5202. doi:10.1038/ncomms6202 ncomms6202 [pii]

17. Bandara V, Michael MZ, Gleadle JM. Hypoxia represses microRNA biogenesis proteins in breast cancer cells. BMC Cancer. 2014;14:533. doi:10.1186/1471-2407-14-533. 1471-2407-14-533 [pii]

18. Klinge CM. miRNAs regulated by estrogens, tamoxifen, and endocrine disruptors and their downstream gene targets. Mol Cell Endocrinol. 2015; doi:10.1016/j.mce.2015.01.035.

19. Grant JS, Morecroft I, Dempsie Y, van Rooij E, MacLean MR, Baker AH. Transient but not genetic loss of miR-451 is protective in the development of pulmonary arterial hypertension. Pulm Circ. 2013;3(4):840–50. doi:10.1086/674751. PC2013009 [pii]

20. Wang L, Guo LJ, Liu J, Wang W, Yuan JX, Zhao L, et al. MicroRNA expression profile of pulmonary artery smooth muscle cells and the effect of let-7d in chronic thromboembolic pulmonary hypertension. Pulm Circ. 2013;3(3):654–64. doi:10.1086/674310.

21. Parikh VN, Jin RC, Rabello S, Gulbahce N, White K, Hale A, et al. MicroRNA-21 integrates pathogenic signaling to control pulmonary hypertension: results of a network bioinformatics approach. Circulation. 2012;125(12):1520–32. doi:10.1161/CIRCULATIONAHA.111.060269.

22. Green DE, Murphy TC, Kang BY, Searles CD, Hart CM. PPARgamma ligands attenuate hypoxia-induced proliferation in human pulmonary artery smooth muscle cells through modulation of microRNA-21. PLoS One 2015;10(7):e0133391. doi:10.1371/journal.pone.0133391 PONE-D-15-13472 [pii].

23. Drake KM, Zygmunt D, Mavrakis L, Harbor P, Wang L, Comhair SA, et al. Altered microRNA processing in heritable pulmonary arterial hypertension: an important role for Smad-8. Am J Respir Crit Care Med. 2011;184(12):1400–8. doi:10.1164/rccm.201106-1130OC. 201106-1130OC [pii]

24. Takahashi H, Goto N, Kojima Y, Tsuda Y, Morio Y, Muramatsu M et al. Downregulation of type II bone morphogenetic protein receptor in hypoxic pulmonary hypertension. Am J Phys Lung Cell Mol Phys 2006;290(3):L450–L458. doi:00206.2005 [pii] 10.1152/ajplung.00206.2005.

25. Morty RE, Nejman B, Kwapiszewska G, Hecker M, Zakrzewicz A, Kouri FM et al. Dysregulated bone morphogenetic protein signaling in monocrotaline-induced pulmonary arterial hypertension. Arterioscler Thromb Vasc Biol 2007;27(5):1072–1078. doi:ATVBAHA.107.141200 [pii] 10.1161/ATVBAHA.107.141200.

26. Atkinson C, Stewart S, Upton PD, Machado R, Thomson JR, Trembath RC, et al. Primary pulmonary hypertension is associated with reduced pulmonary vascular expression of type II bone morphogenetic protein receptor. Circulation. 2002;105(14):1672–8.

27. Davis BN, Hilyard AC, Lagna G, Hata A. SMAD proteins control DROSHA-mediated microRNA maturation. Nature. 2008;454(7200):56–61. doi:10.1038/nature07086. nature07086 [pii]

28. Sarkar J, Gou D, Turaka P, Viktorova E, Ramchandran R, Raj JU. MicroRNA-21 plays a role in hypoxia-mediated pulmonary artery smooth muscle cell proliferation and migration. Am J Phys Lung Cell Mol Phys. 2010;299(6):L861–71. doi:10.1152/ajplung.00201.2010.

29. Polytarchou C, Iliopoulos D, Hatziapostolou M, Kottakis F, Maroulakou I, Struhl K et al. Akt2 regulates all Akt isoforms and promotes resistance to hypoxia through induction of miR-21 upon oxygen deprivation. Cancer Res 2011;71(13):4720–4731. doi:10.1158/0008-5472.CAN-11-0365 0008-5472.CAN-11-0365 [pii].

30. Iannone L, Zhao L, Dubois O, Duluc L, Rhodes CJ, Wharton J, et al. miR-21/DDAH1 pathway regulates pulmonary vascular responses to hypoxia. Biochem J. 2014;462(1):103–12. doi:10.1042/BJ20140486. BJ20140486 [pii]

31. Yang S, Banerjee S, Freitas A, Cui H, Xie N, Abraham E et al. miR-21 regulates chronic hypoxia-induced pulmonary vascular remodeling. Am J Phys Lung Cell Mol Phys 2012;302(6):L521–L529. doi:10.1152/ajplung.00316.2011 ajplung.00316.2011 [pii].

32. Lin Y, Liu X, Cheng Y, Yang J, Huo Y, Zhang C. Involvement of microRNAs in hydrogen peroxide-mediated gene regulation and cellular injury response in vascular smooth muscle cells. J Biol Chem 2009;284(12):7903–7913. doi:10.1074/jbc.M806920200 M806920200 [pii].

33. White K, Dempsie Y, Caruso P, Wallace E, McDonald RA, Stevens H, et al. Endothelial apoptosis in pulmonary hypertension is controlled by a microRNA/programmed cell death 4/caspase-3 axis. Hypertension. 2014;64(1):185–94. doi:10.1161/HYPERTENSIONAHA.113.03037 HYPERTENSIONAHA.113.03037 [pii]

34. Ameshima S, Golpon H, Cool CD, Chan D, Vandivier RW, Gardai SJ, et al. Peroxisome proliferator-activated receptor gamma (PPARgamma) expression is decreased in pulmonary hypertension and affects endothelial cell growth. Circ Res. 2003;92(10):1162–9. doi:10.1161/01.RES.0000073585.50092.14 01.RES.0000073585.50092.14 [pii]

35. Falcetti E, Hall SM, Phillips PG, Patel J, Morrell NW, Haworth SG, et al. Smooth muscle proliferation and role of the prostacyclin (IP) receptor in idiopathic pulmonary arterial hypertension. Am J Respir Crit Care Med. 2010;182(9):1161–70. doi:10.1164/rccm.201001-0011OC 201001-0011OC [pii]

36. Wojciak-Stothard B, Zhao L, Oliver E, Dubois O, Wu Y, Kardassis D, et al. Role of RhoB in the regulation of pulmonary endothelial and smooth muscle cell responses to hypoxia. Circ Res. 2012;110(11):1423–34. doi:10.1161/CIRCRESAHA.112.264473 CIRCRESAHA.112.264473 [pii]

37. Ghatnekar A, Chrobak I, Reese C, Stawski L, Seta F, Wirrig E, et al. Endothelial GATA-6 deficiency promotes pulmonary arterial hypertension. Am J Pathol. 2013;182(6):2391–406. doi:10.1016/j.ajpath.2013.02.039 S0002-9440(13)00218-6 [pii]

38. Chan YC, Banerjee J, Choi SY, Sen CK. miR-210: the master hypoxamir. Microcirculation. 2012;19(3):215–23. doi:10.1111/j.1549-8719.2011.00154.x.

39. Chan SY, Loscalzo J. MicroRNA-210: a unique and pleiotropic hypoxamir. Cell Cycle. 2010;9(6):1072–83. doi:11006 [pii]

40. Gou D, Ramchandran R, Peng X, Yao L, Kang K, Sarkar J, et al. miR-210 has an antiapoptotic effect in pulmonary artery smooth muscle cells during hypoxia. Am J Phys Lung Cell Mol Phys. 2012;303(8):L682–91. doi:10.1152/ajplung.00344.2011.

41. White K, Lu Y, Annis S, Hale AE, Chau BN, Dahlman JE, et al. Genetic and hypoxic alterations of the microRNA-210-ISCU1/2 axis promote iron-sulfur deficiency and pulmonary hypertension. EMBO Mol Med. 2015;7(6):695–713. doi:10.15252/emmm.201404511.

42. Chan SY, Zhang YY, Hemann C, Mahoney CE, Zweier JL, Loscalzo J. MicroRNA-210 controls mitochondrial metabolism during hypoxia by repressing the iron-sulfur cluster assembly proteins ISCU1/2. Cell Metab. 2009;10(4):273–84. doi:10.1016/j.cmet.2009.08.015 S1550-4131(09)00265-4 [pii]

43. Hong S, Paulson QX, Johnson DG. E2F1 and E2F3 activate ATM through distinct mechanisms to promote E1A-induced apoptosis. Cell Cycle. 2008;7(3):391–400.

44. Martinez LA, Goluszko E, Chen HZ, Leone G, Post S, Lozano G, et al. E2F3 is a mediator of DNA damage-induced apoptosis. Mol Cell Biol. 2010;30(2):524–36. doi:10.1128/MCB.00938-09.

45. Jin Y, Pang T, Nelin LD, Wang W, Wang Y, Yan J, et al. MKP-1 is a target of miR-210 and mediate the negative regulation of miR-210 inhibitor on hypoxic hPASMC proliferation. Cell Biol Int. 2015;39(1):113–20. doi:10.1002/cbin.10339.

46. Caruso P, Dempsie Y, Stevens HC, McDonald RA, Long L, Lu R, et al. A role for miR-145 in pulmonary arterial hypertension: evidence from mouse models and patient samples. Circ Res. 2012;111(3):290–300. doi:10.1161/CIRCRESAHA.112.267591 CIRCRESAHA.112.267591 [pii]

47. Shatat MA, Tian H, Zhang R, Tandon G, Hale A, Fritz JS, et al. Endothelial Kruppel-like factor 4 modulates pulmonary arterial hypertension. Am J Respir Cell Mol Biol. 2014;50(3):647–53. doi:10.1165/rcmb.2013-0135OC.

48. Atkins GB, Jain MK. Role of Kruppel-like transcription factors in endothelial biology. Circ Res. 2007;100(12):1686–95. doi:100/12/1686 [pii] 10.1161/01.RES.0000267856.00713.0a

49. Davis-Dusenbery BN, Chan MC, Reno KE, Weisman AS, Layne MD, Lagna G, et al. downregulation of Kruppel-like factor-4 (KLF4) by microRNA-143/145 is critical for modulation of vascular smooth muscle cell phenotype by transforming growth factor-beta and bone morphogenetic protein 4. J Biol Chem. 2011;286(32):28097–110. doi:10.1074/jbc.M111.236950.

50. Cordes KR, Sheehy NT, White MP, Berry EC, Morton SU, Muth AN, et al. miR-145 and miR-143 regulate smooth muscle cell fate and plasticity. Nature. 2009;460(7256):705–10. doi:10.1038/nature08195.

51. Cheng Y, Liu X, Yang J, Lin Y, Xu DZ, Lu Q, et al. MicroRNA-145, a novel smooth muscle cell phenotypic marker and modulator, controls vascular neointimal lesion formation. Circ Res. 2009;105(2):158–66. doi:10.1161/CIRCRESAHA.109.197517 CIRCRESAHA.109.197517 [pii]

52. Hamik A, Lin Z, Kumar A, Balcells M, Sinha S, Katz J, et al. Kruppel-like factor 4 regulates endothelial inflammation. J Biol Chem. 2007;282(18):13769–79. doi:M700078200 [pii] 10.1074/jbc.M700078200

53. Hassoun PM, Mouthon L, Barbera JA, Eddahibi S, Flores SC, Grimminger F, et al. Inflammation, growth factors, and pulmonary vascular remodeling. J Am Coll Cardiol. 2009;54(1 Suppl):S10–9. doi:10.1016/j.jacc.2009.04.006 S0735-1097(09)01208-X [pii]

54. Bonnet S, Rochefort G, Sutendra G, Archer SL, Haromy A, Webster L, et al. The nuclear factor of activated T cells in pulmonary arterial hypertension can be therapeutically targeted. Proc Natl Acad Sci U S A. 2007;104(27):11418–23. doi:0610467104 [pii] 10.1073/pnas.0610467104

55. Bierer R, Nitta CH, Friedman J, Codianni S, de Frutos S, Dominguez-Bautista JA, et al. NFATc3 is required for chronic hypoxia-induced pulmonary hypertension in adult and neonatal mice. Am J Phys Lung Cell Mol Phys. 2011;301(6):L872–80. doi:10.1152/ajplung.00405.2010 ajplung.00405.2010 [pii]

56. Kang K, Peng X, Zhang X, Wang Y, Zhang L, Gao L, et al. MicroRNA-124 suppresses the transactivation of nuclear factor of activated T cells by targeting multiple genes and inhibits the proliferation of pulmonary artery smooth muscle cells. J Biol Chem. 2013;288(35):25414–27. doi:10.1074/jbc.M113.460287 M113.460287 [pii]

57. Wang D, Zhang H, Li M, Frid MG, Flockton AR, McKeon BA, et al. MicroRNA-124 controls the proliferative, migratory, and inflammatory phenotype of pulmonary vascular fibroblasts. Circ Res. 2014;114(1):67–78. doi:10.1161/CIRCRESAHA.114.301633.

58. Gordan JD, Bertout JA, Hu CJ, Diehl JA, Simon MC. HIF-2alpha promotes hypoxic cell proliferation by enhancing c-myc transcriptional activity. Cancer Cell. 2007;11(4):335–47. doi:S1535-6108(07)00059-1 [pii] 10.1016/j.ccr.2007.02.006

59. Itoh T, Nagaya N, Ishibashi-Ueda H, Kyotani S, Oya H, Sakamaki F, et al. Increased plasma monocyte chemoattractant protein-1 level in idiopathic pulmonary arterial hypertension. Respirology. 2006;11(2):158–63. doi:RES [pii] 10.1111/j.1440-1843.2006.00821.x.

60. Bertero T, Lu Y, Annis S, Hale A, Bhat B, Saggar R, et al. Systems-level regulation of microRNA networks by miR-130/301 promotes pulmonary hypertension. J Clin Invest. 2014;124(8):3514–28. doi:10.1172/JCI74773.

61. Bertero T, Cottrill K, Krauszman A, Lu Y, Annis S, Hale A, et al. The microRNA-130/301 family controls vasoconstriction in pulmonary hypertension. J Biol Chem. 2015;290(4):2069–85. doi:10.1074/jbc.M114.617845 M114.617845 [pii]

62. Masri FA, Xu W, Comhair SA, Asosingh K, Koo M, Vasanji A, et al. Hyperproliferative apoptosis-resistant endothelial cells in idiopathic pulmonary arterial hypertension. Am J Phys Lung Cell Mol Phys. 2007;293(3):L548–54. doi:00428.2006 [pii] 10.1152/ajplung.00428.2006

63. Potus F, Graydon C, Provencher S, Bonnet S. Vascular remodeling process in pulmonary arterial hypertension, with focus on miR-204 and miR-126 (2013 Grover Conference series). Pulm Circ. 2014;4(2):175–84. doi:10.1086/675980 PC2013105 [pii]

64. Courboulin A, Paulin R, Giguere NJ, Saksouk N, Perreault T, Meloche J, et al. Role for miR-204 in human pulmonary arterial hypertension. J Exp Med. 2011;208(3):535–48. doi:10.1084/jem.20101812.

65. Meloche J, Pflieger A, Vaillancourt M, Paulin R, Potus F, Zervopoulos S, et al. Role for DNA damage signaling in pulmonary arterial hypertension. Circulation. 2014;129(7):786–97. doi:10.1161/CIRCULATIONAHA.113.006167 CIRCULATIONAHA.113.006167 [pii]

66. Cui RR, Li SJ, Liu LJ, Yi L, Liang QH, Zhu X, et al. MicroRNA-204 regulates vascular smooth muscle cell calcification in vitro and in vivo. Cardiovasc Res. 2012;96(2):320–9. doi:10.1093/cvr/cvs258 cvs258 [pii]

67. Kuhr FK, Smith KA, Song MY, Levitan I, Yuan JX. New mechanisms of pulmonary arterial hypertension: role of Ca(2)(+) signaling. Am J Physiol Heart Circ Physiol. 2012;302(8):H1546–62. doi:10.1152/ajpheart.00944.2011 ajpheart.00944.2011 [pii]

68. He L, Xu J, Chen L, Li L. Apelin/APJ signaling in hypoxia-related diseases. Clin Chim Acta. 2015;451(Pt B):191–8. doi:10.1016/j.cca.2015.09.029 S0009-8981(15)00438-6 [pii]

69. Chandra SM, Razavi H, Kim J, Agrawal R, Kundu RK, de Jesus PV, et al. Disruption of the apelin-APJ system worsens hypoxia-induced pulmonary hypertension. Arterioscler Thromb Vasc Biol. 2011;31(4):814–20. doi:10.1161/ATVBAHA.110.219980.

70. Kim J, Kang Y, Kojima Y, Lighthouse JK, Hu X, Aldred MA, et al. An endothelial apelin-FGF link mediated by miR-424 and miR-503 is disrupted in pulmonary arterial hypertension. Nat Med. 2013;19(1):74–82. doi:10.1038/nm.3040.

71. Chen T, Zhou G, Zhou Q, Tang H, Ibe JC, Cheng H, et al. Loss of microRNA-17 approximately 92 in smooth muscle cells attenuates experimental pulmonary hypertension via induction of PDZ and LIM domain 5. Am J Respir Crit Care Med. 2015;191(6):678–92. doi:10.1164/rccm.201405-0941OC.

72. Brock M, Trenkmann M, Gay RE, Michel BA, Gay S, Fischler M, et al. Interleukin-6 modulates the expression of the bone morphogenic protein receptor type II through a novel STAT3-microRNA cluster 17/92 pathway. Circ Res. 2009;104(10):1184–91. doi:10.1161/CIRCRESAHA.109.197491.

73. Steiner MK, Syrkina OL, Kolliputi N, Mark EJ, Hales CA, Waxman AB. Interleukin-6 overexpression induces pulmonary hypertension. Circ Res. 2009;104(2):236–44. 28p following 44. doi:10.1161/CIRCRESAHA.108.182014 CIRCRESAHA.108.182014 [pii]

74. Pullamsetti SS, Doebele C, Fischer A, Savai R, Kojonazarov B, Dahal BK, et al. Inhibition of microRNA-17 improves lung and heart function in experimental pulmonary hypertension. Am J Respir Crit Care Med. 2012;185(4):409–19. doi:10.1164/rccm.201106-1093OC.

75. Brock M, Samillan VJ, Trenkmann M, Schwarzwald C, Ulrich S, Gay RE, et al. AntagomiR directed against miR-20a restores functional BMPR2 signalling and prevents vascular remodelling in hypoxia-induced pulmonary hypertension. Eur Heart J. 2014;35(45):3203–11. doi:10.1093/eurheartj/ehs060 ehs060 [pii]

76. Brock M, Haider TJ, Vogel J, Gassmann M, Speich R, Trenkmann M, et al. The hypoxia-induced microRNA-130a controls pulmonary smooth muscle cell proliferation by directly targeting CDKN1A. Int J Biochem Cell Biol. 2015;61:129–37. doi:10.1016/j.biocel.2015.02.002 S1357-2725(15)00045-X [pii]

77. Li XJ, Ren ZJ, Tang JH. MicroRNA-34a: a potential therapeutic target in human cancer. Cell Death Dis. 2014;5:e1327.doi:10.1038/cddis.2014.270 cddis2014270 [pii]

78. Diaz MR, Vivas-Mejia PE. Nanoparticles as drug delivery systems in cancer medicine: emphasis on RNAi-containing nanoliposomes. Pharmaceuticals (Basel). 2013;6(11):1361–80. doi:10.3390/ph6111361 ph6111361 [pii]

79. Janssen HL, Reesink HW, Lawitz EJ, Zeuzem S, Rodriguez-Torres M, Patel K, et al. Treatment of HCV infection by targeting microRNA. N Engl J Med. 2013;368(18):1685–94. doi:10.1056/NEJMoa1209026.

80. Kao SC, Fulham M, Wong K, Cooper W, Brahmbhatt H, MacDiarmid J, et al. A significant metabolic and radiological response after a novel targeted microRNA-based treatment approach in malignant pleural mesothelioma. Am J Respir Crit Care Med. 2015;191(12):1467–9. doi:10.1164/rccm.201503-0461LE.

81. Hydbring P, Badalian-Very G. Clinical applications of microRNAs. F1000Res. 2013;2:136. doi:10.12688/f1000research.2–136.v3

82. Wang H, Jiang Y, Peng H, Chen Y, Zhu P, Huang Y. Recent progress in microRNA delivery for cancer therapy by non-viral synthetic vectors. Adv Drug Deliv Rev. 2015;81:142–60. doi:10.1016/j.addr.2014.10.031 S0169-409X(14)00239-7 [pii]

83. Wiggins JF, Ruffino L, Kelnar K, Omotola M, Patrawala L, Brown D, et al. Development of a lung cancer therapeutic based on the tumor suppressor microRNA-34. Cancer Res. 2010;70(14):5923–30. doi:10.1158/0008-5472.CAN-10-0655 0008-5472.CAN-10-0655 [pii]

84. Bader AG, Brown D, Stoudemire J, Lammers P. Developing therapeutic microRNAs for cancer. Gene Ther. 2011;18(12):1121–6. doi:10.1038/gt.2011.79 gt201179 [pii]

85. Peng B, Chen Y, Leong KW. MicroRNA delivery for regenerative medicine. Adv Drug Deliv Rev. 2015;88:108–22. doi:10.1016/j.addr.2015.05.014 S0169-409X(15)00109-X [pii]

86. Ebert MS, Neilson JR, Sharp PA. MicroRNA sponges: competitive inhibitors of small RNAs in mammalian cells. Nat Methods. 2007;4(9):721–6. doi:nmeth1079 [pii] 10.1038/nmeth1079

87. Ebert MS, Sharp PA. MicroRNA sponges: progress and possibilities. RNA. 2010;16(11):2043–50. doi:10.1261/rna.2414110 rna.2414110 [pii]

88. Montgomery RL, Hullinger TG, Semus HM, Dickinson BA, Seto AG, Lynch JM, et al. Therapeutic inhibition of miR-208a improves cardiac function and survival during heart failure. Circulation. 2011;124(14):1537–47. doi:10.1161/CIRCULATIONAHA.111.030932 CIRCULATIONAHA.111.030932 [pii]

89. Li Z, Rana TM. Therapeutic targeting of microRNAs: current status and future challenges. Nat Rev Drug Discov. 2014;13(8):622–38. doi:10.1038/nrd4359 nrd4359 [pii]

90. Alastalo TP, Li M, Perez Vde J, Pham D, Sawada H, Wang JK, et al. Disruption of PPARgamma/beta-catenin-mediated regulation of apelin impairs BMP-induced mouse and human pulmonary arterial EC survival. J Clin Invest. 2011;121(9):3735–46. doi:10.1172/JCI43382.

91. Sarrion I, Milian L, Juan G, Ramon M, Furest I, Carda C, et al. Role of circulating miRNAs as biomarkers in idiopathic pulmonary arterial hypertension: possible relevance of miR-23a. Oxidative Med Cell Longev. 2015;2015:792846. doi:10.1155/2015/792846.

92. Newman MA, Hammond SM. Emerging paradigms of regulated microRNA processing. Genes Dev. 2010;24(11):1086–92. doi:10.1101/gad.1919710 24/11/1086 [pii].

93. Lal A, Navarro F, Maher CA, Maliszewski LE, Yan N, O'Day E, et al. miR-24 Inhibits cell proliferation by targeting E2F2, MYC, and other cell-cycle genes via binding to "seedless" 3'UTR microRNA recognition elements. Mol Cell. 2009;35(5):610–25. doi:10.1016/j.molcel.2009.08.020 S1097-2765(09)00600-5 [pii]

94. Arechavala-Gomeza V, Graham IR, Popplewell LJ, Adams AM, Aartsma-Rus A, Kinali M, et al. Comparative analysis of antisense oligonucleotide sequences for targeted skipping of exon 51 during dystrophin pre-mRNA splicing in human muscle. Hum Gene Ther. 2007;18(9):798–810. doi:10.1089/hum.2006.061.

95. Kerkmann M, Costa LT, Richter C, Rothenfusser S, Battiany J, Hornung V, et al. Spontaneous formation of nucleic acid-based nanoparticles is responsible for high interferon-alpha induction by CpG-A in plasmacytoid dendritic cells. J Biol Chem. 2005;280(9):8086–93. doi:M410868200 [pii] 10.1074/jbc.M410868200.

96. Rivera RM, Bennett LB. Epigenetics in humans: an overview. Curr Opin Endocrinol Diabetes Obes. 2010;17(6):493–9. doi:10.1097/MED.0b013e3283404f4b.

97. Ventura A, Young AG, Winslow MM, Lintault L, Meissner A, Erkeland SJ, et al. Targeted deletion reveals essential and overlapping functions of the miR-17 through 92 family of miRNA clusters. Cell. 2008;132(5):875–86. doi:10.1016/j.cell.2008.02.019 S0092-8674(08)00267-5 [pii]

98. Dakhlallah D, Batte K, Wang Y, Cantemir-Stone CZ, Yan P, Nuovo G, et al. Epigenetic regulation of miR-17~92 contributes to the pathogenesis of pulmonary fibrosis. Am J Respir Crit Care Med. 2013;187(4):397–405. doi:10.1164/rccm.201205-0888OC rccm.201205-0888OC [pii]

99. Ji R, Cheng Y, Yue J, Yang J, Liu X, Chen H, et al. MicroRNA expression signature and antisense-mediated depletion reveal an essential role of microRNA in vascular neointimal lesion formation. Circ Res. 2007;100(11):1579–88. doi:CIRCRESAHA.106.141986 [pii] 10.1161/CIRCRESAHA.106.141986.

100. Li Y, Yan L, Zhang W, Hu N, Chen W, Wang H, et al. MicroRNA-21 inhibits platelet-derived growth factor-induced human aortic vascular smooth muscle cell proliferation and migration through targeting activator protein-1. Am J Transl Res. 2014;6(5):507–16.

101. Kang BY, Park KK, Green DE, Bijli KM, Searles CD, Sutliff RL, et al. Hypoxia mediates mutual repression between microRNA-27a and PPARgamma in the pulmonary vasculature. PLoS One. 2013;8(11):e79503.doi:10.1371/journal.pone.0079503 PONE-D-13-24907 [pii]

102. Bi R, Bao C, Jiang L, Liu H, Yang Y, Mei J, et al. MicroRNA-27b plays a role in pulmonary arterial hypertension by modulating peroxisome proliferator-activated receptor gamma dependent Hsp90-eNOS signaling and nitric oxide production. Biochem Biophys Res Commun. 2015;460(2):469–75. doi:10.1016/j.bbrc.2015.03.057 S0006-291X(15)00492-1 [pii]

103. Elia L, Quintavalle M, Zhang J, Contu R, Cossu L, Latronico MV, et al. The knockout of miR-143 and -145 alters smooth muscle cell maintenance and vascular homeostasis in mice: correlates with human disease. Cell Death Differ. 2009;16(12):1590–8. doi:10.1038/cdd.2009.153 cdd2009153 [pii]

104. Deng L, Blanco FJ, Stevens H, Lu R, Caudrillier A, McBride M, et al. MicroRNA-143 activation regulates smooth muscle and endothelial cell crosstalk in pulmonary arterial hypertension. Circ Res. 2015;117(10):870–83. doi:10.1161/CIRCRESAHA.115.306806 CIRCRESAHA.115.306806 [pii]

105. Horita HN, Simpson PA, Ostriker A, Furgeson S, Van Putten V, Weiser-Evans MC, et al. Serum response factor regulates expression of phosphatase and tensin homolog through a microRNA network in vascular smooth muscle cells. Arterioscler Thromb Vasc Biol. 2011;31(12):2909–19. doi:10.1161/ATVBAHA.111.233585 ATVBAHA.111.233585 [pii]

106. Ghosh G, Subramanian IV, Adhikari N, Zhang X, Joshi HP, Basi D, et al. Hypoxia-induced microRNA-424 expression in human endothelial cells regulates HIF-alpha isoforms and promotes angiogenesis. J Clin Invest. 2010;120(11):4141–54. doi:10.1172/JCI42980 42980 [pii]

Chapter 4
Sex Hormones

Kaori Oshima and Masahiko Oka

Abstract Males and females are biologically distinct, and certain pathological conditions affect both sexes differently. Obvious sex difference exists in pulmonary arterial hypertension (PAH). The major sex difference is female sex hormones, especially estrogens, and therefore, the roles of estrogens have been intensively studied in PAH. The incidence of PAH in females is higher than in males, suggesting a female-specific risk factor. However, a general notion that estrogens are cardiovascular protective, and their protective effects demonstrated in animal models, resulted in the emerging concept of "estrogen paradox" in PAH. Later, it was found that female PAH patients live longer, suggesting the survival benefit of estrogens. Questions that need to be answered are (1) Why is PAH more prevalent in females despite the protective effects of estrogens? and (2) Why do female PAH patients show better survival despite the higher incidence of the syndrome? Even with the rigorous research efforts to answer these paradoxical questions, the field has not come to a consensus. This chapter summarizes the current leading theories for the estrogen paradox in PAH.

Keywords Pulmonary arterial hypertension • Estrogen paradox

K. Oshima
Department of Pharmacology, College of Medicine, University of South Alabama, Mobile, AL 36688, USA

Center for Lung Biology, College of Medicine, University of South Alabama, Mobile, AL 36688, USA

M. Oka (✉)
Department of Pharmacology, College of Medicine, University of South Alabama, Mobile, AL 36688, USA

Center for Lung Biology, College of Medicine, University of South Alabama, Mobile, AL 36688, USA

Department of Internal Medicine, College of Medicine, University of South Alabama, Mobile, AL 36688, USA
e-mail: moka@southalabama.edu

© Springer Science+Business Media Singapore 2017
Y. Fukumoto (ed.), *Diagnosis and Treatment of Pulmonary Hypertension*,
DOI 10.1007/978-981-287-840-3_4

4.1 Estrogen Paradox in PAH

It has long been recognized that the prevalence of PAH is higher in females than in males. Although the ratio of female to male varies depending on subgroups of PAH, epidemiological studies from various countries consistently demonstrate this female predominance in PAH [1–3]. A recent study showed that among male PAH patients, a higher level of estrogens was associated with PAH [4]. Higher female incidence in PAH is not found in pediatric, prepuberty patients [5]. These data collectively suggest that female sex hormones, such as estrogens, have disadvantageous effects and play a role in PAH pathogenesis.

However, it is a general consensus that estrogens are cardiovascular protective. The incidence of atherosclerotic diseases is low in premenopausal females, while it increases after menopause, and postmenopausal use of estrogens is associated with reduced risk of cardiovascular disease [6]. Postmenopausal women also have increased risk of developing PAH [7], which suggests a protective effect of estrogens. Studies with two classical animal models, chronic hypoxia- and monocrotaline-induced pulmonary hypertension, have consistently shown protective effects of estrogens [8–10]. The protective effect of estrogens in hypoxic humans is indirectly supported by the male predominance in the incidence of high altitude-induced pulmonary hypertension [11].

These studies in humans and animals suggest a protective effect of estrogens, which is contrary to the epidemiological data in PAH, which points to an opposite effect of estrogens. These conflicting results led to the concept, "estrogen paradox" [12–14].

Although classical experimental models consistently showed protective effect of estrogens, they presented with limited pathological phenotypes and did not fully recapitulate the human PAH. Therefore, various animal models were developed in recent years in an attempt to obtain a better understanding of the pathogenesis of PAH. The studies with transgenic animal models are unfortunately inconclusive and more confusing, showing protective or detrimental effects of estrogens in PAH. In the Sugen/hypoxia-exposed rat model of PAH, which closely mimics the human hemodynamic profile as well as the pulmonary vascular histopathology [15, 16], the difference between sexes in hemodynamic severity and PAH characteristics is also inconclusive [17, 18]. The data from studies of recent animal models are generally contradictory, and perhaps this reflects the differential effects of estrogens that can be exerted depending on the initiating stimuli for PAH. It also highlights the need for a better animal model that consistently demonstrates higher incidence and better outcome in females, similarly to the human PAH.

The estrogen paradox became more complicated when it was reported that female PAH patients have better survival [19] while male sex is associated with increased risk of death [2, 20]. These findings suggest estrogens have a beneficial effect in PAH, which appears contradictory to the epidemiological finding which indicates that estrogens are a risk factor.

This estrogen paradox in PAH, i.e., females have higher prevalence but longer survival, has been a focus of numerous studies. They have investigated how estrogens exert harmful effects in the pulmonary circulation and how they provide survival benefit in female PAH patients. The exact mechanisms of these sex differences are unclear, and the field has not come to a consensus on whether estrogens are protective or harmful in PAH. This chapter summarizes current understanding of effects of the major female sex steroids, estrogens, on the PAH pathophysiology and the sex difference.

4.2   Published Theories for the Estrogen Paradox in PAH

The current knowledge on estrogens and the leading hypotheses on the estrogen paradox based on numerous studies are described below.

4.2.1   How Estrogens Exert Harmful Effects to the Pulmonary Circulation

4.2.1.1   Altered Estrogen Receptor (ER) Signaling

Altered estrogen receptor (ER) signaling is thought to contribute to PAH pathology. Estrogens exert their effects mainly via two types of ERs, ERα and ERβ, which mediate various genomic pathways [21]. In the pulmonary circulation, both ERα and ERβ are present and active in humans and rats [22, 23]. Multiple studies demonstrate favorable effects of estrogens, including upregulation of endothelial nitric oxide synthase and prostacyclin synthase in the lungs via those receptors [24, 25]. Estrogen signaling can also be mediated via a G-protein-coupled membrane receptor, GPR30, whose primary function is to activate non-genomic pathways to elicit acute effects of estrogens [12]. The relative proportion of each receptor and additionally their alternative splicing variants affect the overall effect of complex estrogen signaling [14].

In systemic vasculature, single-nucleotide polymorphisms (SNPs) in genes encoding ERα or ERβ are associated with development of myocardial infarction, hypertension, left ventricular hypertrophy, and stroke [12]. Genome-wide RNA expression profiling in the lungs indicated the upregulation of estrogen receptor 1 (ESR1), which encodes ERα, in an idiopathic PAH cohort compared to idiopathic fibrosis and normal cohorts, both in males and females [26]. The ESR1 abnormality is also associated with increased risk of developing pulmonary hypertension in patients with advanced liver disease [27]. The significance of the ERs increases because non-estrogen ligands can also trigger ER activation in the absence of estrogens [14]. This genetic factor may predispose certain populations to increased risk of developing PAH.

Studies in animal models have yielded conflicting results as to which receptor contributes to the PAH pathogenesis. 17β-Estradiol (E2), which is the most important estrogen in premenopausal females, demonstrated a protective effect in the chronic hypoxia model, and this was dependent on both ERs [12, 28]. The protective effect of E2 in the monocrotaline model was mediated by ERβ [10]. On the other hand, in female rats of the same model, downregulation of lung ERα was observed, while no change was found in ERβ [29]. These results indicate that the roles of each receptor may depend on sex and pulmonary hypertensive stimulus. In addition, ER function may be altered as a consequence of mutations in other genes or environment of the vasculature. For example, pulmonary microvascular endothelial cells with BMPR2 mutation showed dysregulation of ERα trafficking [30], which would affect the relative abundance and location of ERα. Hypoxia increased the expression of ERβ, but not ERα, in male rats [31].

Given the genetic alterations observed in human PAH patients, one possibility is that the altered ER signaling contributes to PAH pathogenesis, potentially as an additional "hit" for the onset of PAH, although the cause-and-effect relationship for this clinical observation is still unclear.

4.2.1.2 Altered Estrogen Metabolites

It has been suggested that an imbalance of estrogen metabolites may explain the estrogen paradox in PAH. Estrogens and their metabolites can elicit various effects that may oppose each other. A distinct feature that separates PAH from other forms of pulmonary hypertension is the extensive pulmonary vascular remodeling. The pathogenesis of this remodeling process is unclear, but antiapoptotic, proproliferative, and angiogenic cells and inflammation are implicated in the disease process. Estrogens and estrogen metabolites are known to play a role in the modulation of these cellular phenotypes and the environment, and, therefore, protective or harmful effects of estrogens and their metabolites are primarily evaluated based on these cellular behaviors.

Simplified estrogen metabolism is shown in Fig. 4.1. 17β-Estradiol (E2) is synthesized from precursors by aromatase [14]. E2 is metabolized to 2-hydroxyestradiol (2-OHE2) and 4-hydroxyestradiol (4-OHE2) by the enzyme CYP1A1 and CYP1B1 [12]. These hydroxyestradiols are quickly converted to 2-methoxyestradiol (2-ME2) and 4-methoxyestradiol (4-ME2) by the enzyme, catechol-O-methyltransferase (COMT) [14]. Estrone (E1) is the primary estrogen during menopause and has a weaker estrogenic activity than E2 [32]. E1 is also synthesized from precursors, as well as reversibly converted from E2 by 17β-hydroxysteroid dehydrogenase [12]. E1 subsequently is metabolized to 16α-hydroxyestrone (16α-OHE1) by CYP1B1 [12].

An increased level of CYP1B1 is found in the lungs of idiopathic and heritable PAH patients as well as in various animal models of pulmonary hypertension, including chronic hypoxia- and Sugen/hypoxia-exposed rats [33]. This leads to increased levels of 16α-OHE1, which has innate effects of antiapoptosis,

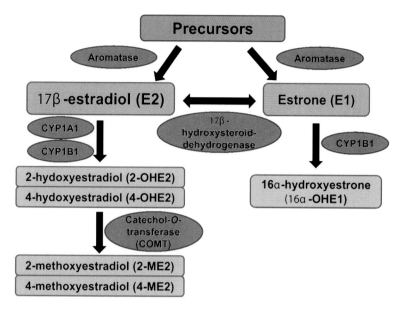

Fig. 4.1 The simplified estrogen metabolism (modified from Lahm et al. (12)). *CYP* Cytochrome P-450

proproliferation, and pro-inflammation [12]. These properties suggest detrimental effects in pulmonary vascular remodeling by propagating undesirable cellular phenotypes. The unfavorable effects of 16α-OHE1 are demonstrated by studies in CYP1B1-null mice and in chronic hypoxia- and Sugen/hypoxia-exposed rats [33].

In heritable PAH, the higher activity of CYP1B1 results in a higher penetrance of PAH. Among the carriers of BMPR2 mutation, wild-type homozygous genotype of CYP1B1 was associated with lower urinary 2-OHE2/16α-OHE1, suggesting a shift toward proproliferative antiapoptotic metabolites [34]. In addition, high concentrations of E2 and 16α-OHE1 reduce BMPR2 gene expression [30]. Therefore, increased activity of CYP1B1 and a subsequent increase of 16α-OHE1 levels appear to facilitate PAH pathogenesis.

An increased level of CYP1B1 also shifts the pathway toward more synthesis of 2-ME2. 2-ME2 has antiproliferative and proapoptotic properties that suggest a protective role against vascular remodeling [13]. The beneficial effects of 2-ME2 are shown in the monocrotaline, bleomycin, and Sugen/hypoxia animal models [35–37]. However, this theory of estrogen metabolites is challenged due to the weak affinity of 2-ME2 for the receptors [38] and to the study that showed that treatment with E2 attenuated pulmonary hypertension in the presence of a COMT inhibitor, which inhibits the synthesis of 2-ME2 [28].

Among patients with severe liver disease, SNPs in aromatase are associated with development of PAH [27], which suggests a protective role of E2. On the other hand, an increase in aromatase is reported in human PAH, as well as in the chronic hypoxia- and Sugen/hypoxia-exposed models, and the inhibition of aromatase has been shown to have therapeutic effect in both rat models [17].

Taken together, altered estrogen metabolism in the pulmonary circulation can shift the cellular phenotypes from protective to harmful effects of estrogens in PAH pathology. The enzymes that modulate estrogen metabolism are present in vascular cells, which suggest that the local concentrations of the estrogen metabolites likely differ from circulating levels and contribute to cellular modulation [13]. Therefore, the effects of estrogen metabolites should be investigated in a more detailed and specific manner.

4.2.1.3   Microenvironment

The effect of E2 depends on the microenvironment of the target tissue/organ, affected by environmental and genetic background. This may contribute to the conflicting data among studies and the estrogen paradox.

One critical variable that contributes to the environment is the timing of E2 participation in relation to progression status of the disorder. A study on atherosclerosis showed a protective effect of E2 in mild atherosclerotic patients and a harmful effect in advanced atherosclerotic patients [39]. As demonstrated in epidemiological studies in PAH, the patient age has significant effects on the hemodynamic profiles and survival [19, 40]. Environmental changes in the pulmonary circulation, such as oxygen tension, are also important. In pulmonary arterial endothelial cells, E2 decreased VEGF expression upon exposure to hypoxia, while it had no effect on normoxic cells [28]. Genetic background is another key factor to the microenvironment. The genetic alterations that affect estrogen signaling and metabolism, such as SNPs in ESR1, aromatase, and CYP1B1, directly influence the estrogen signaling and metabolism. As seen in the higher penetrance of pulmonary hypertension in BMPR2 mutation carriers, the effects of estrogens are also affected by other genetic alterations. The effects of estrogens depend on the target vascular layers (media vs. intima) and the condition of endothelium (intact/quiescent vs. dysfunctional), as well as the concentrations of estrogens [13]. Therefore, the effects of estrogens are dictated by various factors that compose the microenvironment.

4.2.2   How Estrogens Exert Survival Benefit in Female PAH Patients

4.2.2.1   Cardiac Protective Effect of Estrogens

The estrogen paradox may be partly explained by the organ-specific effect of estrogens. The hypothesis is that estrogens may be harmful to the pulmonary arteries, but protective in the heart. Since a major determinant of survival in PAH is right heart function [20], the better cardiac function provided by E2 effects benefits female

PAH patients. Right ventricular function, defined by right ventricular ejection fraction, was better in female PAH patients and was improved with PAH-specific therapies in female patients, while males did not benefit [41, 42]. Exogenous hormone therapy is associated with better right ventricular systolic function [43]. In the Sugen/hypoxia rat model, female rats developed significantly less cardiac fibrosis [44], and exogenous E2 treatment improved right heart function [18]. On the other hand, female PAH patients tend to have more severe vascular remodeling and inflammation in pulmonary arteries [45]. In the Sugen/hypoxia model, female rats developed more intimal, angio-proliferative lesions compared to males [44]. These results may indicate the potential roles of estrogens in exacerbating the vascular remodeling while protecting the heart function in PAH.

4.3 The Perspective

The overall effect of estrogens is determined by numerous factors such as age, genetic background, oxygen tension, cell types, cell condition, concentration of estrogens, expression levels of ERs, estrogen metabolites, co-regulators of estrogens, and organs [46]. Therefore, whether estrogens are protective or detrimental as an end result depends on the balance of all the components in the target tissue/organ.

One of the key features of estrogens is that they apparently exhibit opposite effects depending on the timing/progression of the disorder (i.e., whether the disease was already established or not). Estrogens are protective if present at the time of a disease onset, but ineffective when administered in later stages of the pathology. This is supported by studies of atherosclerosis and Alzheimer's disease, as well as of balloon injury-induced carotid artery stenosis [46]. It is, therefore, important to fully elucidate exactly what factors determine how estrogens behave, protective or detrimental, in the hypertensive pulmonary circulation. Development of animal models of PAH that recapitulate human pathology and epidemiology may be required to settle this issue.

Additionally, a recent large clinical study has surprisingly revealed that young female PAH patients (<45 years) have better hemodynamic profiles as compared to men [40]. Although more detailed subcategorized analyses of these epidemiological data are needed, such as longitudinal follow-up studies focusing on sex and hormonal status, the implication of this observation could be that estrogens are beneficial, even in the damaged pulmonary circulation in PAH. Then, the question is why PAH is more frequent but less severe in females, or if there is any specific stimuli/stimulus that favors females to trigger less severe PAH. This could be a very critical issue in this field that needs to be carefully addressed in the future.

4.4   Conclusion

The "estrogen paradox" is not limited to the PAH field. It is now clear that the effects of estrogens in the cardiovascular system are not only beneficial but also detrimental based on the conflicting results of hormone replacement therapy [39, 47]. Estrogens modulate various aspects of the pulmonary circulation, such as vascular tone, cellular proliferation, apoptosis, angiogenesis, as well as inflammatory status, and their effects can be either good or bad depending on various factors. Unfortunately, the current understanding of the roles of estrogens in PAH is incomplete, and many more studies are needed to define their exact roles. Altered estrogen metabolism, altered estrogen signaling, and the microenvironment are likely contributing to the conflicting and paradoxical effects of estrogens. It is thus critical to perform thorough, rigorous studies of the diverse and complex estrogen pharmacology.

Acknowledgment We thank Dr. Ivan F. McMurtry for the critical reading and suggestions for this chapter.

References

1. Badesch DB, Raskob GE, Elliott CG, Krichman AM, Farber HW, Frost AE, et al. Pulmonary arterial hypertension: baseline characteristics from the REVEAL Registry. Chest. 2010;137(2):376–87. Epub 2009/10/20
2. Olsson KM, Delcroix M, Ghofrani HA, Tiede H, Huscher D, Speich R, et al. Anticoagulation and survival in pulmonary arterial hypertension: results from the Comparative, Prospective Registry of Newly Initiated Therapies for Pulmonary Hypertension (COMPERA). Circulation. 2014;129(1):57–65. Epub 2013/10/02
3. Alves Jr JL, Gavilanes F, Jardim C, Fernandes CJ, Morinaga LT, Dias B, et al. Pulmonary arterial hypertension in the southern hemisphere: results from a registry of incident Brazilian cases. Chest. 2015;147(2):495–501. Epub 2014/10/16
4. Ventetuolo CE, Baird GL, Barr RG, DA B, JS F, NS H, et al. Higher estradiol and lower dehydroepiandrosterone-sulfate levels are associated with pulmonary arterial hypertension in men. Am J Respir Crit Care Med. 2015; Epub 2015/12/15
5. van Loon RL, Roofthooft MT, Hillege HL, ten Harkel AD, van Osch-Gevers M, Delhaas T, et al. Pediatric pulmonary hypertension in the Netherlands: epidemiology and characterization during the period 1991 to 2005. Circulation. 2011;124(16):1755–64. Epub 2011/09/29
6. Mendelsohn ME, Karas RH. The protective effects of estrogen on the cardiovascular system. N Engl J Med. 1999;340(23):1801–11. Epub 1999/06/11
7. Scorza R, Caronni M, Bazzi S, Nador F, Beretta L, Antonioli R, et al. Post-menopause is the main risk factor for developing isolated pulmonary hypertension in systemic sclerosis. Ann N Y Acad Sci. 2002;966:238–46. Epub 2002/07/13
8. Rabinovitch M, Gamble WJ, Miettinen OS, Reid L. Age and sex influence on pulmonary hypertension of chronic hypoxia and on recovery. Am J Physiol. 1981;240(1):H62–72. Epub 1981/01/01
9. Farhat MY, Chen MF, Bhatti T, Iqbal A, Cathapermal S, Ramwell PW. Protection by oestradiol against the development of cardiovascular changes associated with monocrotaline pulmonary hypertension in rats. Br J Pharmacol. 1993;110(2):719–23. Epub 1993/10/01

10. Umar S, Iorga A, Matori H, Nadadur RD, Li J, Maltese F, et al. Estrogen rescues preexisting severe pulmonary hypertension in rats. Am J Respir Crit Care Med. 2011;184(6):715–23. Epub 2011/06/28

11. Aldashev AA, Sarybaev AS, Sydykov AS, Kalmyrzaev BB, Kim EV, Mamanova LB, et al. Characterization of high-altitude pulmonary hypertension in the Kyrgyz: association with angiotensin-converting enzyme genotype. Am J Respir Crit Care Med. 2002;166(10):1396–402. Epub 2002/10/31

12. Lahm T, Tuder RM, Petrache I. Progress in solving the sex hormone paradox in pulmonary hypertension. Am J Physiol Lung Cell Mol Physiol. 2014;307(1):L7–26. Epub 2014/05/13

13. Tofovic SP. Estrogens and development of pulmonary hypertension: interaction of estradiol metabolism and pulmonary vascular disease. J Cardiovasc Pharmacol. 2010;56(6):696–708. Epub 2010/10/01

14. Austin ED, Lahm T, West J, Tofovic SP, Johansen AK, Maclean MR, et al. Gender, sex hormones and pulmonary hypertension. Pulm Circ. 2013;3(2):294–314. Epub 2013/09/10

15. Toba M, Alzoubi A, O'Neill KD, Gairhe S, Matsumoto Y, Oshima K, et al. Temporal hemodynamic and histological progression in Sugen5416/hypoxia/normoxia-exposed pulmonary arterial hypertensive rats. Am J Physiol Heart Circ Physiol. 2014;306(2):H243–50. Epub 2013/11/19

16. Abe K, Toba M, Alzoubi A, Ito M, Fagan KA, Cool CD, et al. Formation of plexiform lesions in experimental severe pulmonary arterial hypertension. Circulation. 2010;121(25):2747–54. Epub 2010/06/16

17. Mair KM, Wright AF, Duggan N, Rowlands DJ, Hussey MJ, Roberts S, et al. Sex-dependent influence of endogenous estrogen in pulmonary hypertension. Am J Respir Crit Care Med. 2014;190(4):456–67. Epub 2014/06/24

18. Frump AL, Goss KN, Vayl A, Albrecht M, Fisher A, Tursunova R, et al. Estradiol improves right ventricular function in rats with severe angioproliferative pulmonary hypertension: effects of endogenous and exogenous sex hormones. Am J Physiol Lung Cell Mol Physiol. 2015;308(9):L873–90. Epub 2015/02/26

19. Shapiro S, Traiger GL, Turner M, McGoon MD, Wason P, Barst RJ. Sex differences in the diagnosis, treatment, and outcome of patients with pulmonary arterial hypertension enrolled in the registry to evaluate early and long-term pulmonary arterial hypertension disease management. Chest. 2012;141(2):363–73. Epub 2011/07/16

20. Benza RL, Miller DP, Gomberg-Maitland M, Frantz RP, Foreman AJ, Coffey CS, et al. Predicting survival in pulmonary arterial hypertension: insights from the Registry to Evaluate Early and Long-Term Pulmonary Arterial Hypertension Disease Management (REVEAL). Circulation. 2010;122(2):164–72. Epub 2010/06/30

21. Umar S, Rabinovitch M, Eghbali M. Estrogen paradox in pulmonary hypertension: current controversies and future perspectives. Am J Respir Crit Care Med. 2012;186(2):125–31. Epub 2012/05/09

22. Hamidi SA, Dickman KG, Berisha H, Said SI. 17beta-estradiol protects the lung against acute injury: possible mediation by vasoactive intestinal polypeptide. Endocrinology. 2011;152(12):4729–37. Epub 2011/10/20

23. Mollerup S, Jorgensen K, Berge G, Haugen A. Expression of estrogen receptors alpha and beta in human lung tissue and cell lines. Lung Cancer. 2002;37(2):153–9. Epub 2002/07/26

24. Lahm T, Crisostomo PR, Markel TA, Wang M, Wang Y, Tan J, et al. Selective estrogen receptor-alpha and estrogen receptor-beta agonists rapidly decrease pulmonary artery vasoconstriction by a nitric oxide-dependent mechanism. Am J Physiol Regul Integr Comp Physiol. 2008;295(5):R1486–93. Epub 2008/10/04

25. Sherman TS, Chambliss KL, Gibson LL, Pace MC, Mendelsohn ME, Pfister SL, et al. Estrogen acutely activates prostacyclin synthesis in ovine fetal pulmonary artery endothelium. Am J Respir Cell Mol Biol. 2002;26(5):610–6. Epub 2002/04/24

26. Rajkumar R, Konishi K, Richards TJ, Ishizawar DC, Wiechert AC, Kaminski N, et al. Genomewide RNA expression profiling in lung identifies distinct signatures in idiopathic

pulmonary arterial hypertension and secondary pulmonary hypertension. Am J Physiol Heart Circ Physiol. 2010;298(4):H1235–48. Epub 2010/01/19

27. Roberts KE, Fallon MB, Krowka MJ, Brown RS, Trotter JF, Peter I, et al. Genetic risk factors for portopulmonary hypertension in patients with advanced liver disease. Am J Respir Crit Care Med. 2009;179(9):835–42. Epub 2009/02/17

28. Lahm T, Albrecht M, Fisher AJ, Selej M, Patel NG, Brown JA, et al. 17beta-Estradiol attenuates hypoxic pulmonary hypertension via estrogen receptor-mediated effects. Am J Respir Crit Care Med. 2012;185(9):965–80. Epub 2012/03/03

29. Yuan P, Wu WH, Gao L, Zheng ZQ, Liu D, Mei HY, et al. Oestradiol ameliorates monocrotaline pulmonary hypertension via NO, prostacyclin and endothelin-1 pathways. Eur Respir J. 2013;41(5):1116–25. Epub 2012/09/01

30. Fessel JP, Chen X, Frump A, Gladson S, Blackwell T, Kang C, et al. Interaction between bone morphogenetic protein receptor type 2 and estrogenic compounds in pulmonary arterial hypertension. Pulm Circ. 2013;3(3):564–77. Epub 2014/03/13

31. Mona S, Jordan W, Angelia DL, Marjorie A, Kelly S, Irina P, et al. Hypoxia increases expression of estrogen receptor (ER)-Beta in vivo and in vitro. A107 pulmonary hypertension associated with hypoxia and paranchymal lung disease. Am Thorac Soc. 2013:A2257

32. Kuijper EA, Ket JC, Caanen MR, Lambalk CB. Reproductive hormone concentrations in pregnancy and neonates: a systematic review. Reprod Biomed Online. 2013;27(1):33–63. Epub 2013/05/15

33. White K, Johansen AK, Nilsen M, Ciuclan L, Wallace E, Paton L, et al. Activity of the estrogen-metabolizing enzyme cytochrome P450 1B1 influences the development of pulmonary arterial hypertension. Circulation. 2012;126(9):1087–98. Epub 2012/08/04

34. Austin ED, Cogan JD, West JD, Hedges LK, Hamid R, Dawson EP, et al. Alterations in oestrogen metabolism: implications for higher penetrance of familial pulmonary arterial hypertension in females. Eur Respir J. 2009;34(5):1093–9. Epub 2009/04/10

35. Tofovic SP, Rafikova O. Preventive and therapeutic effects of 2-Methoxyestradiol, but not estradiol, in severe occlusive pulmonary arterial hypertension in female rats. A51 experimental models of pulmonary hypertension. Am Thorac Soc. 2009:A1802.

36. Tofovic SP, Salah EM, Mady HH, Jackson EK, Melhem MF. Estradiol metabolites attenuate monocrotaline-induced pulmonary hypertension in rats. J Cardiovasc Pharmacol. 2005;46(4):430–7. Epub 2005/09/15

37. Tofovic SP, Zhang X, Jackson EK, Zhu H, Petrusevska G. 2-methoxyestradiol attenuates bleomycin-induced pulmonary hypertension and fibrosis in estrogen-deficient rats. Vascul Pharmacol. 2009;51(2–3):190–7. Epub 2009/06/23

38. Tofovic SP, Zhang X, Jackson EK, Dacic S, Petrusevska G. 2-Methoxyestradiol mediates the protective effects of estradiol in monocrotaline-induced pulmonary hypertension. Vascul Pharmacol. 2006;45(6):358–67. Epub 2006/07/29

39. Mendelsohn ME, Karas RH. Molecular and cellular basis of cardiovascular gender differences. Science. 2005;308(5728):1583–7. Epub 2005/06/11

40. Ventetuolo CE, Praestgaard A, Palevsky HI, Klinger JR, Halpern SD, Kawut SM. Sex and haemodynamics in pulmonary arterial hypertension. Eur Respir J. 2014;43(2):523–30. Epub 2013/08/21

41. Jacobs W, van de Veerdonk MC, Trip P, de Man F, Heymans MW, Marcus JT, et al. The right ventricle explains sex differences in survival in idiopathic pulmonary arterial hypertension. Chest. 2014;145(6):1230–6. Epub 2013/12/07

42. Kawut SM, Al-Naamani N, Agerstrand C, Rosenzweig EB, Rowan C, Barst RJ, et al. Determinants of right ventricular ejection fraction in pulmonary arterial hypertension. Chest. 2009;135(3):752–9. Epub 2008/10/14

43. Ventetuolo CE, Ouyang P, Bluemke DA, Tandri H, Barr RG, Bagiella E, et al. Sex hormones are associated with right ventricular structure and function: The MESA-right ventricle study. Am J Respir Crit Care Med. 2011;183(5):659–67. Epub 2010/10/05

44. Rafikova O, Rafikov R, Meadows ML, Kangath A, Jonigk D, Black SM. The sexual dimorphism associated with pulmonary hypertension corresponds to a fibrotic phenotype. Pulm Circ. 2015;5(1):184–97. Epub 2015/05/21

45. Stacher E, Graham BB, Hunt JM, Gandjeva A, Groshong SD, McLaughlin VV, et al. Modern age pathology of pulmonary arterial hypertension. Am J Respir Crit Care Med. 2012;186(3):261–72. Epub 2012/06/09

46. Straub RH. The complex role of estrogens in inflammation. Endocr Rev. 2007;28(5):521–74. Epub 2007/07/21

47. Phillips GB. Is atherosclerotic cardiovascular disease an endocrinological disorder? The estrogen-androgen paradox. J Clin Endocrinol Metab. 2005;90(5):2708–11. Epub 2005/02/03

Chapter 5
Rho-Kinase as a Therapeutic Target for Pulmonary Hypertension

Kimio Satoh, Koichiro Sugimura, and Hiroaki Shimokawa

Abstract Pulmonary vascular remodeling contributes to the development of pulmonary vascular resistance in patients with pulmonary hypertension (PH). The development of PH involves a multiple genetic, molecular, and humoral abnormalities, in which fibroblasts, vascular smooth muscle and endothelial cells, and inflammatory cells play a crucial role. A series of studies demonstrated the important roles of Rho-kinase in the cardiovascular system. The RhoA/Rho-kinase pathway plays important roles in many cellular functions, including contraction, motility, proliferation, and apoptosis, and its excessive activity induces oxidative stress. Furthermore, the important role of Rho-kinase has been demonstrated in the pathogenesis of many cardiovascular diseases including PH. Additionally, cyclophilin A is secreted by vascular smooth muscle cells, inflammatory cells, and activated platelets in a Rho-kinase-dependent manner, playing important roles in a wide range of cardiovascular diseases. Therefore, the RhoA/Rho-kinase pathway plays crucial roles in both physiological and pathological conditions and is an important therapeutic target in cardiovascular medicine. Here, we will review the recent advances regarding the importance of Rho-kinases in the development of PH and as a therapeutic target.

Keywords Cardiovascular system • Inflammation • Oxidative stress • Rho-kinase

5.1 Introduction

Inflammation contributes to the pathogenesis of pulmonary arterial hypertension (PAH), which is characterized by pulmonary vascular remodeling [1]. Endothelial cell dysfunction, vascular smooth muscle cell (VSMC) proliferation, perivascular inflammation, and bone morphogenetic protein receptor 2 (BMPR2) mutation are

K. Satoh, M.D., Ph.D. • K. Sugimura, M.D., Ph.D. • H. Shimokawa, M.D., Ph.D. (✉)
Department of Cardiovascular Medicine, Tohoku University Graduate School of Medicine,
1-1 Seiryomachi, Aoba-ku, Sendai, Miyagi 980-8574, Japan
e-mail: shimo@cardio.med.tohoku.ac.jp

© Springer Science+Business Media Singapore 2017
Y. Fukumoto (ed.), *Diagnosis and Treatment of Pulmonary Hypertension*,
DOI 10.1007/978-981-287-840-3_5

important in the development of PAH, which leads to right ventricular failure and premature death [1]. Hypoxia promotes VSMC proliferation and chronic hypoxic exposure of mice induces pulmonary vascular remodeling [2]. Pulmonary vascular inflammation plays a crucial role for the development of hypoxia-induced pulmonary hypertension (PH) [3, 4], for which Rho-kinase plays a crucial role [5–7]. Additionally, Rho-kinase promotes secretion of cyclophilin A (CyPA) from VSMCs, and extracellular CyPA stimulates VSMC proliferation in vivo [8]. Extracellular CyPA induces endothelial cell adhesion molecule expression, induces apoptosis, and is a chemoattractant for inflammatory cells [9]. Basigin (Bsg) is an extracellular CyPA receptor [10] and is an essential receptor for malaria, which disrupts nitric oxide metabolism and causes harmful endothelial activation, including the Rho/Rho-kinase activation [11]. Therefore, the Rho-kinase/CyPA/Bsg signaling may contribute to the development of PH. In this chapter, we will review the recent progress in the understanding of Rho-kinase signaling pathway in the development of PH, which is a novel therapeutic target in patients with PAH.

5.1.1   Roles of Rho-Kinases in the Cardiovascular System

Rho-kinases (Rho-kinase α/ROKα/ROCK 2 and Rho-kinase β/ROKβ/ROCK 1) were identified as the effectors of the small GTP-binding protein, RhoA, independently by the three research groups [12–14]. During the last 20 years, significant progress has been made in the understanding of the molecular mechanisms and therapeutic importance of Rho-kinases in the cardiovascular system. The Rho family of small G proteins comprises 20 members of ubiquitously expressed proteins in mammals, including RhoA, Rac1, and Cdc42 [15, 16]. Among them, RhoA acts as a molecular switch that cycles between an inactive GDP-bound and an active GTP-bound conformation interacting with downstream targets. Rho-kinases play important roles in many intracellular signaling pathways [17, 18].

5.1.2   Functional Differences Between ROCK1 and ROCK2

To elucidate the functions of the ROCK isoforms in vivo, ROCK1- and ROCK2-deficient mice have been generated [19, 20]. Importantly, ROCK1-deficient mice were born with their eyelids opened [19], whereas ROCK2-deficient mice presented placental dysfunction and fetal death [20, 21]. Thus, the role of ROCK2, the main isoform in the cardiovascular system, remained to be fully elucidated in vivo. In order to address this point, we developed tissue-specific knockout mice for ROCK1 and ROCK2. Using VSMC-specific ROCK2 knockout mice, we demonstrated that in VSMC, ROCK2 plays a crucial role in the development of hypoxia-induced PH [5]. These mutant mice revealed normal growth and body weight under physiological conditions. However, in wild-type mice, chronic hypoxia significantly increased ROCK2 expression and ROCK activity in the lung tissues and caused PH and right ventricular hypertrophy, all of which were suppressed in the VSMC-specific ROCK2 knockout mice [5].

5.1.3 Roles of Rho-Kinase in VSMC Function

Rho-kinase has been implicated in the pathogenesis of cardiovascular diseases, in part by promoting VSMC proliferation [22–24]. Rho-kinase plays an important role in mediating various cellular functions, not only VSMC contraction [25, 26] but also actin cytoskeleton organization [27], adhesion, and cytokinesis [16]. Thus, Rho-kinase plays a crucial role for the development of cardiovascular disease through inflammation, EC damage, VSMC contraction, and proliferation. Rho-kinase inhibitors have excellent vasodilator activity and can induce vasodilation especially when the vasoconstrictor tone is increased by a variety of mechanisms, including enhanced calcium entry through activation of G protein-coupled receptors, ventilator hypoxia, and NOS inhibition [28].

5.1.4 Pathological Roles of Rho-Kinase in the Cardiovascular System

Accumulating evidence indicated that Rho-kinase plays important roles in the pathogenesis of a wide range of cardiovascular diseases [16, 29, 30]. Indeed, the RhoA/Rho-kinase pathway not only mediates VSMC hypercontraction but also promotes cardiovascular diseases by enhancing ROS production [15, 31, 32]. The beneficial effects of long-term inhibition of Rho-kinase for the treatment of cardiovascular disease have been demonstrated in various animal models such as coronary artery spasm, arteriosclerosis, restenosis, ischemia/reperfusion injury, hypertension, PH, stroke, and cardiac hypertrophy/heart failure [15, 16, 26, 29]. Gene transfer of dominant-negative Rho-kinase reduced neointimal formation of the coronary artery in pigs [33]. Long-term treatment with a Rho-kinase inhibitor suppressed neointimal formation after vascular injury in vivo [34, 35], monocyte chemoattractant protein (MCP)-1-induced vascular lesion formation [36], constrictive remodeling [37, 38], in-stent restenosis [39], and development of cardiac allograft vasculopathy [40].

5.1.5   Rho-Kinase-Mediated Development of Cardiovascular Diseases

In EC, Rho-kinase downregulates eNOS [41] and substantially activates pro-inflammatory pathways, including enhanced expression of adhesion molecules. The expression of Rho-kinase is accelerated by inflammatory stimuli such as AngII and IL-1β [42] and by remnant lipoproteins in human coronary VSMC [43]. Rho-kinase also upregulates NAD(P)H oxidases and augments AngII-induced ROS production [44–46].

Several growth factors are secreted by VSMC in response to oxidative stress. Among them, CyPA has been identified as a protein that is secreted by VSMC, inflammatory cells, and activated platelets in a Rho-kinase-dependent manner [47–49]. Secreted extracellular CyPA stimulates ERK1/ERK2 in VSMC, contributing to ROS production and creating a vicious cycle for ROS augmentation [50, 51]. Rho-kinase, a downstream effector of RhoA, mediates myosin II activation via phosphorylation and inactivation of myosin II light chain phosphatase [17]. Myosin II-mediated vesicle transport is required for CyPA secretion from VSMC in a Rho-kinase- dependent manner. Moreover, extracellular CyPA activates platelets via basigin (CD147)-mediated phosphoinositide-3-kinase (PI3K)/Akt signaling, leading to enhanced adhesion and thrombus formation [52, 53]. Moreover, thrombin suppresses eNOS in EC via Rho-kinase pathway [54]. Thus, CyPA and Rho-kinase function in concert, leading to the development of vascular diseases. Indeed, CyPA may be a key mediator of Rho-kinase that generates a vicious cycle for ROS augmentation, affecting EC, VSMC, and inflammatory cells [49].

Importantly, CyPA plays a crucial role in the translocation of Nox enzymes, such as p47phox [55], contributing to VSMC proliferation and vascular diseases [56]. Since ROS production by Nox enzymes activates other oxidase systems, CyPA and Nox enzymes amplify ROS formation in a synergistic manner, leading to augmentation of oxidative stress. Additionally, CyPA secretion from VSMCs requires ROS production, RhoA/Rho-kinase activation [30]. Thus, both intracellular and extracellular CyPA contribute to ROS production in the three-legged race with Rho-kinase activation. Furthermore, basigin has been identified as an extracellular receptor for CyPA in inflammatory cells [57] and VSMCs [58]. Further knowledge of the extracellular CyPA receptors on vascular cells will contribute to the development of novel therapies for cardiovascular diseases.

5.1.6   Rho-Kinase in Pulmonary Hypertension

Rho-kinase is involved in the pathogenesis of PH as it is associated with hypoxic exposure, endothelial dysfunction, VSMC proliferation, enhanced ROS production, and inflammatory cell migration [59]. Pulmonary vascular dysfunction plays a crucial role in the development of hypoxia-induced PH [3, 4], for which Rho-kinase plays a crucial role [5–7]. Long-term treatment with fasudil suppresses the development of monocrotaline-induced PH in rats [60] and hypoxia-induced PH in mice [61]. Furthermore, we have recently demonstrated the crucial role of ROCK2 in the development of hypoxia-induced PH using VSMC-specific ROCK2 knockout mice [5]. Consistently, we observed Rho-kinase activation in patients with pulmonary arterial hypertension (PAH) [62]. Furthermore, fasudil significantly reduced pulmonary vascular resistance in patients with PAH [63, 64].

Since CyPA secretion is regulated by Rho-kinase [50, 65], we further tested the hypothesis that CyPA contributes to the development of PH in mice and humans [58]. Importantly, we demonstrated that extracellular CyPA and its receptor, basigin (Bsg, CD147), are crucial for hypoxia-induced PH as they induce growth factor secretion, inflammatory cell recruitment, and VSMC proliferation [58]. Based on these findings, we proposed a novel mechanism for hypoxia-induced PH in which hypoxia induces growth-promoting genes in VSMCs through a CyPA/Bsg-dependent pathway [58].

These results suggest that extracellular CyPA and vascular Bsg are crucial for PH development and could be potential therapeutic targets. Intravenous injection of a number of different Rho-kinase inhibitors reduces pulmonary arterial pressure even under resting conditions [66]. These results suggest that Rho-kinase plays a physiological role in the maintenance of baseline vasoconstrictor tone in the pulmonary and systemic vascular beds and is involved in the development of PH. Furthermore, we demonstrated that the combination therapy with fasudil and sildenafil showed synergistic effects through inhibition of Rho-kinase activity for the treatment of PH in rats [6].

5.1.7 Rho-Kinase as a Therapeutic Target

Rho-kinase inhibitors, fasudil [67], and Y-27632 [68] have been developed and proved to inhibit Rho-kinase activity in a competitive manner with ATP at the Rho-binding site [69]. Hydroxyfasudil, a major active metabolite of fasudil, exerts a more specific inhibitory effect on Rho-kinase [44, 70]. The role of the Rho-kinase pathway has been emerging, and the indications of Rho-kinase inhibitors have been expanding in cardiovascular medicine [15, 16, 29–31]. Currently, many pharmaceutical companies and manufacturers have strong interests in the RhoA/Rho-kinase signaling and the development of its inhibitors [26, 29, 31]. Among them, Akama et al. performed a kinome-wide screen to investigate the members of the benzoxaborole family and identified Rho-kinase as a target [71, 72]. Based on the role of Rho-kinase in disease processes that include smooth muscle contraction, fibrosis, and inflammation, the target and therapeutic applications for Rho-kinase inhibitors are mainly in the field of cardiovascular diseases. However, our recent study demonstrated a crucial role for Rho-kinase in cardiac development [73], which may warn against the use of Rho-kinase inhibitors during pregnancy. Until date, we demonstrated that several medications, including statins, calcium channel blockers, and eicosapentaenoic acid (EPA), have an indirect inhibitory effect on Rho-kinase [16, 30]. Thus, the higher doses of these drugs during pregnancy might potentially cause the development of congenital heart diseases [74].

5.1.8 Conclusions

Rho-kinase is substantially involved in the pathogenesis of PH and Rho-kinase inhibitors may be useful for the treatment of PH.

References

1. Michelakis ED. Pulmonary arterial hypertension: yesterday, today, tomorrow. Circ Res. 2014;115(1):109–14.
2. Stenmark KR, Fagan KA, Frid MG. Hypoxia-induced pulmonary vascular remodeling: cellular and molecular mechanisms. Circ Res. 2006;99(7):675–91.
3. Satoh K, Kagaya Y, Nakano M, Ito Y, Ohta J, Tada H, et al. Important role of endogenous erythropoietin system in recruitment of endothelial progenitor cells in hypoxia-induced pulmonary hypertension in mice. Circulation. 2006;113(11):1442–50.
4. Satoh K, Fukumoto Y, Nakano M, Sugimura K, Nawata J, Demachi J, et al. Statin ameliorates hypoxia-induced pulmonary hypertension associated with down-regulated stromal cell-derived factor-1. Cardiovasc Res. 2009;81(1):226–34.
5. Shimizu T, Fukumoto Y, Tanaka S, Satoh K, Ikeda S, Shimokawa H. Crucial role of ROCK2 in vascular smooth muscle cells for hypoxia-induced pulmonary hypertension in mice. Arterioscler Thromb Vasc Biol. 2013;33(12):2780–91.
6. Elias-Al-Mamun M, Satoh K, Tanaka S, Shimizu T, Nergui S, Miyata S, et al. Combination therapy with fasudil and sildenafil ameliorates monocrotaline-induced pulmonary hypertension and survival in rats. Circ J. 2014;78(4):967–76.
7. Ikeda S, Satoh K, Kikuchi N, Miyata S, Suzuki K, Omura J, et al. Crucial role of Rho-kinase in pressure overload-induced right ventricular hypertrophy and dysfunction in mice. Arterioscler Thromb Vasc Biol. 2014;34(6):1260–71.
8. Satoh K, Matoba T, Suzuki J, O'Dell MR, Nigro P, Cui Z, et al. Cyclophilin A mediates vascular remodeling by promoting inflammation and vascular smooth muscle cell proliferation. Circulation. 2008;117(24):3088–98.
9. Nigro P, Satoh K, O'Dell MR, Soe NN, Cui Z, Mohan A, et al. Cyclophilin A is an inflammatory mediator that promotes atherosclerosis in apolipoprotein E-deficient mice. J Exp Med. 2011;208(1):53–66.
10. Yurchenko V, Zybarth G, O'Connor M, Dai WW, Franchin G, Hao T, et al. Active site residues of cyclophilin A are crucial for its signaling activity via CD147. J Biol Chem. 2002;277(25):22959–65.
11. Miller LH, Ackerman HC, Su XZ, Wellems TE. Malaria biology and disease pathogenesis: insights for new treatments. Nat Med. 2013;19(2):156–67.
12. Matsui T, Amano M, Yamamoto T, Chihara K, Nakafuku M, Ito M, et al. Rho-associated kinase, a novel serine/threonine kinase, as a putative target for small GTP binding protein Rho. EMBO J. 1996;15(9):2208–16.
13. Leung T, Chen XQ, Manser E, Lim L. The p160 RhoA-binding kinase ROKα is a member of a kinase family and is involved in the reorganization of the cytoskeleton. Mol Cell Biol. 1996;16(10):5313–27.

14. Ishizaki T, Maekawa M, Fujisawa K, Okawa K, Iwamatsu A, Fujita A, et al. The small GTP-binding protein Rho binds to and activates a 160 kDa Ser/Thr protein kinase homologous to myotonic dystrophy kinase. EMBO J. 1996;15(8):1885–93.
15. Shimokawa H. 2014 Williams Harvey lecture: importance of coronary vasomotion abnormalities -from bench to bedside. Eur Heart J. 2014;35(45):3180–93.
16. Shimokawa H, Takeshita A. Rho-kinase is an important therapeutic target in cardiovascular medicine. Arterioscler Thromb Vasc Biol. 2005;25(9):1767–75.
17. Kimura K, Ito M, Amano M, Chihara K, Fukata Y, Nakafuku M, et al. Regulation of myosin phosphatase by Rho and Rho-associated kinase (Rho-kinase). Science. 1996;273(5272):245–8.
18. Amano M, Ito M, Kimura K, Fukata Y, Chihara K, Nakano T, et al. Phosphorylation and activation of myosin by Rho-associated kinase (Rho-kinase). J Biol Chem. 1996;271(34):20246–9.
19. Shimizu Y, Thumkeo D, Keel J, Ishizaki T, Oshima H, Oshima M, et al. ROCK-I regulates closure of the eyelids and ventral body wall by inducing assembly of actomyosin bundles. J Cell Biol. 2005;168(6):941–53.
20. Thumkeo D, Keel J, Ishizaki T, Hirose M, Nonomura K, Oshima H, et al. Targeted disruption of the mouse Rho-associated kinase 2 gene results in intrauterine growth retardation and fetal death. Mol Cell Biol. 2003;23(14):5043–55.
21. Noma K, Rikitake Y, Oyama N, Yan G, Alcaide P, Liu PY, et al. ROCK1 mediates leukocyte recruitment and neointima formation following vascular injury. J Clin Invest. 2008;118(5):1632–44.
22. Alexander RW. Theodore Cooper memorial lecture. Hypertension and the pathogenesis of atherosclerosis. Oxidative stress and the mediation of arterial inflammatory response: a new perspective. Hypertension. 1995;25(2):155–61.
23. Omar HA, Cherry PD, Mortelliti MP, Burke-Wolin T, Wolin MS. Inhibition of coronary artery superoxide dismutase attenuates endothelium-dependent and -independent nitrovasodilator relaxation. Circ Res. 1991;69(3):601–8.
24. Baas AS, Berk BC. Differential activation of mitogen-activated protein kinases by H_2O_2 and O_2^- in vascular smooth muscle cells. Circ Res. 1995;77(1):29–36.
25. Shimokawa H. Cellular and molecular mechanisms of coronary artery spasm: lessons from animal models. Jpn Circ J. 2000;64(1):1–12.
26. Shimokawa H. Rho-kinase as a novel therapeutic target in treatment of cardiovascular diseases. J Cardiovasc Pharmacol. 2002;39(3):319–27.
27. Amano M, Chihara K, Kimura K, Fukata Y, Nakamura N, Matsuura Y, et al. Formation of actin stress fibers and focal adhesions enhanced by Rho-kinase. Science. 1997;275(5304):1308–11.
28. Wang J, Weigand L, Foxson J, Shimoda LA, Sylvester JT. Ca^{2+} signaling in hypoxic pulmonary vasoconstriction: effects of myosin light chain and Rho-kinase antagonists. Am J Physiol Lung Cell Mol Physiol. 2007;293(3):L674–85.
29. Shimokawa H, Rashid M. Development of Rho-kinase inhibitors for cardiovascular medicine. Trends Pharmacol Sci. 2007;28(6):296–302.
30. Satoh K, Fukumoto Y, Shimokawa H. Rho-kinase: important new therapeutic target in cardiovascular diseases. Am J Physiol Heart Circ Physiol. 2011;301(2):H287–96.
31. Shimokawa H, Satoh K. 2015 ATVB plenary lecture: translational research on Rho-kinase in cardiovascular medicine. Arterioscler Thromb Vasc Biol. 2015;35(8):1756–69.
32. Shimokawa H, Sunamura S, Satoh K. RhoA/Rho-kinase in the cardiovascular system. Circ Res. 2016;118:352–66.
33. Eto Y, Shimokawa H, Hiroki J, Morishige K, Kandabashi T, Matsumoto Y, et al. Gene transfer of dominant negative Rho-kinase suppresses neointimal formation after balloon injury in pigs. Am J Physiol Heart Circ Physiol. 2000;278(6):H1744–50.

34. Sawada N, Itoh H, Ueyama K, Yamashita J, Doi K, Chun TH, et al. Inhibition of Rho-associated kinase results in suppression of neointimal formation of balloon-injured arteries. Circulation. 2000;101(17):2030–3.
35. Shibata R, Kai H, Seki Y, Kato S, Morimatsu M, Kaibuchi K, et al. Role of Rho-associated kinase in neointima formation after vascular injury. Circulation. 2001;103(2):284–9.
36. Miyata K, Shimokawa H, Kandabashi T, Higo T, Morishige K, Eto Y, et al. Rho-kinase is involved in macrophage-mediated formation of coronary vascular lesions in pigs in vivo. Arterioscler Thromb Vasc Biol. 2000;20(11):2351–8.
37. Shimokawa H, Ito A, Fukumoto Y, Kadokami T, Nakaike R, Sakata M, et al. Chronic treatment with interleukin-1β induces coronary intimal lesions and vasospastic responses in pigs in vivo. The role of platelet-derived growth factor. J Clin Invest. 1996;97(3):769–76.
38. Shimokawa H, Morishige K, Miyata K, Kandabashi T, Eto Y, Ikegaki I, et al. Long-term inhibition of Rho-kinase induces a regression of arteriosclerotic coronary lesions in a porcine model in vivo. Cardiovasc Res. 2001;51(1):169–77.
39. Matsumoto Y, Uwatoku T, Oi K, Abe K, Hattori T, Morishige K, et al. Long-term inhibition of Rho-kinase suppresses neointimal formation after stent implantation in porcine coronary arteries: involvement of multiple mechanisms. Arterioscler Thromb Vasc Biol. 2004;24(1):181–6.
40. Hattori T, Shimokawa H, Higashi M, Hiroki J, Mukai Y, Tsutsui H, et al. Long-term inhibition of Rho-kinase suppresses left ventricular remodeling after myocardial infarction in mice. Circulation. 2004;109(18):2234–9.
41. Takemoto M, Sun J, Hiroki J, Shimokawa H, Liao JK. Rho-kinase mediates hypoxia-induced downregulation of endothelial nitric oxide synthase. Circulation. 2002;106(1):57–62.
42. Hiroki J, Shimokawa H, Higashi M, Morikawa K, Kandabashi T, Kawamura N, et al. Inflammatory stimuli upregulate Rho-kinase in human coronary vascular smooth muscle cells. J Mol Cell Cardiol. 2004;37(2):537–46.
43. Oi K, Shimokawa H, Hiroki J, Uwatoku T, Abe K, Matsumoto Y, et al. Remnant lipoproteins from patients with sudden cardiac death enhance coronary vasospastic activity through upregulation of Rho-kinase. Arterioscler Thromb Vasc Biol. 2004;24(5):918–22.
44. Higashi M, Shimokawa H, Hattori T, Hiroki J, Mukai Y, Morikawa K, et al. Long-term inhibition of Rho-kinase suppresses angiotensin II-induced cardiovascular hypertrophy in rats in vivo: effect on endothelial NAD(P)H oxidase system. Circ Res. 2003;93(8):767–75.
45. Satoh K, Godo S, Saito H, Enkhjargal B, Shimokawa H. Dual roles of vascular-derived reactive oxygen species-with a special reference to hydrogen peroxide and cyclophilin A. J Mol Cell Cardiol. 2014;73C:50–6.
46. Shimokawa H, Satoh K. Light and dark of reactive oxygen species for vascular function. J Cardiovasc Pharmacol. 2015;65(5):412–8.
47. Jin ZG, Melaragno MG, Liao DF, Yan C, Haendeler J, Suh YA, et al. Cyclophilin A is a secreted growth factor induced by oxidative stress. Circ Res. 2000;87(9):789–96.
48. Liao DF, Jin ZG, Baas AS, Daum G, Gygi SP, Aebersold R, et al. Purification and identification of secreted oxidative stress-induced factors from vascular smooth muscle cells. J Biol Chem. 2000;275(1):189–96.
49. Satoh K. Cyclophilin A in cardiovascular homeostasis and diseases. Tohoku J Exp Med. 2015;235(1):1–15.
50. Satoh K, Nigro P, Berk BC. Oxidative stress and vascular smooth muscle cell growth: a mechanistic linkage by cyclophilin A. Antioxid Redox Signal. 2010;12(5):675–82.
51. Satoh K, Shimokawa H, Berk BC. Cyclophilin A: promising new target in cardiovascular therapy. Circ J. 2010;74(11):2249–56.
52. Seizer P, Ungern-Sternberg SN, Schonberger T, Borst O, Munzer P, Schmidt EM, et al. Extracellular cyclophilin A activates platelets via EMMPRIN (CD147) and PI3K/Akt signaling, which promotes platelet adhesion and thrombus formation in vitro and in vivo. Arterioscler Thromb Vasc Biol. 2015;35(3):655–63.
53. Seizer P, Gawaz M, May AE. Cyclophilin A and EMMPRIN (CD147) in cardiovascular diseases. Cardiovasc Res. 2014;102(1):17–23.

54. Eto M, Barandier C, Rathgeb L, Kozai T, Joch H, Yang Z, et al. Thrombin suppresses endothelial nitric oxide synthase and upregulates endothelin-converting enzyme-1 expression by distinct pathways: role of Rho/ROCK and mitogen-activated protein kinase. Circ Res. 2001;89(7):583–90.

55. Soe NN, Sowden M, Baskaran P, Smolock EM, Kim Y, Nigro P, et al. Cyclophilin A is required for angiotensin II-induced p47phox translocation to caveolae in vascular smooth muscle cells. Arterioscler Thromb Vasc Biol. 2013;33(9):2147–53.

56. Lassegue B, San MA, Griendling K. Biochemistry, physiology, and pathophysiology of NADPH oxidases in the cardiovascular system. Circ Res. 2012;110:1364–90.

57. Pushkarsky T, Zybarth G, Dubrovsky L, Yurchenko V, Tang H, Guo H, et al. CD147 facilitates HIV-1 infection by interacting with virus-associated cyclophilin A. Proc Natl Acad Sci U S A. 2001;98(11):6360–5.

58. Satoh K, Satoh T, Kikuchi N, Omura J, Kurosawa R, Suzuki K, et al. Basigin mediates pulmonary hypertension by promoting inflammation and vascular smooth muscle cell proliferation. Circ Res. 2014;115(8):738–50.

59. Fukumoto Y, Shimokawa H. Rho-kinase inhibitors. Handb Exp Pharmacol. 2013;218:351–63.

60. Abe K, Shimokawa H, Morikawa K, Uwatoku T, Oi K, Matsumoto Y, et al. Long-term treatment with a Rho-kinase inhibitor improves monocrotaline-induced fatal pulmonary hypertension in rats. Circ Res. 2004;94(3):385–93.

61. Abe K, Tawara S, Oi K, Hizume T, Uwatoku T, Fukumoto Y, et al. Long-term inhibition of Rho-kinase ameliorates hypoxia-induced pulmonary hypertension in mice. J Cardiovasc Pharmacol. 2006;48(6):280–5.

62. Doe Z, Fukumoto Y, Takaki A, Tawara S, Ohashi J, Nakano M, et al. Evidence for Rho-kinase activation in patients with pulmonary arterial hypertension. Circ J. 2009;73(9):1731–9.

63. Fukumoto Y, Matoba T, Ito A, Tanaka H, Kishi T, Hayashidani S, et al. Acute vasodilator effects of a Rho-kinase inhibitor, fasudil, in patients with severe pulmonary hypertension. Heart. 2005;91(3):391–2.

64. Fukumoto Y, Yamada N, Matsubara H, Mizoguchi M, Uchino K, Yao A, et al. Double-blind, placebo-controlled clinical trial with a Rho-kinase inhibitor in pulmonary arterial hypertension. Circ J. 2013;77(10):2619–25.

65. Suzuki J, Jin ZG, Meoli DF, Matoba T, Berk BC. Cyclophilin A is secreted by a vesicular pathway in vascular smooth muscle cells. Circ Res. 2006;98(6):811–7.

66. Dhaliwal JS, Casey DB, Greco AJ, Badejo Jr AM, Gallen TB, Murthy SN, et al. Rho kinase and Ca^{2+} entry mediate increased pulmonary and systemic vascular resistance in L-NAME-treated rats. Am J Physiol Lung Cell Mol Physiol. 2007;293(5):L1306–13.

67. Asano T, Ikegaki I, Satoh S, Suzuki Y, Shibuya M, Takayasu M, et al. Mechanism of action of a novel antivasospasm drug, HA1077. J Pharmacol Exp Ther. 1987;241(3):1033–40.

68. Uehata M, Ishizaki T, Satoh H, Ono T, Kawahara T, Morishita T, et al. Calcium sensitization of smooth muscle mediated by a Rho-associated protein kinase in hypertension. Nature. 1997;389(6654):990–4.

69. Davies SP, Reddy H, Caivano M, Cohen P. Specificity and mechanism of action of some commonly used protein kinase inhibitors. Biochem J. 2000;351(Pt 1):95–105.

70. Shimokawa H, Seto M, Katsumata N, Amano M, Kozai T, Yamawaki T, et al. Rho-kinase-mediated pathway induces enhanced myosin light chain phosphorylations in a swine model of coronary artery spasm. Cardiovasc Res. 1999;43(4):1029–39.

71. Akama T, Dong C, Virtucio C, Sullivan D, Zhou Y, Zhang YK, et al. Linking phenotype to kinase: identification of a novel benzoxaborole hinge-binding motif for kinase inhibition and development of high-potency Rho-kinase inhibitors. J Pharmacol Exp Ther. 2013;347(3):615–25.

72. Akama T, Dong C, Virtucio C, Freund YR, Chen D, Orr MD, et al. Discovery and structure-activity relationships of 6-(benzoylamino)benzoxaboroles as orally active anti-inflammatory agents. Bioorg Med Chem Lett. 2013;23(21):5870–3.

73. Ellawindy A, Satoh K, Sunamura S, Kikuchi N, Suzuki K, Minami T, et al. Rho-Kinase inhibition during early cardiac development causes arrhythmogenic right ventricular cardiomyopathy in mice. Arterioscler Thromb Vasc Biol. 2015;35(10):2172–84.
74. Wei L, Roberts W, Wang L, Yamada M, Zhang S, Zhao Z, et al. Rho kinases play an obligatory role in vertebrate embryonic organogenesis. Development. 2001;128(15):2953–62.

Chapter 6

The Unique Property of the Pulmonary Artery Regarding the Smooth Muscle Effects of Proteinase-Activated Receptor 1: The Possible Contribution to the Pathogenesis of Pulmonary Hypertension

Katsuya Hirano

Abstract Pulmonary hypertension is characterized by the progressive elevation of pulmonary vascular resistance. Vasoconstriction, vascular remodeling, and thrombus formation are the major contributing factors for increased vascular resistance. Thrombotic arteriopathy and increased coagulability are associated with pulmonary hypertension. Anticoagulation therapy exerts beneficial effects which improve the survival of patients. The coagulation system may contribute to the pathogenesis and pathophysiology of pulmonary hypertension. Proteinase-activated receptor 1 (PAR_1) mediates the vascular effects of thrombin. In systemic circulation, PAR_1 predominantly exerts endothelial effects in normal arteries, while the smooth muscle effects, such as vasoconstriction and vascular remodeling, are limited. In contrast, the pulmonary artery has a unique property with regard to the smooth muscle effects of PAR_1. PAR_1 induces vasoconstriction, even in normal arteries. Rho-associated coiled-coil-containing protein kinase and reactive oxygen species contribute to the PAR_1-mediated pulmonary vasoconstriction. Accordingly, PAR_1 is suggested to play a critical role in the pathogenesis and pathophysiology of pulmonary hypertension, by contributing to vasoconstriction and vascular remodeling. PAR_1 is therefore a potential new therapeutic target for the treatment of pulmonary hypertension. However, the pathological contribution of PAR_1 to pulmonary hypertension remains to be established in future investigations.

Keywords Thrombin • Receptor • Smooth muscle • Pulmonary artery

K. Hirano (✉)
Department of Cardiovascular Physiology, Faculty of Medicine, Kagawa University,
1750-1 Ikenobe, Miki-cho, Kita-gun, Kagawa 761-0793, Japan
e-mail: khirano@med.kagawa-u.ac.jp

© Springer Science+Business Media Singapore 2017
Y. Fukumoto (ed.), *Diagnosis and Treatment of Pulmonary Hypertension*,
DOI 10.1007/978-981-287-840-3_6

6.1 Proteinase-Activated Receptor Family

The proteinase-activated receptors (PARs) form a unique family of G protein-coupled receptors, which belong to the δ group of class A rhodopsin receptors [1–3]. The first member, PAR_1, was cloned from a cDNA library of megakaryocytes, which are a precursor of platelets, as a thrombin receptor which mediates platelet activation [4]. Four subtypes, PAR_1-PAR_4, are currently known. Of these, PAR_1, PAR_3, and PAR_4 serve as receptors for thrombin [1, 2]. PAR_1 and PAR_3 contain amino acid sequences which are similar to those seen in the thrombin-binding domain of hirudin; thus, they are high-affinity receptors for thrombin [1]. PAR_3 is considered to lack signaling activity by itself, but functions a cofactor of PAR_1 or PAR_4. PAR_3 modulates the signaling activity of PAR_1 or facilitates the thrombin activation of the low-affinity receptor PAR_4 [1, 5]. Accordingly, PAR_1 plays an important role as a high-affinity, signaling receptor for thrombin. In the vascular system, the most relevant agonists are the proteinases which are involved in blood coagulation and fibrinolysis, such as thrombin, factors VIIa and Xa, plasmin, and activated protein C [1, 2]. The PARs are therefore thought to play critical roles under pathological situations in which coagulation-fibrinolysis activity increases and thereby contribute to the pathogenesis and pathophysiology of various vascular diseases, including atherosclerosis, hypertension, cerebral vasospasm, and pulmonary hypertension.

6.1.1 The Activation and Signaling of the PARs

The PARs are activated by a unique mechanism. The activation depends on the proteolytic cleavage of the N-terminal extracellular domain of the receptor molecule (Fig. 6.1). This cleavage unveils a cryptic ligand region, which in turn activates the receptor [1, 2]. The canonical activation sites for human PAR_1, PAR_2, and PAR_4 are R41/S42, R36/S37, and R47/G48, and the minimal sequences of the ligand region are SFLLRN, SLIGKV, and GYPGQV, respectively [6]. The synthetic peptides that correspond to (but which are not necessarily identical to) the ligand region are capable of activating the relevant receptors without receptor cleavage. Such peptides are referred to as PAR-activating peptides.

Noncanonical cleavage has also been shown to activate receptor signaling [7–9]. The noncanonical cleavage sites of human PAR_1 are R46/N47 for activated protein C, D39/P40 for matrix metalloproteinase 1, S42/F43 for matrix metalloproteinase 3, L45/R46 for elastase, and A36/T37 for proteinase 3 [9]. In this case, it causes biased signaling [7–9]. The canonical activation of PAR_1 by thrombin causes G_q/Ca^{2+} signaling, $G_{12/13}$/RhoA signaling, and β-arrestin/ERK signaling [7–9]. In contrast, activated protein C activates β-arrestin/Rac and Akt signaling, matrix metalloproteinase 1 activates $G_{12/13}$/RhoA and MAP kinase signaling, matrix metalloproteinase 3 activates G_q/Ca^{2+} and ERK signaling, and elastase and proteinase 3 activate G_i/MAP kinase signaling [9].

Fig. 6.1 Activation of a proteinase-activated receptor
The agonist proteinase cleaves the N-terminal extracellular region, thereby unveiling a cryptic ligand region, which in turn interacts with and activates the receptor

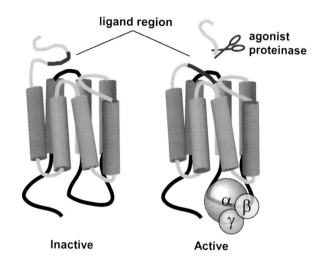

6.1.2 The Vascular Effects of PAR₁ Under Physiological Conditions

The interaction between coagulation factors and the vessel wall plays a critical role in the pathology of vascular diseases. The PARs are some of the most important molecules mediating this interaction. In endothelial cells, thrombin causes endothelium-dependent relaxation or contraction [1, 2, 6]. Nitric oxide (NO), prostacyclin, and hyperpolarization mediate the relaxant response, while prostaglandin H_2, thromboxane A_2, and endothelin-1 mediate the contractile response [2, 6]. Thrombin also causes migration, proliferation, angiogenesis, barrier dysfunction, pro-inflammatory conversion of the phenotype, and the production of cytokines and reactive oxygen species (ROS) in endothelial cells [1, 2, 10]. The phenotypic conversion of endothelial cells is characterized by an increase in the expression of vascular cell adhesion molecule 1, intercellular adhesion molecule 1, and plasminogen activator inhibitor 1 and tissue factor and a decrease in the expression of endothelial NO synthase. In smooth muscle, thrombin causes contraction, migration, proliferation, and the production of extracellular matrix, cytokines, endothelin-1, and ROS [1, 2, 10].

In normal arteries of the systemic circulation, the most frequently observed vasomotor effect of thrombin is an endothelium-dependent relaxation [2]. Smooth muscle contraction has been reported in the some types of arteries, such as the guinea pig aorta, the rabbit aorta, and the canine coronary artery [2]. No contractile effect has been observed in many other types of arteries including the rat aorta [11], the rabbit femoral artery [12], the rabbit mesenteric artery [13], the rabbit basilar artery [14, 15], the porcine coronary artery [16], or the porcine renal interlobar artery [17]. As a result, the endothelial effects of PAR₁ predominantly occur in normal arteries of the systemic circulation, while the smooth muscle effects are limited. These vascular effects of PAR₁ are consistent with its exclusive expression in endothelial cells in normal human arteries [18].

6.1.3   The Upregulation and Impaired Desensitization of PAR₁ in Smooth Muscle Under Pathological Conditions Affecting Systemic Circulation

The smooth muscle effects of PAR$_1$, such as contraction, migration, proliferation, and the production of extracellular matrix, become apparent due to an increase in the activity of PAR$_1$ under pathological conditions [2]. Increases in PAR$_1$ activity can be attributed to either an increase in expression or the impairment of receptor desensitization [2, 18–20]. During the development of atherosclerotic lesions in the human coronary artery, the endothelium-dependent relaxant effect of PAR$_1$ decreases and eventually disappears, while the smooth muscle contractile effect becomes predominant in accordance with the upregulation of PAR$_1$ expression [18, 19]. The PAR$_1$ upregulation and increased contractile effect are observed in various pathological situations [2, 21], including balloon injury and subarachnoid hemorrhage [12, 14, 15]. However, the mechanism underlying the upregulation of the receptor may differ according to the situation. In the case of subarachnoid hemorrhage, thrombin is suggested to induce the upregulation of PAR$_1$ by activating PAR$_1$ itself, because a thrombin inhibitor and PAR$_1$ antagonist have been shown to prevent the upregulation or increased activity [14, 22].

Once activated, PAR$_1$ is then subjected to phosphorylation, β-arrestin binding, endocytosis, and lysosomal degradation [21]. Since the activation of PAR$_1$ is an irreversible process that depends on the proteolytic removal of the extracellular region, these processes which occur after PAR$_1$ activation play an important role in the negative regulation and eventual termination of the signaling activity of activated PAR$_1$. It is conceivable that PAR$_1$ obtains sustained signaling activity, when these receptor desensitization mechanisms are impaired. In fact, the thrombin-induced contraction has been shown to persist after the termination of thrombin stimulation in the basilar artery isolated from a model of subarachnoid hemorrhage [15, 22, 23]. Furthermore, the administration of antioxidative agents (vitamin C and tempol) in combination with a thrombin inhibitor prevented the impairment of receptor desensitization during subarachnoid hemorrhage.

6.2   The Vasoconstrictor Effect of Thrombin in the Pulmonary Artery

6.2.1   The Unique Property of the Pulmonary Artery in Regard to the Vasoconstrictor Effects of PAR₁

Thrombin and PAR$_1$-activating peptide not only cause endothelium-dependent relaxation but also smooth muscle contraction in the porcine pulmonary artery, even under physiological conditions [24, 25]. The contractile response to PAR$_1$ agonists is consistently observed in various species, including the pig [24–27], sheep [28], guinea pig [29], and mouse [30]. The vasoconstrictor effect of thrombin was shown to be abrogated in PAR_1 knockout mice [30]. The observation of the consistent vasoconstrictor effect of PAR_1 in the normal pulmonary artery is in clear contrast to that seen with the majority of normal arteries of the systemic circulation, which exhibit endothelium-dependent relaxant response, but not a contractile response, to thrombin.

Furthermore, an isometric tension study demonstrated that the main pulmonary artery (external diameter: approximately 2 cm), the left pulmonary artery (external diameter: approximately 1 cm), proximal (corresponding to the segmental branch; external diameter: approximately 4 mm) and distal (corresponding to the subsegmental branch or a more distal branch; external diameter: approximately 1–2 mm) branches of the intrapulmonary artery exhibited a similar responsiveness to thrombin when normalized to the level seen with high K^+-depolarization [24]. These observations suggest that the relative responsiveness to thrombin was similar along the vasculature of the pulmonary artery, at least from the main pulmonary artery through the distal branch of the intrapulmonary artery. However, it remains to be established whether a similar responsiveness to thrombin can be extrapolated to the more distal precapillary arterioles, which play an essential role as a main site of the lesions which contribute to the pathogenesis and pathophysiology of pulmonary hypertension.

6.2.2 The Mechanisms Underlying PAR₁-Mediated Pulmonary Vasoconstriction

The contraction of vascular smooth muscle is primarily regulated by the Ca^{2+}-dependent reversible phosphorylation of the 20-kDa regulatory myosin light chain (MLC) [31]. However, the quantitative relationship between the degree of Ca^{2+} signaling and the extent of the contraction depends on the types of contractile stimulants or relaxant agents that are used [32]. The agonist stimulation generates a greater degree of contraction for a given degree of Ca^{2+} signaling in comparison to that seen with membrane depolarization. This phenomenon is referred to as an increase in the myofilament sensitivity to Ca^{2+} [32, 33]. The regulation of MLC phosphatase activity plays a critical role in the regulation of the myofilament Ca^{2+} sensitivity [32, 33]. The phosphorylation of a regulatory subunit of MLC phosphatase, named myosin phosphatase target subunit 1 (MYPT1), or an inhibitor protein of MLC phosphatase, named 17-kDa PKC-potentiated inhibitory protein of type 1 protein phosphatase (CPI-17), causes the inactivation of the MLC phosphatase activity, thereby enhancing the myofilament Ca^{2+} sensitivity [32, 33]. Rho-associated coiled-coil-containing protein kinase (ROCK), zipper-interacting kinase, and integrin-linked kinase play a major role in phosphorylating MYPT1 or CPI-17 and therefore regulate myofilament Ca^{2+} sensitivity [32, 33]. As a result, the canonical mechanisms regulating the smooth muscle contraction consist of the Ca^{2+}-dependent MLC phosphorylation and regulation of myofilament Ca^{2+} sensitivity.

In the presence of extracellular Ca^{2+}, thrombin and PAR_1-activating peptide induced the sustained elevation of the cytosolic Ca^{2+} concentrations ($[Ca^{2+}]_i$) and MLC phosphorylation in the porcine distal intrapulmonary artery [24, 25]. Furthermore, both PAR_1 agonists induced the contraction at the fixed level of $[Ca^{2+}]_i$ in membrane-permeabilized preparations of the porcine distal intrapulmonary artery [24]. This observation indicates that PAR_1 activation causes an increase in the myofilament Ca^{2+} sensitization. The thrombin-induced MLC phosphorylation, the increase in the myofilament Ca^{2+} sensitivity, and the contraction are all inhibited by a ROCK inhibitor (Y27632), while thrombin induces the phosphorylation of MYPT1 at the ROCK phosphorylation site [24, 25]. As a result, the PAR_1-mediated contraction appears to be attributable to the canonical mechanism of smooth muscle contraction (Fig. 6.2). Namely, PAR_1 activation causes Ca^{2+}-dependent MLC phosphorylation as well as the activation of ROCK activity, which then phosphorylates MYPT1, inhibits the MLC phosphatases activity, and increases the myofilament Ca^{2+} sensitivity.

In the absence of extracellular Ca^{2+}, both thrombin and PAR_1-activating peptide induce sustained contraction to a similar or greater extent than that seen in the presence of extracellular Ca^{2+} [25]. However, this contraction is not associated with any increase in $[Ca^{2+}]_i$ or MLC phosphorylation [25]. A noncanonical mechanism is therefore suggested to be involved in this contraction. Hydrogen peroxide also causes Ca^{2+} and MLC phosphorylation-independent contraction in the absence of extracellular Ca^{2+}, while pretreatment with N-acetyl-L-cysteine inhibits the PAR_1-mediated contraction in the absence of extracellular Ca^{2+} [25]. In fact, PAR_1 agonists only induce ROS production in the absence of extracellular Ca^{2+} [25]. These observations suggest that the PAR_1-mediated contraction seen in the absence of extracellular Ca^{2+} is mediated by ROS (Fig. 6.2). Although the precise mechanism through which ROS cause smooth muscle contraction remains to be elucidated, ROCK inhibitor inhibits the PAR_1-mediated ROS production and the contraction that is seen in the absence of extracellular Ca^{2+} [25]. In line with this fact, thrombin induces the phosphorylation of MYPT1 at the ROCK phosphorylation site in the absence of extracellular Ca^{2+}, which supports the activation of ROCK (Fig. 6.2) [25].

It should be noted that PAR_1 agonists induce ROS production in the presence of extracellular Ca^{2+}, when the activity of glutathione peroxidase (GPx), one of scavenger enzymes against ROS, is inhibited [25]. The GPx activity is in fact suppressed in vitamin D–deficient hypocalcemic rats [34], suggesting the dependence of the GPx activity on extracellular Ca^{2+}. It is conceivable that the contribution of ROS to the PAR_1-mediated vasoconstrictor effect becomes apparent in the absence of extracellular Ca^{2+} due to the suppression of scavenger activity (represented by GPx) (Fig. 6.2). In other words, although PAR_1 is capable of producing ROS irrespective of the presence or absence of extracellular Ca^{2+}, the contribution of an ROS-mediated noncanonical mechanism to the vasoconstriction in the presence of extracellular Ca^{2+} is cloaked due to the preserved ROS scavenging activity (Fig. 6.2). The production of ROS may increase, and the scavenging activity may decrease under the pathological

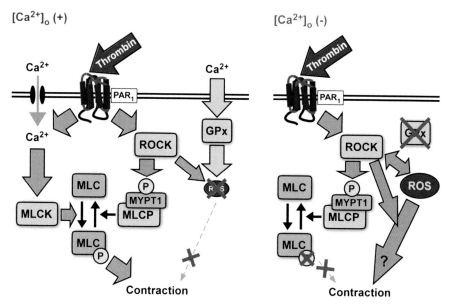

Fig. 6.2 The mechanisms underlying thrombin-induced pulmonary vasoconstriction
The schematic illustration summarizes the mechanisms of the thrombin-induced pulmonary vaso-constriction based on previous observations [24, 25]. The contraction seen in the presence of extra-cellular Ca^{2+} ($[Ca^{2+}]_o$) is dependent on Ca^{2+} and myosin light chain (MLC) phosphorylation, while that seen in the absence of $[Ca^{2+}]_o$ is independent of Ca^{2+} and MLC phosphorylation, but dependent on reactive oxygen species (ROS). Rho-associated coiled-coil-containing protein kinase (ROCK) phosphorylates myosin phosphatase target subunit 1 (MYPT1) of MLC phosphatase (MLCP), thereby inactivating MLCP and augmenting MLC phosphorylation in the presence of $[Ca^{2+}]_o$. ROCK induces ROS production and also contributes to the ROS-dependent, Ca^{2+} and MLC phosphorylation-independent contraction in the absence of $[Ca^{2+}]_o$. However, the mechanism by which ROS causes smooth muscle contraction remains unknown (?). Abbreviations: *GPx* glutathi-one peroxidase, *MLCK* MLC kinase. The *yellow circles* containing the letter "P" indicate the phosphorylated form of protein

situation of pulmonary hypertension [35–37]. Furthermore, the activity of ROCK is elevated in the rat model of monocrotaline-induced pulmonary hypertension and in patients with idiopathic pulmonary arterial hypertension [38, 39]. It is therefore hypothesized that both canonical and noncanonical mechanisms contribute to the vasoconstriction in pathological pulmonary hypertension.

6.3 The Possible Involvement of PAR₁ in the Pathogenesis of Pulmonary Hypertension

Pulmonary hypertension is characterized by a progressive increase in pulmonary vascular resistance. Vasoconstriction, vascular remodeling, and thrombus formation are major pathological findings that contribute to an increase in vascular resistance (Fig. 6.3). Thrombus formation and thrombotic pulmonary arteriopathy are

Fig. 6.3 The proposed role of PAR$_1$ in the pathogenesis and pathophysiology of pulmonary hypertension **The coagulation system contributes to the increase in pulmonary vascular resistance by inducing obstructive lesions and by inducing vasoconstriction and vascular remodeling via PAR$_1$ activation**

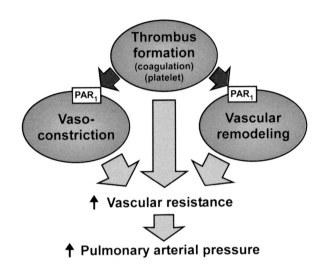

commonly observed in patients with pulmonary hypertension [40, 41]. Increased coagulability is also observed in patients with pulmonary hypertension [42, 43]. Five out of seven clinical studies (one prospective and six retrospective case-control studies) demonstrated the beneficial effect of anticoagulation therapy in improving the survival of patients with pulmonary hypertension [44]. The recent large-scale COMPERA study with 1283 patients with pulmonary arterial hypertension also demonstrated that anticoagulation treatment significantly improved the 3-year survival of idiopathic pulmonary arterial hypertension patients [45]. However, the REVEAL registry failed to demonstrate a significant improvement in the survival of 187 patients who received anticoagulation therapy [46]. The therapeutic effects of anticoagulation therapy remain controversial [44–46].

PAR$_1$ causes contraction, migration, proliferation, and the production of extra-cellular matrix, endothelin-1, cytokines, and ROS in vascular smooth muscle. These effects have the potential to induce vasoconstriction and vascular remodeling thereby contributing to the pathogenesis and pathophysiology of pulmonary hypertension (Fig. 6.3). The unique property of the pulmonary artery regarding the smooth muscle effect of PAR$_1$ may therefore play a fundamental role in the coagulation system and PAR$_1$ to contribute to the pathogenesis of pulmonary hypertension. The involvement of ROCK and ROS in PAR$_1$-mediated pulmonary vasoconstriction also supports the potential contribution of PAR$_1$ to the pathogenesis and pathophysiology of pulmonary hypertension, because it is associated with increases in ROCK activity and ROS production. Moreover, it is possible that the expression of PAR$_1$ is upregulated and that the desensitization mechanism is impaired in pulmonary hypertension as is observed in pathological conditions that affect the systemic circulation.

However, the role of PAR$_1$ in the pathogenesis and pathophysiology of pulmonary hypertension still remains to be investigated. In animal models, investigations on the preventive effects of pharmacological intervention with PAR$_1$ antagonists or the genetic knockout of PAR_1 are expected to provide plausible answers to this question. If the pathological role of PAR_1 is established, it may lead to a paradigm shift in the understanding of the pathogenesis and pathophysiology of pulmonary hypertension, especially in regard to the role of thrombus formation. Namely, thrombus formation contributes to the pathogenesis and pathophysiology of pulmonary hypertension, by not only causing occlusive lesions of pulmonary artery but also by inducing vasoconstriction and vascular remodeling via PAR_1 (Fig. 6.3). In that case, PAR_1 would be a potentially useful therapeutic target for the treatment of pulmonary hypertension.

References

1. Coughlin SR. Thrombin signalling and protease-activated receptors. Nature. 2000;407:258–64.
2. Hirano K. The roles of proteinase-activated receptors in the vascular physiology and pathophysiology. Arterioscler Thromb Vasc Biol. 2007;27:27–36.
3. Fredriksson R, Lagerstrom MC, Lundin LG, Schioth HB. The G-protein-coupled receptors in the human genome form five main families. Phylogenetic analysis, paralogon groups, and fingerprints. Mol Pharmacol. 2003;63:1256–72.
4. Vu TK, Hung DT, Wheaton VI, Coughlin SR. Molecular cloning of a functional thrombin receptor reveals a novel proteolytic mechanism of receptor activation. Cell. 1991;64:1057–68.
5. McLaughlin JN, Patterson MM, Malik AB. Protease-activated receptor-3 (PAR_3) regulates PAR_1 signaling by receptor dimerization. Proc Natl Acad Sci U S A. 2007;104:5662–7.
6. Hirano K, Kanaide H. Role of protease-activated receptors in the vascular system. J Atheroscler Thromb. 2003;10:211–25.
7. Adams MN, Ramachandran R, Yau MK, Suen JY, Fairlie DP, Hollenberg MD, et al. Structure, function and pathophysiology of protease activated receptors. Pharmacol Ther. 2011;130:248–82.
8. Ramachandran R, Noorbakhsh F, Defea K, Hollenberg MD. Targeting proteinase-activated receptors: therapeutic potential and challenges. Nat Rev Drug Discov. 2012;11:69–86.
9. Zhao P, Metcalf M, Bunnett NW. Biased signaling of protease-activated receptors. Front Endocrinol. 2014;5 doi:10.3389/fendo.2014.00067.
10. Macfarlane SR, Seatter MJ, Kanke T, Hunter GD, Plevin R. Proteinase-activated receptors. Pharmacol Rev. 2001;53:245–82.
11. Aman M, Hirano M, Kanaide H, Hirano K. Upregulation of proteinase-activated receptor-2 and increased response to trypsin in endothelial cells after exposure to oxidative stress in rat aortas. J Vasc Res. 2010;47:494–506.
12. Fukunaga R, Hirano K, Hirano M, Niiro N, Nishimura J, Maehara Y, et al. Upregulation of proteinase-activated receptors and hypercontractile responses precede development of arterial lesions after balloon injury. Am J Physiol Heart Circ Physiol. 2006;291:H2388–95.
13. Shiga N, Hirano K, Hirano M, Nishimura J, Nawata H, Kanaide H. Long-term inhibition of RhoA attenuates vascular contractility by enhancing endothelial NO production in an intact rabbit mesenteric artery. Circ Res. 2005;96:1014–21.
14. Kai Y, Hirano K, Maeda Y, Nishimura J, Sasaki T, Kanaide H. Prevention of the hypercontractile response to thrombin by proteinase-activated receptor-1 antagonist in subarachnoid hemorrhage. Stroke. 2007;38:3259–65.

15. Maeda Y, Hirano K, Kai Y, Hirano M, Suzuki SO, Sasaki T, et al. Up-regulation of proteinase-activated receptor 1 and increased contractile responses to thrombin after subarachnoid haemorrhage. Br J Pharmacol. 2007;152:1131–9.

16. Mizuno O, Hirano K, Nishimura J, Kubo C, Kanaide H. Mechanism of endothelium-dependent relaxation induced by thrombin in the pig coronary artery. Eur J Pharmacol. 1998;351:67–77.

17. Derkach DN, Ihara E, Hirano K, Nishimura J, Takahashi S, Kanaide H. Thrombin causes endothelium-dependent biphasic regulation of vascular tone in the porcine renal interlobar artery. Br J Pharmacol. 2000;131:1635–42.

18. Nelken NA, Soifer SJ, O'Keefe J, Vu TK, Charo IF, Coughlin SR. Thrombin receptor expression in normal and atherosclerotic human arteries. J Clin Invest. 1992;90:1614–21.

19. Ku DD, Dai J. Expression of thrombin receptors in human atherosclerotic coronary arteries leads to an exaggerated vasoconstrictory response in vitro. J Cardiovasc Pharmacol. 1997;30:649–57.

20. Hirano K, Hirano M. Current perspective on the role of the thrombin receptor in cerebral vasospasm after subarachnoid hemorrhage. J Pharmacol Sci. 2010;114:127–33.

21. Hirano K, Yufu T, Hirano M, Nishimura J, Kanaide H. Physiology and pathophysiology of proteinase-activated receptors (PARs): regulation of the expression of PARs. J Pharmacol Sci. 2005;97:31–7.

22. Kameda K, Kikkawa Y, Hirano M, Matsuo S, Sasaki T, Hirano K. Combined argatroban and anti-oxidative agents prevents increased vascular contractility to thrombin and other ligands after subarachnoid haemorrhage. Br J Pharmacol. 2012;165:106–19.

23. Kikkawa Y, Kameda K, Hirano M, Sasaki T, Hirano K. Impaired feedback regulation of the receptor activity and the myofilament Ca^{2+} sensitivity contributes to increased vascular reactiveness after subarachnoid hemorrhage. J Cereb Blood Flow Metab. 2010;30:1637–50.

24. Maki J, Hirano M, Hoka S, Kanaide H, Hirano K. Thrombin activation of proteinase-activated receptor 1 potentiates the myofilament Ca^{2+} sensitivity and induces vasoconstriction in porcine pulmonary arteries. Br J Pharmacol. 2010;159:919–27.

25. Maki J, Hirano M, Hoka S, Kanaide H, Hirano K. Involvement of reactive oxygen species in thrombin-induced pulmonary vasoconstriction. Am J Respir Crit Care Med. 2010;182:1435–44.

26. Glusa E, Paintz M. Relaxant and contractile responses of porcine pulmonary arteries to a thrombin receptor activating peptide (TRAP). Naunyn Schmiedebergs Arch Pharmacol. 1994;349:431–6.

27. Glusa E, Bretschneider E, Paintz M. Contractile effects of thrombin in porcine pulmonary arteries and the influence of thrombin inhibitors. Naunyn Schmiedebergs Arch Pharmacol. 1994;349:101–6.

28. Garcia-Szabo R, Kern DF, Malik AB. Pulmonary vascular response to thrombin: effects of thromboxane synthetase inhibition with OKY-046 and OKY-1581. Prostaglandins. 1984;28:851–66.

29. Lum H, Andersen TT, Fenton 2nd JW, Malik AB. Thrombin receptor activation peptide induces pulmonary vasoconstriction. Am J Physiol. 1994;266:C448–54.

30. Vogel SM, Gao X, Mehta D, Ye RD, John TA, Andrade-Gordon P, et al. Abrogation of thrombin-induced increase in pulmonary microvascular permeability in PAR-1 knockout mice. Physiol Genomics. 2000;4:137–45.

31. Hartshorne DJ. Biochemistry of the contractile process in smooth muscle. In: Johnson LR, editor. Physiology of the Gastrointestinal Tract. 2nd ed. New York: Raven Press; 1987. p. 423–82.

32. Hirano K. Current topics in the regulatory mechanism underlying the Ca^{2+} sensitization of the contractile apparatus in vascular smooth muscle. J Pharmacol Sci. 2007;104:109–15.

33. Somlyo AP, Somlyo AV. Ca^{2+} sensitivity of smooth muscle and nonmuscle myosin II: modulated by G proteins, kinases, and myosin phosphatase. Physiol Rev. 2003;83:1325–58.

34. Pahuja DN, Mitra AG, Deshpande UR, Nadkarni GD. The role of calcium in the modulation of the hepatic anti-oxidant defence system. J Trace Elem Electrolytes Health Dis. 1993;7:71–4.
35. Bowers R, Cool C, Murphy RC, Tuder RM, Hopken MW, Flores SC, et al. Oxidative stress in severe pulmonary hypertension. Am J Respir Crit Care Med. 2004;169:764–9.
36. Irodova NL, Lankin VZ, Konovalova GK, Kochetov AG, Chazova IE. Oxidative stress in patients with primary pulmonary hypertension. Bull Exp Biol Med. 2002;133:580–2.
37. Fike CD, JC S, MR K, Zhang Y, JL A. Reactive oxygen species from NADPH oxidase contribute to altered pulmonary vascular responses in piglets with chronic hypoxia-induced pulmonary hypertension. Am J Physiol Lung Cell Mol Physiol. 2008;295:L881–8.
38. Abe K, Shimokawa H, Morikawa K, Uwatoku T, Oi K, Matsumoto Y, et al. Long-term treatment with a Rho-kinase inhibitor improves monocrotaline-induced fatal pulmonary hypertension in rats. Circ Res. 2004;94:385–93.
39. Doe Z, Fukumoto Y, Takaki A, Tawara S, Ohashi J, Nakano M, et al. Evidence for Rho-kinase activation in patients with pulmonary arterial hypertension. Circ J. 2009;73:1731–9.
40. Fuster V, Steele PM, Edwards WD, Gersh BJ, McGoon MD, Frye RL. Primary pulmonary hypertension: natural history and the importance of thrombosis. Circulation. 1984;70:580–7.
41. Johnson SR, Granton JT, Mehta S. Thrombotic arteriopathy and anticoagulation in pulmonary hypertension. Chest. 2006;130:545–52.
42. Tournier A, Wahl D, Chaouat A, Max JP, Regnault V, Lecompte T, et al. Calibrated automated thrombography demonstrates hypercoagulability in patients with idiopathic pulmonary arterial hypertension. Thromb Res. 2010;126:e418–22.
43. Welsh CH, Hassell KL, Badesch DB, Kressin DC, Marlar RA. Coagulation and fibrinolytic profiles in patients with severe pulmonary hypertension. Chest. 1996;110:710–7.
44. Johnson SR, Mehta S, Granton JT. Anticoagulation in pulmonary arterial hypertension: a qualitative systematic review. Eur Respir J. 2006;28:999–1004.
45. Olsson KM, Delcroix M, Ghofrani HA, Tiede H, Huscher D, Speich R, et al. Anticoagulation and survival in pulmonary arterial hypertension: results from the Comparative, Prospective Registry of Newly Initiated Therapies for Pulmonary Hypertension (COMPERA). Circulation. 2014;129:57–65.
46. Preston IR, Roberts KE, Miller DP, Sen GP, Selej M, Benton WW, et al. Effect of warfarin treatment on survival of patients with pulmonary arterial hypertension (PAH) in the Registry to Evaluate Early and Long-term PAH disease management (REVEAL). Circulation. 2015;132:2403–11.

Chapter 7
Animal Models with Pulmonary Hypertension

Kohtaro Abe

Abstract Pulmonary arterial hypertension (PAH) comprises a multifactorial group of pulmonary vascular disorders that frequently lead to right heart failure and premature death. Histologically, patients with severe PAH have combinations of small pulmonary arterial medial and adventitial thickening, occlusive neointima, and complex plexiform lesions. Despite recent advances in treatments targeting those remodeled pulmonary arteries, the mortality in severe PAH is still high. To explore the novel treatment for severe PAH, better understandings of the pathogenesis of these lesions are needed. Numerous studies to investigate the pathogenic cellular and molecular mechanisms have been done using conventional animal models (i.e., chronically hypoxic and monocrotaline-injected rats) of pulmonary hypertension (PH). Although these animal models have contributed to provide important mechanistic insights for the development of the treatments, they do not develop the histological hallmarks of PAH, plexiform lesions. This chapter provides an overview of the histological characteristics observed in humans with pulmonary hypertension and preclinical models and discusses the better model to be used for investigating the pathogenesis of PAH and preclinical drug evaluations.

Keywords Pulmonary hypertension • Animal model • Vascular endothelial growth factor (VEGF) • Plexiform lesions

7.1 Pathological Findings of Pulmonary Vascular Lesions in Human PAH

Pulmonary arterial hypertension (PAH: World Health Organization Group 1 pulmonary hypertension) is frequently severe and leads to right heart failure and death [1]. The major contributing factors to increase pulmonary arterial resistance and pressure include sustained vasoconstriction, in situ thrombus, and progressive vascular

K. Abe (✉)
Department of Cardiovascular Medicine, Kyushu University Graduate School of Medicine,
3-1-1, Maidashi, Higashi-ku 812-8582, Fukuoka, Japan
e-mail: koabe@cardiol.med.kyushu-u.ac.jp

© Springer Science+Business Media Singapore 2017
Y. Fukumoto (ed.), *Diagnosis and Treatment of Pulmonary Hypertension*,
DOI 10.1007/978-981-287-840-3_7

Table 7.1 Histological features of grades of hypertensive pulmonary vascular lesions (Heath-Edwards classification)

	Grades of hypertensive pulmonary vascular lesions					
	1	2	3	4	5	6
Types of media of arteries/arterioles	Hypertrophied ──────────────────────────────→					
				Some generalized dilatation ──────→		
				Local dilatation lesions ──────→		
						NA→
Types of intimal reaction	None ──→					
		Cellular ──────────────────────────────→				
			Fibrous and fibroelastic ──────────→			
			Plexiform lesion ──────────→			

NA necrotizing arteritis

remodeling [2, 3]. Particularly, vascular remodeling is thought to be a major player to narrow small pulmonary arteries in patients with advanced PAH. In 1958, Heath and Edwards classified six grades of hypertensive pulmonary arterial lesions according to histological features in media and intimal areas in 69 patients primarily with congenital heart disease-associated pulmonary hypertension (previously known as secondary pulmonary hypertension). [4]. As shown in Table 7.1, a medial muscular pulmonary artery is hypertrophied toward vascular lumen (grade 1) at the early stage of PAH. As advance in pulmonary hypertension, proliferation of intimal cells in arterioles and small muscular arteries raises a fibrous thickening from a cellular thickening (grades 2 and 3). At the late stage, the plexiform lesions (grade 4) appear with neointimal lesions. Of note, this study also indicated the indistinguishable lesions in two patients with primary pulmonary hypertension (currently known as idiopathic PAH). These remodeled pulmonary arteries obviously contribute to increases in pulmonary arterial resistance and pressure in PAH. Numerous studies using lung tissue samples from patients have been done for better understandings of the pathogenesis and developing novel treatments of PAH. However, these clinical studies include the following critical limitations. First, it is essentially impossible to obtain the lung samples at the early-stage patients, because, in most cases, only a single lung specimen becomes available at the time of transplant or at autopsy. Second, it is also impossible to obtain serial lung tissue samples for detailed assessment of the lung vascular morphology/pathobiology because of its invasiveness. Third, it is impossible to exclude the effects of treatments (i.e., a high dose of intravenous epoprostenol) on the cellular and molecular signaling, because most of the end-stage patients have received various treatments [5]. Therefore, a novel experimental model that precisely simulates the clinical PAH phenotype is needed to solve these problems.

7.2 Conventional Animal Models with Pulmonary Hypertension

In order to investigate the pathogenesis of PAH, several animal models with pulmonary hypertension have been utilized [6]. The most frequently used animal models are the chronic hypoxia- and monocrotaline-exposed rodents. It is true that these conventional models have contributed to the better understanding of the pathogenesis of PAH and provided valuable information to the subsequent clinical studies. However, they do not adequately replicate human PAH.

7.2.1 Monocrotaline

Monocrotaline is a toxic pyrrolizidine alkaloid made from the plant *Crotalaria spectabilis* [7, 8]. Rats are most commonly used since mice cannot convert monocrotaline into the monocrotaline pyrrole due to the lack of the hepatic metabolism by cytochrome *P-450*. Generally, an adult male rat is administered with a single injection of monocrotaline (typically 60 mg/kg subcutaneously or intraperitoneally), then leading to high pulmonary arterial pressures within 3 weeks and a death of unknown cause. Although the mechanisms that monocrotaline causes pulmonary hypertension have not been fully understood, it is widely thought that endothelial injury and accumulation of inflammatory cells caused by monocrotaline may play an important role in the development of vascular remodeling [6, 7, 8]. However, this model presents only increased vascular wall thickness medial wall thickness (grade 1) but not neointimal lesions, which are frequently observed in the late stage of human PAH. In addition, monocrotaline directly causes myocarditis with significant liver and kidney damages, suggesting that the multiple organ failure is a possible cause of death in this model [9, 10]. Thus, monocrotaline-exposed rats do not seem to replicate idiopathic PAH in human, even though they have severe pulmonary hypertension.

7.2.2 Chronic Hypoxia

Various types of animals develop mild to moderate pulmonary hypertension after a couple of weeks under hypoxic (typically 10 % O_2) or hypobaric conditions [6, 11]. Generally, rats and mice exposed to 3-week hypoxia present only increased vascular wall thickness (grade 1). However, there is no evidence of right heart failure in chronic hypoxia-exposed animals [6]. Thus, this model does not also seem to adequately replicate severe PAH.

7.3   Other Animal Models with Pulmonary Hypertension

7.3.1   Fawn-Hooded Rats

Fawn-hooded rats spontaneously present severe pulmonary hypertension and extent of medial hypertrophy, which are further developed in the mild hypoxia of Denver's high altitude [12, 13]. However, they develop not only pulmonary but also systemic hypertension, which is not typical in human PAH.

7.3.2   Mice Overexpressing S100A4/Mts1

S100A4/Mts1, a member of the S100 family of calcium-binding proteins, was initially found in metastatic mouse mammary adenocarcinoma cells [14]. Transgenic mice overexpressing S100A4/Mts1 develop pulmonary arterial changes resembling human neointimal lesions leading to occlusion of the arterial lumen [15]. The plexiform-like lesions were also observed in this mice model. However, surprisingly, there was no evidence of medical wall thickness and severe pulmonary hypertension.

7.3.3   Mice Overexpressing IL-6

Several reports have indicated that serum levels of interleukin-6 (IL-6) were elevated and that the expression in the lungs was increased in patients with PAH [16]. Mice, which overexpress IL-6, were reported to develop pulmonary hypertension, which was enhanced by chronic exposure to hypoxia [17]. Of note, this animal model demonstrates not only medical wall thickness but also intimal occlusive lesions. However, there was no evidence of plexiform lesion formations.

7.3.4   Murine Models with BMPR2 Mutations

Bone morphogenetic protein receptor type 2 (BMPR2] mutations are found in approximately 80 % of cases of heritable PAH and approximately 20 % of idiopathic PAH patients [18, 19]. Since the function of the BMPR2 receptor serves as an internal brake against TGF-β signaling, loss of BMPR2 function activate TGF-β signaling, resulting in various proliferative and inflammatory responses. Compared to wild-type mice, transgenic mice with heterozygous BMPR2 mutations develop increased wall thickness with mild pulmonary hypertension under normoxic condition [20]. When BMPR2 deficiency mice are exposed to hypoxia for 3–5 weeks, they showed further increases in RV systolic pressure and medial thickness of small pulmonary arteries without intimal lesions [20, 21]. These results suggest that the BMPR2 mutation alone may be insufficient to generate severe pulmonary hypertension.

7.4 What Do We Need to Establish the Preclinical Model Resembling Human Pathologic Findings?

As summarized in Table 7.2, there are no models that replicate human severe PAH with occlusive intimal and complex plexiform lesions. Therefore, some investigators attempted to modify these models to develop pulmonary vascular lesions. Tanaka et al. have reported that monocrotaline-exposed rats with a subclavian to pulmonary artery anastomosis develop neointimal changes [22]. White et al. have also demonstrated that monocrotaline given to left pneumonectomized young rats caused severe pulmonary hypertension accompanied by development of occlusive intimal lesions [23]. These results suggest that at least two "hits" (monocrotaline pulse excessive shear stress) are necessary for the development of intimal lesions of small pulmonary arteries. Interestingly, the model reported by White presented perivascular plexiform-like lesions. The majority of cells in these lesions, which are comprised by α-smooth muscle actin- and vascular endothelial growth factor (VEGF)-positive cells, are highly proliferative. Also, these lesions include disorganized vascular channels lined by von Willebrand factor (an endothelial marker)-positive cells. The similar features of these lesions are observed in vascular lesions of human PAH. On the other hand, there is a major difference in time course of lesion formation between White's model and human PAH. In contrast to the development of plexiform lesions in advanced and severe stages of human PAH, the plexiform-like lesion in pneumonectomized rats develops very early (within 1 week) before the establishment of severe pulmonary hypertension.

Table 7.2 Histological characteristics in conventional animal models with pulmonary hypertension

Models	Species	Pulmonary hypertension	Medial hypertrophy	Intimal lesions	Plexiform lesions
Chronic hypoxia	R, M, D, G, P, S	Low	Yes	No	No
MCT	R, D, S	High	Yes	No	No
MCT/pneumonectomy	R, D, S	High	Yes	Yes	Yes or no
Fawn-hooded	R	High	Yes	No	No
S100A4/Mts4 overexpressing	M	Low	Yes	Yes	No
IL-6 overexpressing	M	Low	Yes	Yes	No
BMPR2+/−	M	Low	Yes	No	No
Systemic shunt	R, D, P, S	High	Yes	Yes	Yes or no

Grade is characterized MCT, monocrotaline; SERT, serotonin transporter; BMPR2, bone morphogenetic protein receptor type 2; "yes" characteristic is present; "no" characteristic is not present
R rats, M mice, D dos, G guinea pigs, P pigs, S sheep

7.5   Preclinical Animal Model with Severe PH and Complex Occlusive Lesion Formation

In 2001, Tuder et al. have reported that VEGF and VEGF receptor-2 are overexpressed in both intimal and plexiform lesions in human PAH [24]. They initially hypothesized that the blockade of VEGF signaling by VEGF receptor blocker Sugen(SU)5416, semaxinib, might attenuate the development of pulmonary hypertension in chronic hypoxia-exposed rats (Sugen5416/hypoxia/normoxia-exposed rats) [25]. However, unexpectedly, this "two-hit" rats present severe pulmonary hypertension and occlusive intimal lesion 3 weeks after SU5416 injection, unlike chronic hypoxia-exposed alone rats [25]. Although it is not totally clear how VEGF blockade accelerates pulmonary hypertension and occlusive intimal lesion in chronic hypoxia-exposed rats, Taraseviciene-Stewart et al. proposed the possible mechanisms as the following [25, 26]. The initial blockade of VEGF by SU5416 causes endothelial cell apoptosis in pulmonary arteries, and then majority of cells are killed. However, survived apoptosis-resistant endothelial cells are proliferated to occlude the vascular lumen under hypoxic condition, which is assumed to increase shear stress on the surface of inner cells. Interestingly, high pulmonary arterial pressure induced by the combination of SU5416 and hypoxia is sustained even after return to normoxia. They concluded that by 5 weeks (3 weeks of chronic hypoxia and 2 weeks of reexposure to normoxia) after the SU5416 injection, this "two-hit" model, but neither SU5416 nor hypoxia alone, develops severe progressive PAH associated with formation of occlusive neointimal lesions in small pulmonary arteries and arterioles. However, the plexiform lesions characteristic of human severe PAH have not been observed 5-week time point after SU5416 injection [26, 27].

We have previously reported that the later stages (i.e., 13–14 weeks after the SU5416 injection) of the SU5416/hypoxia/normoxia-exposed rats would develop plexiform lesions with progressive pulmonary hypertension (Fig. 7.1a) [28]. As shown in Fig. 7.1b, RV systolic pressure (RVSP, a marker of systolic pulmonary arterial pressure) initially increased time dependently, and it appeared to reach its maximum (>100 mmHg) around 5 weeks after SU5416 injection and stayed at about the same high level thereafter. At the 3- to 5-week time point, cardiac index (CI) decreased to approximately 50 % of normal and tended to further decrease at the 8- and 13-week time points. Reflecting the increases in RVSP and the reductions in CI, estimated total pulmonary resistance index (TPRI) estimated by dividing RVSP by CI showed a progressive increase from 1 to 13 weeks (Fig. 7.1c) [29]. There was no significant elevation in systemic arterial pressure. Serial histological examination revealed that SU5416/hypoxia/normoxia-exposed rats time dependently demonstrated various forms of vascular remodeling without lung parenchymal abnormalities (Fig. 7.2a). Following Heath-Edwards classification, medial wall hypertrophy (grade 1) and neointimal thickening (grades 2 and 3) appeared from 3- to 5-week time points after the SU5416 injection. At 13–14 weeks after the

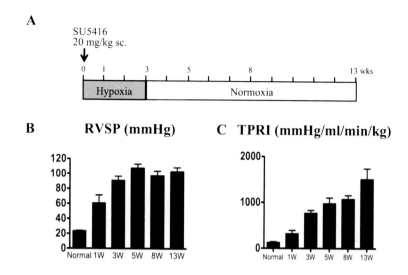

Fig. 7.1 SU5416/normoxia/hypoxia-exposed PAH rats. Protocol of SU5416/normoxia/hypoxia model (**a**), temporal changes in right ventricular systolic pressure (RVSP) (**b**) and total pulmonary resistance index (TPVRI) (**c**) in Sugen5416/hypoxia/normoxia-exposed rats at 1, 3, 5, 8, and 13 weeks after the Sugen5416 injection (Modified from Abe [28] and Toba [29])

SU5416 injection, rats developed severe PAH accompanied by concentric laminar neointimal and complex plexiform lesions (grade 4) strikingly similar to that observed in human severe PAH. Unfortunately, mice with the combination of SU5416 and hypoxia failed to develop severe pulmonary hypertension and complex plexiform lesion [30]. The reason for the difference between the rat and murine models is unknown.

The mortality rate of SU5416/hypoxia/normoxia-exposed SD rats was low despite of low cardiac function. This result is uncommon in human PAH with RV dysfunction. However, this mortality rate was significantly worsening in Fischer344 with the combination of SU5416 and hypoxia, even though the severities of both pulmonary hypertension and RV function are similar between SD and Fischer 344 rats [31, 32]. In addition, the mortality rate in SU5416/hypoxia/normoxia-exposed SD rats increases after treadmill exercise [33], probably because complete resting state may prevent the death associated with RV heart failure in this model. Thus, some modifications of this model are needed to replicate time course of human PAH.

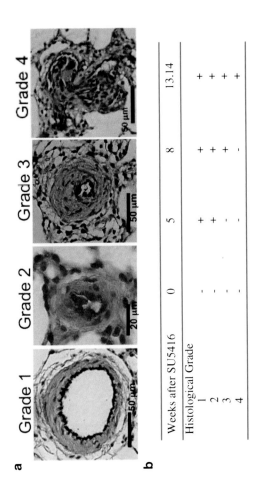

Fig. 7.2 Pulmonary arterial lesions in SU5416/normoxia/hypoxia-exposed PAH rats. Representative photomicrograph showing sequential changes of pulmonary vascular lesions following Heath-Edwards classification in various stages of SU5416/normoxia/hypoxia-exposed PAH rats (**a**) and timing in sequential appearances of difference grades of pulmonary arterial lesions (**b**). High-magnification photomicrograph showing medial wall thickness (grade 1), cellular intimal reaction/proliferation (grade 2), concentric laminar neointimal lesion (grade 3), and plexiform lesion (grade 4). von Willebrand factor stained (Modified from Abe [28])

7.6   Conclusion

This chapter reviewed the similarities and differences among various models and human PAH from the point of view of pathophysiological findings. Numerous animal models have been investigated since the monocrotaline-exposed rat was firstly described in 1967 [7]. It is true that these animal models have provided variable mechanisms of the development and maintenance of PAH. However, there is no perfect animal PAH models mimicking human severe PAH. We should understand this fact, when we plan to translate preclinical data to clinical.

Acknowledgment and Funding   We thank Dr. Masahiko Oka for helpful editorial comments. This work was supported by Grants-in-Aid for Scientific Research from the Japan Society for the Promotion Science (20588107).

References

1. Simonneau G, Robbins IM, Beghetti M, Channick RN, Delcroix M, Denton CP, et al. Updated clinical classification of pulmonary hypertension. J Am Coll Cardiol. 2009;54:S43–54.
2. Stacher E, Graham BB, Hunt JM, Gandjeva A, Groshong SD, McLaughlin VV, et al. Modern age pathology of pulmonary arterial hypertension. Am J Respir Crit Care Med. 2012;186:261–72.
3. Wagenvoort CA. Plexogenic arteriopathy. Thorax. 1994;49:S39–45.
4. Heath D, Edwards JE. The pathology of hypertensive pulmonary vascular disease: a description of six grades of structural changes in the pulmonary arteries with special reference to congenital cardiac septal defects. Circulation. 1958;18:533–47.
5. Galiè N, Corris PA, Frost A, Girgis RE, Granton J, Jing ZC, et al. Updated treatment algorithm of pulmonary arterial hypertension. J Am Coll Cardiol. 2013;62(25 Suppl):D60–72.
6. Stenmark KR, Meyrick B, Galie N, Mooi WJ, McMurtry IF. Animal models of pulmonary arterial hypertension: the hope for etiological discovery and pharmacological cure. Am J Physiol Lung Cell Mol Physiol. 2009;297:L1013–32.
7. Kay JM, Harris P, Heath D. Pulmonary hypertension produced in rats by ingestion of *Crotalaria spectabilis* seeds. Thorax. 1967;22(2):176–9.
8. Wilson DW, Segall HJ, Pan LC, Lamé MW, Estep JE, Morin D. Mechanisms and pathology of monocrotaline pulmonary toxicity. Crit Rev Toxicol. 1992;22(5–6):307–25.
9. Gomez-Arroyo JG, Farkas L, Alhussaini AA, Farkas D, Kraskauskas D, Voelkel NF, Bogaard HJ. The monocrotaline model of pulmonary hypertension in perspective. Am J Physiol Lung Cell Mol Physiol. 2012;302(4):L363–9.
10. Kurozumi T, Tanaka K, Kido M, Shoyama Y. Monocrotaline-induced renal lesions. Mol Pathol. 1983;39(3):377–86.
11. Herget J, Suggett AJ, Leach E, Barer GR. Resolution of pulmonary hypertension and other features induced by chronic hypoxia in rats during complete and intermittent normoxia. Thorax. 1978;33(4):468–73.
12. Sato K, Webb S, Tucker A, Rabinovitch M, O'Brien RF, McMurtry IF, Stelzner TJ. Factors influencing the idiopathic development of pulmonary hypertension in the fawn hooded rat. Am Rev Respir Dis. 1992;145(4 Pt 1):793–7.
13. Nagaoka T, Gebb SA, Karoor V, Homma N, Morris KG, McMurtry IF, Oka M. Involvement of RhoA/Rho kinase signaling in pulmonary hypertension of the fawn-hooded rat. J Appl Physiol. 2006;100(3):996–1002.

14. Ebralidze A, Tulchinsky E, Grigorian M, Afanasyeva A, Senin V, Revazova E, Lukanidin E. Isolation and characterization of a gene specifically expressed in different metastatic cells and whose deduced gene product has a high degree of homology to a Ca2+−binding protein family. Genes Dev. 1989;3:1086–93.

15. Greenway S, van Suylen RJ, Du Marchie Sarvaas G, Kwan E, Ambartsumian N, Lukanidin E, Rabinovitch M. S100A4/Mts1 produces murine pulmonary artery changes resembling plexogenic arteriopathy and is increased in human plexogenic arteriopathy. Am J Pathol. 2004;164:253–62.

16. Humbert M, Monti G, Brenot F, Sitbon O, Portier A, Grangeot-Keros L, Duroux P, Galanaud P, Simonneau G, Emilie D. Increased interleukin-1 and interleukin-6 serum concentrations in severe primary pulmonary hypertension. Am J Respir Crit Care Med. 1995;151(5):1628–31.

17. Steiner MK, Syrkina OL, Kolliputi N, Mark EJ, Hales CA, Waxman AB. Interleukin-6 overexpression induces pulmonary hypertension. Circ Res. 2009;104(2):236–44.

18. Deng Z, Morse JH, Slager SL, Cuervo N, Moore KJ, Venetos G, Kalachikov S, Cayanis E, Fischer SG, Barst RJ, Hodge SE, Knowles JA. Familial primary pulmonary hypertension (gene PPH1) is caused by mutations in the bone morphogenetic protein receptor-II gene. Am J Hum Genet. 2000;67(3):737–44.

19. Elliott CG. Genetics of pulmonary arterial hypertension: current and future implications. Semin Respir Crit Care Med. 2005;26(4):365–71.

20. Beppu H, Ichinose F, Kawai N, Jones RC, Yu PB, Zapol WM, Miyazono K, Li E, Bloch KD. BMPR-II heterozygous mice have mild pulmonary hypertension and an impaired pulmonary vascular remodeling response to prolonged hypoxia. Am J Physiol Lung Cell Mol Physiol. 2004;287(6):L1241–7.

21. Frank DB, Lowery J, Anderson L, Brink M, Reese J, de Caestecker M. Increased susceptibility to hypoxic pulmonary hypertension in Bmpr2 mutant mice is associated with endothelial dysfunction in the pulmonary vasculature. Am J Physiol Lung Cell Mol Physiol. 2008;294(1):L98–109.

22. Tanaka Y, Schuster DP, Davis EC, Patterson GA, Botney MD. The role of vascular injury and hemodynamics in rat pulmonary artery remodeling. J Clin Invest. 1996;98(2):434–42.

23. White RJ, Meoli DF, Swarthout RF, Kallop DY, Galaria II, Harvey JL, Miller CM, Blaxall BC, Hall CM, Pierce RA, Cool CD, Taubman MB. Plexiform-like lesions and increased tissue factor expression in a rat model of severe pulmonary arterial hypertension. Am J Physiol Lung Cell Mol Physiol. 2007;293:L583–90.

24. Tuder RM, Chacon M, Alger L, Wang J, Taraseviciene-Stewart L, Kasahara Y, Cool CD, Bishop AE, Geraci M, Semenza GL, Yacoub M, Polak JM, Voelkel NF. Expression of angiogenesis-related molecules in plexiform lesions in severe pulmonary hypertension: evidence for a process of disordered angiogenesis. J Pathol. 2001;195(3):367–74.

25. Taraseviciene-Stewart L, Kasahara Y, Alger L, Hirth P, Mc Mahon G, Waltenberger J, Voelkel NF, Tuder RM. Inhibition of the VEGF receptor 2 combined with chronic hypoxia causes cell death-dependent pulmonary endothelial cell proliferation and severe pulmonary hypertension. FASEB J. 2001;15:427–38.

26. Sakao S, Taraseviciene-Stewart L, Lee JD, Wood K, Cool CD, Voelkel NF. Initial apoptosis is followed by increased proliferation of apoptosis-resistant endothelial cells. FASEB J. 2005;19(9):1178–80.

27. Oka M, Homma N, Taraseviciene-Stewart L, Morris KG, Kraskauskas D, Burns N, Voelkel NF, McMurtry IF. Rho kinase-mediated vasoconstriction is important in severe occlusive pulmonary arterial hypertension in rats. Circ Res. 2007;100:923–9.

28. Abe K, Toba M, Alzoubi A, Ito M, Fagan KA, Cool CD, Voelkel NF, McMurtry IF, Oka M. Formation of plexiform lesions in experimental severe pulmonary arterial hypertension. Circulation. 2010;121:2747–54.

29. Toba M, Alzoubi A, O'Neill KD, Gairhe S, Matsumoto Y, Oshima K, Abe K, Oka M, McMurtry IF. Temporal hemodynamic and histological progression in Sugen5416/hypoxia/normoxia-exposed pulmonary arterial hypertensive rats. Am J Physiol Heart Circ Physiol. 2014;306(2):H243–50.

30. Ciuclan L, Bonneau O, Hussey M, Duggan N, Holmes AM, Good R, Stringer R, Jones P, Morrell NW, Jarai G, Walker C, Westwick J, Thomas M. A novel murine model of severe pulmonary arterial hypertension. Am J Respir Crit Care Med. 2011;184(10):1171–82.
31. Jiang B, Deng Y, Suen C, Taha M, Chaudhary KR, Courtman DW, Stewart DJ. Marked strain-specific differences in the SU5416 rat model of severe pulmonary arterial hypertension. Am J Respir Cell Mol Biol. 2016;54(4):461–8.
32. Alzoubi A, Almalouf P, Toba M, O'Neill K, Qian X, Francis M, Taylor MS, Alexeyev M, McMurtry IF, Oka M, Stevens T. TRPC4 inactivation confers a survival benefit in severe pulmonary arterial hypertension. Am J Pathol. 2013;183(6):1779–88.
33. Bogaard HJ, Natarajan R, Mizuno S, Abbate A, Chang PJ, Chau VQ, Hoke NN, Kraskauskas D, Kasper M, Salloum FN, Voelkel NF. Adrenergic receptor blockade reverses right heart remodeling and dysfunction in pulmonary hypertensive rats. Am J Respir Crit Care Med. 2010;182:652–60.

Chapter 8
Human Pathology

Hatsue Ishibashi-Ueda and Keiko Ohta-Ogo

Abstract The vascular histopathology of the patients with pulmonary hypertension is very important for the understanding of the pathogenesis, disease severity, and expectance of prognosis. The clinical symptoms and signs of pulmonary arterial hypertension (PAH) are similar even among various types of etiologies. The vascular pathology of PAH also shows common expressions among primary PAH and secondary PAH. The histology is usually corresponding to hemodynamically affected location of pulmonary vascular bed, i.e., precapillary, capillary, or postcapillary. Primary causes of precapillary disturbance include cardiac left-to-right shunt and pulmonary embolism. Postcapillary pulmonary hypertension (PH) includes mitral stenosis or left ventricular failure. Some types of pulmonary arterial remodeling such as medial hypertrophy and intimal cellular thickening due to PAH are considered to be the occurring reverse remodeling after adequate therapies. Here, according to the classification proposed at the 2013 World Symposium on Pulmonary Hypertension held in Nice, histopathological expressions about PAH are presented, and the recognition of pulmonary vascular changes may help to use diagnostic imaging modality such as MRI and angiography for the therapy for PAH.

Keywords Histopathology • Complex lesions • Plexiform lesion

8.1 Introduction

The pulmonary vessel morphology is quite different from that of systemic circulation because of hemodynamics. Some types of pulmonary vascular changes are not seen in systemic vessels. The disease of persistent pulmonary hypertension (PH) usually shows morphological changes. The location of underlying principle diseases of pulmonary vessels may be divided in precapillary, capillary, and postcapillary parts. Especially, the pulmonary arteries can change the morphology based on the degree and duration of pulmonary artery pressure. These findings were already

H. Ishibashi-Ueda (✉) • K. Ohta-Ogo
Department of Pathology, National Cerebral and Cardiovascular Center,
5-7-1, Fujishiro-dai, Suita, Osaka 565-8565, Japan
e-mail: hueda@ncvc.go.jp

Table 8.1 Modification of pathological classification of vasculopathies of pulmonary hypertension, consensus from the 3rd World Symposium on PAH in Venice, 2003 [3]

1. Pulmonary arteriopathy (pre- and intra-acinar arteries)
Subsets
Pulmonary arteriopathy with isolated medial hypertrophy
Pulmonary arteriopathy with medial hypertrophy and intimal thickening (cellular, fibrotic)
Concentric laminar
Eccentric, concentric nonlaminar
Pulmonary arteriopathy with plexiform and/or dilation lesions or arteritis
Pulmonary arteriopathy with isolated arteritis
1a. As above but with coexisting venous-venular changes (cellular and/or fibrotic intimal thickening, muscularization)
The presence of the following changes should be noted:
Adventitial thickening; thrombotic lesions (fresh, organized, recanalized, colander lesion); necrotizing or lympho-monocytic arteritis; elastic artery changes (fibrotic or atheromatous intimal plaques, elastic laminae degeneration); bronchial vessel changes, ferruginous incrustation, calcifications, foreign body emboli, organized infarct perivascular lymphocytic infiltrates
2. Pulmonary occlusive venopathy, PVO (veins of various size and venules) with or without coexisting arteriopathy (formerly pulmonary veno-occlusive disease, PVOD)
Histopathologic features:
Venous changes: intimal thickening/obstruction (cellular, fibrotic), obstructive fibrous luminal septa (recanalization)
Adventitial thickening (fibrotic), muscularization, iron and calcium incrustation with foreign body reaction:
Capillary changes: dilated, congested capillaries; angioma-like lesions
Interstitial changes: edema, fibrosis, hemosiderosis, lymphocytic infiltrates
Others: dilated lymphatics, alveoli with hemosiderin-laden macrophages, type II cell hyperplasia
3. Pulmonary microvasculopathy, PM (formerly pulmonary capillary hemangioma, PCH) with or without coexisting arteriopathy and/or venopathy
Histopathologic features:
Microvessel changes: localized capillary proliferations within pulmonary interstitium, obstructive capillary proliferation in veins and venular walls
Venous-venular intimal fibrosis
Interstitial changes: edema, fibrosis, hemosiderosis
Others: dilated lymphatics, alveoli with hemosiderin-laden macrophages, type II cell hyperplasia
4. Unclassifiable

well known as a Heath and Edwards classification. They classified morphological characteristics in 1958 using grades 1–6, mainly focusing on the thickening of the pulmonary artery wall, for the decision of the surgical indications for pulmonary arterial hypertension in congenital heart disease (CHD) with a left-to-right shunt [1]. In the Heath-Edwards classification grade, the famous plexiform lesions correspond not only to CHD but also to grade 4. In grades 5 and 6, there are complex lesions with grade 4 changes, such as vasculitis, fibrinoid changes, and hemorrhage, and the clinical severity is said not to differ between these three grades. In 1970, Wagenvoort reported severe PH in CHD as plexogenic arteriopathy. Wagenvoort [2] also observed these plexiform lesions in idiopathic pulmonary hypertension and reported that they occur during the terminal period of pulmonary hypertension. In recent years, post-lung transplant outcomes have quite improved, and also medication therapy for PH has advanced, making this refractory disease receive global attention and become an attractive topic for medical researchers. Furthermore, as more numbers of the patients with corrected CHD in childhood are reaching adulthood in these days, the complication of pulmonary hypertension is also an important issue among adult CHD. In 2003, during the 3rd World Symposium on Pulmonary Arterial Hypertension held in Venice, Italy, clinical classifications and new classifications for pulmonary histopathology were also presented from the pathologists group (Table 8.1) [3]. They proposed the disease concept of primary pulmonary hypertension (PPH) as pulmonary arterial hypertension (PAH) and suggested that descriptions be used histopathologically for pulmonary artery lesion sites and the presence of concomitant inflammatory findings. In this chapter, we simplify these classifications and provide an outline of the pathology of pulmonary artery lesions focusing on PAH in accordance with the updated clinical classification presented at the 5th World Symposium on Pulmonary Hypertension held in Nice, France, in 2013 (see Chap. 7. Animal Models with Pulmonary Hypertension) [4] and the Japanese Circulation Society guidelines [5].

8.2 Pathological Classification

8.2.1 Group 1: Pulmonary Arterial Hypertension (PAH) Caused by Increased Pulmonary Artery Pressure

Under the condition of increased pulmonary artery pressure, pathological lesions commonly appear as usually muscular hypertrophy of media in the precapillary part, i.e., peripheral pulmonary small arteries and arterioles that are ≤500 μm in diameter. Histopathological appearance of pulmonary arteries shows no difference in group 1, from 1.1 to 1.3. The traditional Heath-Edwards grades (1–6) [1] are often used for pathological assessment. The Heath-Edwards grades 1, 2, and 3 are considered reversible pathological alterations with the treatment of PAH. However, the clinical status of cases with pulmonary pathology showing Heath-Edwards grades 4, 5, and 6 is almost the same severity, and histopathological changes at this stage are generally believed to be irreversible. Elastica van Gieson staining is helpful for assessment of medial hypertrophy or intimal thickening.

8.2.1.1   Group 1–1.1. Idiopathic PAH

Isolated Medial Hypertrophy (Corresponds to Heath-Edwards Grade 1)

In muscular arteries with diameters of 100–500 μm, increased pulmonary artery pressure causes medial smooth muscle cell proliferation, leading to medial hypertrophy of pulmonary arteries (Fig. 8.1a). Furthermore, a newly formed muscular layer at the arteriolar or precapillary level (20–70 μm) where there is almost no smooth muscle layer presents in a normal condition (muscularization of arteriole) [6]. Marked medial hypertrophy is observed in muscular arteries 100–500 μm in diameter, but these lesions are said to be the result of vasoconstriction and dilation according to pulmonary artery high pressure. This medial hypertrophy is expected as reversible lesion through the improvement of pulmonary hypertension [7].

Combined Intimal Thickening and Medial Hypertrophy (Corresponds to Heath-Edwards Grades 2 and 3)

Concentric intimal thickening is also involved in addition to the aforementioned medial hypertrophy of the pulmonary artery (Fig. 8.1b). Regarding the intimal components, cellular intimal thickening occurs due to increases in cellular components including α-actin-positive smooth muscle cells (Fig. 8.1c) and myofibroblasts, while fibrotic intimal thickening occurs due to increases in the elastin fibers, collagen fibers, and extracellular matrix (Fig. 8.1d, e, f). Pathological changes of the cellular intimal thickening may be reversible; however, fibrous intimal thickening with replacement of cellular components of smooth muscle cells, i.e., intimal fibrosis, may not completely resolve. Concentric intimal fibrous thickening is also encountered in some connective tissue disease.

Complex Lesions

In addition to the abovementioned medial and intimal thickening, complex lesions include plexiform lesions (Heath-Edwards grade 4) (Fig. 8.2a, b), dilatation lesions (Heath-Edwards grade 5) (Fig. 8.2c, d), and arteritis, sometimes arteritis associated with fibrinoid necrosis (Heath-Edwards grade 6) (Fig. 8.2e, f). Moreover, these lesions frequently occur in some kinds of combination, rather than independently. Plexiform lesions in particular are well known as irreversible lesions.

1. Plexiform lesions occur in a branch of muscular arteries and ramificate roughly perpendicularly from the main trunk of the peripheral pulmonary muscular arteries. Capillary proliferation resembles the plexus within the renal glomeruli (Fig. 8.2b). Distal branches of the plexiform lesions are usually markedly dilated. Plexiform lesions should be distinguished from recanalization of organized thrombus in peripheral arteries. The multiple capillary channels may be accom-

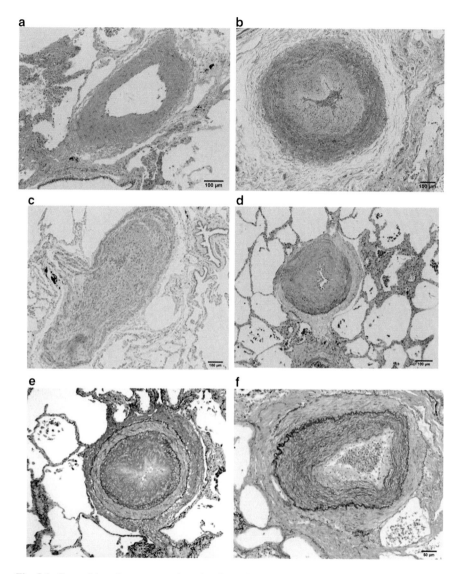

Fig. 8.1 Reversible pulmonary arteriopathy. Constrictive lesions. (**a**) Medial muscular hypertrophy of medium-sized pulmonary artery (*PA*). Heath-Edwards grade 1. H&E stain, X100. (**b**) Medial hypertrophy and cellular intimal thickening of PA. Heath-Edwards grade 2. H&E stain, X100. (**c**) Proliferating spindle cells in intima and media show positive α-smooth muscle actin immunohistochemistry, X100. (**d–f**) Medial hypertrophy and fibrotic intimal thickening of PA. Heath-Edwards grade 3. (**d**) Hyalinized intimal thickening and medial hypertrophy of preacinar PA. Masson's trichrome stain, X100. (**e**) Concentric laminar and fibrotic intimal thickening. EVG stain, X200. (**f**) Concentric multilayer and laminar intimal thickening. Elastica-Masson stain, X200

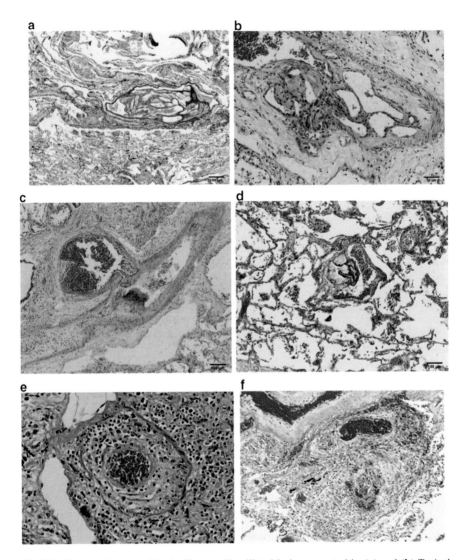

Fig. 8.2 Complex lesions with plexiform and/or dilated lesions or arteritis. (**a**) and (**b**) Typical plexiform lesion, Heath-Edwards grade 4 at branching site of PA. (**a**) Elastica-Masson stain, X100. (**b**): Fibrin thrombi in glomoid plexiform lesion, H&E stain, X200. (**c**) Heath-Edwards grade 5, dilated lesion of branching site of PA, H&E stain, X100. (**d**) Heath-Edwards grade 5, dilated PA located at distal part of plexiform lesion, H&E stain, X100. (**e**) and (**f**) Heath-Edwards grade 6, arteritis. (**e**) Mononuclear cell infiltration destroying PA wall. H&E stain, X200. (**f**) Arteritis with fibrinoid necrosis of PA. Masson's trichrome stain, X100

panied by proliferation of endothelial cells. These vessels become aneurysmal dilatation or convoluted. These are known as angiomatoid lesions and might be shunts between the pulmonary arteries and veins. The plexiform lesions may appear not only in idiopathic PAH but also in various conditions, such as CHD (1.4.4), portal hypertension, collagen disorders (1.4.1), and HIV infection (1.4.2).

2. Dilatation lesions mean aneurysm-like dilated vessels that have taken on tortuous lesions like veins and are frequently observed in distal part of plexiform lesions (Fig. 8.2c, d). This is also presumed to be as a result of the shunt between arterioles and veins.

3. Pulmonary arteritis (Fig. 8.2e) and fibrinoid necrosis (Fig. 8.2f) might also be precursors of plexiform lesions. This lesion always accompanies with destructive inflammatory cell infiltrations in arteries. However, arteritis is also observed in connective tissue disease, so other complex lesions may appear after arteritis.

8.2.1.2 Group 1–1.4 Associated PAH (A-PAH)

Group 1–1.4.1 PAH Associated with Connective Tissue Disease [8–11]

Pulmonary manifestations of various histological types may occur in connective tissue disease (CTD). In systemic lupus erythematosus (SLE) and mixed connective tissue disease (MCTD), there are some common histopathological lesions in the idiopathic group 1.1–1.3, and proliferation of the myointimal cells and fibrous thickening occur in the pulmonary arteries, causing luminal stenosis. They may sometimes present with plexiform lesions. Furthermore, arteritis due to CTD and necrotizing arteritis might develop plexiform lesions.

Pulmonary hypertension is said to be a complication in approximately 10 % of cases of systemic sclerosis (SSc) and localized sclerosis [12, 13]. It is relatively common for pulmonary fibrosis related to interstitial edema to cause thickening of the alveolar wall, which in turn causes thickening of the medial of the pulmonary arterioles present in the alveolar wall. Progression of pulmonary hypertension then occurs due to luminal obstruction by intimal fibrosis [9–11]. Even cases of SSc without pulmonary fibrosis sometimes present with obstruction of the capillaries, peripheral pulmonary arterioles (precapillaries), or pulmonary postcapillary venules or veins which are similar to pulmonary veno-occlusive disease (PVOD). In cases of SSc, Heath-Edwards grade 4 or higher such as plexiform lesions is rarely observed. CREST (calcinosis, Raynaud's phenomenon, esophageal dysfunction, sclerodactyly, and telangiectasia) syndrome is often complicated with pulmonary hypertension.

Group 1–1.4.4. Pulmonary Hypertension Associated with CHD

Pulmonary hypertension in CHD is due to large blood volume and high blood pressure by a left-to-right shunt such as ventricular septal defects (VSD), atrial septal defect (ASD), and patent ductus arteriosus (PDA). Direct blood pressure load promotes the medial thickening of the pulmonary arteries and arterioles accompanied with smooth muscle and elastic fiber proliferation. The obstructive pulmonary artery lesions in CHD appear earlier in VSD and PDA. The intimal lesions readily occur in pulmonary muscular arteries and pulmonary arterioles up to 200 μm in diameter, and fibrous thickening of the intima progresses in a concentric pattern. Medial and intimal stenotic lesion may still be capable of reverse remodeling or adaptation. Due to continuous severe hypertension, vascular changes such as plexogenic arteriopathy may occur. The Heath-Edwards classification was originally used to classify the extent of obstructive pulmonary vascular lesions [1] when determining surgical indications for CHD. Findings corresponding to Heath-Edwards grades 1–3 such as medial thickening, cellular thickening of the intima, early intimal fibrous thickening, and elastic fibrosis are said to be reversible and may regress postoperatively. However, progressive obstructive pulmonary vascular lesions such as plexiform lesions are said to be irreversible. The shunting CHD where the short circuits on the left and right become predominant is known as Eisenmenger syndrome and presents with obstructive pulmonary artery lesions. In addition, there is residual pulmonary hypertension postoperatively, and in some cases, progression of the obstructive pulmonary artery lesions such as plexiform and angiomatoid lesion may be observed [14].

8.2.2   Group 1': Pulmonary Veno-occlusive Disease (PVOD)/ Pulmonary Occlusive Venopathy (PVO)

Conventional primary pulmonary hypertension includes rare disorders such as pulmonary veno-occlusive disease (PVOD) (Fig. 8.3a–d) and pulmonary capillary hemangiomatosis (PCH)/pulmonary microvasculopathy (PM) (Fig. 8.3e, f). Pathologic characteristics of PCH are found in 73 % of PVOD patients, and inversely, pathologic characteristic of PVOD is found in 80 % of PCH patients [15]. The definite diagnosis of PVOD needs histological evaluation. PVOD involves obstructive lesions that primarily damage the peripheral pulmonary veins including interlobular veins [15, 16]. Obstructive intimal fibrosis of pulmonary veins is also recognized. Medial thickening of pulmonary veins may resemble muscular arteries accompanied with intimal and external elastic layers (Fig. 8.3a). The pulmonary veins sometimes become arterialized. Increases in pulmonary artery pressure cause medial and intimal thickening of the pulmonary arteries, but plexiform lesions are rarely seen. Venous occlusion is also observed within the interlobular pleura (Fig. 8.3b). Diffuse capillary congestion (Fig. 8.3c) and capillary proliferation more than three layers due to venous obstruction (Fig. 8.3e, f), which are hemangiomatous lesions, are sometimes seen. A lot of hemosiderin-laden macrophages are observed within the alveoli due to alveolar hemorrhage caused by rupture of the dilated capillaries (Fig. 8.3d). Interstitial edema and lymphatic duct dilatation are also recognized. Lymphadenopathy mediastinum sometimes occurs. Muscular pulmonary arteries show medial hypertrophy. The etiology of the disease is not clear. However, pulmonary venous occlusions are sometimes seen in the associated conditions such as systemic sclerosis, bone marrow transplantation, and antiphospholipid syndrome.

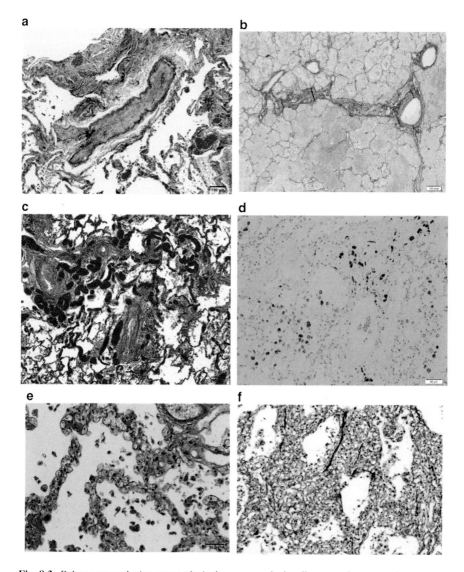

Fig. 8.3 Pulmonary occlusive venopathy/pulmonary occlusive disease: pulmonary microvenopathy/pulmonary capillary hemangioma (PCH). (**a**) Venous obstruction by fibrous intimal thickening and medial hypertrophy of arterialized pulmonary vein. Elastica-Masson stain, X200. (**b**) Septal fibrosis and lumen occlusion of venules complicating alveolar hemorrhage. EVG stain, X100. (**c**) Marked dilatation of capillaries of peri-stenotic PA. H&E stain, X50. (**d**) Hemosiderin-laden macrophages in alveolar space, Perl iron stain, X200. (**e**) and (**f**) More than three-layer capillary proliferation of alveolar septa in PCH. (**e**) H&E stain, X200. (**f**) Victoria blue and silver stain, X100

8.2.3 Group 2: Pulmonary Hypertension Caused by Left Heart Failure

In acquired cardiac disease, such as mitral valve stenosis and regurgitation, pulmonary hypertension is caused by increase pulmonary venous pressure associated with medial thickening of the pulmonary arterioles and medial and intimal thickening of the pulmonary veins. Dilation of the pulmonary capillaries, edema, and alveolar hemorrhage occur, and dilation of the lymphatic ducts and lymph node enlargement are also observed.

8.2.4 Group 3 Pulmonary Hypertension Due to Pulmonary Disease and Hypoxia

The most frequent pulmonary diseases associated with PH are emphysema, pulmonary fibrosis, and their combination (combined pulmonary fibrosis and emphysema, CPFE). Morphologic changes of hypoxic pulmonary hypertension are mainly medial hypertrophy affecting arteriolae smaller than 100 μm in diameter in addition to pathological parenchymal changes of primary diseases. Eccentric intimal fibrosis caused by organized thrombi may also be observed. In bronchiectasis, shunt formation by means of anastomosis of the pulmonary arterioles and bronchial arteries is commonly observed.

8.2.5 Group 4 Chronic Thromboembolic Pulmonary Hypertension (CTEPH) [17, 18]

Since the Dana Point 2008 world congress classification system, chronic pulmonary thromboembolism has been called as chronic thromboembolic pulmonary hypertension (CTEPH). It does not have an etiology originating in the pulmonary artery itself, which is not similar to PAH. Underlying diseases include deep vein thrombosis (DVT) and coagulopathy such as positive antiphospholipid antibodies and deficiency of protein C and protein S, causing recurrent pulmonary thromboembolism resulting in obstruction of medium-sized pulmonary arteries. Most of the pulmonary artery lesions in CTEPH show thrombi that flow from the deep veins via the pulmonary arteries and occlude the segmental and subsegmental arteries. These obstructive lesions sometimes continue from the main pulmonary artery and cause intimal thickening, and the intimal thickening starts mainly from the segmental arteries (Fig. 8.4a, b, c). Web-like structure or colander lesions are often found in organized thromboemboli as a result of recanalization [19] (Fig. 8.4d, e, f). In rare cases, thrombus formation may only be observed in more peripheral pulmonary arteries, and clinical differentiation from idiopathic PAH may be difficult. If there is

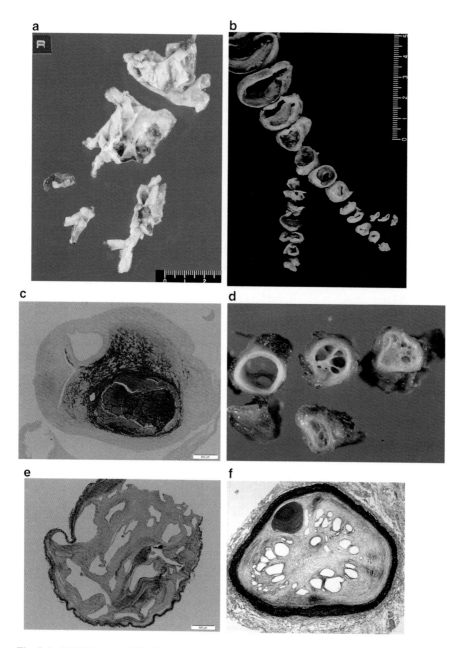

Fig. 8.4 CTEPH. (**a**) and (**b**) Photomacrographs of surgical specimens of pulmonary endarterectomy. (**c**) Lobar artery stenosed by thromboemboli. Masson's trichrome stain, X50. (**d**) Recanalized segmental artery, closeup EVG stain, X100. (**e**) and (**f**) Microscopic features of recanalized segmental artery with multiple lumens, so-called colander lesion, EVG stain, X50

only occlusion of the terminal artery branches, then surgical endarterectomy becomes difficult. Diffuse intimal thickening is often observed at sites in the pulmonary artery where there is no thrombotic obstruction. The dilated pulmonary trunk and the left and right main pulmonary arteries take on an aneurysmal shape, and intramural thrombus formation frequently occurs. In some cases with CTEPH, pulmonary infarcts develop. There is also sometimes obstruction of the pulmonary vein. This finding is rarely observed in idiopathic PAH.

8.3   Conclusions

This chapter described the pathology of pulmonary hypertension in accordance with the international classifications presented at the 5th World Symposium on Pulmonary Hypertension held in Nice, in 2013 (see Chap. 7. Animal Model) [4]. Precapillary PH affects the pulmonary arterial side. Mild to moderate PH are associated with histologic changes such as medial hypertrophy and intimal cellular thickening. Severe PH may develop plexiform lesions. Postcapillary PH including PVOD and left cardiac failure often demonstrates venous medial hypertrophy, luminal occlusion of pulmonary veins by intimal thickening, capillary congestion, and PCH-like capillary proliferation.

Besides lung pathological changes, persistent pulmonary hypertension affects other related organs. Significant right ventricular hypertrophy of the heart is always observed; however, when pulmonary hypertension improves, reverse remodeling of the right ventricle may occur, and moreover, chronic congestion of the liver may also develop. The pathology data that we have accumulated to date will be helpful for clinicians until advances in imaging technology can make it possible to understand tissue changes with diagnostic imaging more easily in the future [20].

References

1. Heath D, Edwards JE. The pathology of hypertensive pulmonary vascular disease. A description of six grades of structural changes in the pulmonary arteries with special references to congenital cardiac septal defects. Circulation. 1958;18(4 Part 1):533–47.
2. Wagenvoort CA, et al. Pathology of pulmonary hypertension. In: Wagenvoort CA, Wagenvoort N, editors. New York: Wiley; 1977. p. 69–75(a), p. 185–195(b), p. 143–176(c).
3. Pietra GG, Capron F, Stewart S, Leone O, Humbert M, Robbins IM, et al. Pathologic assessment of vasculopathies in pulmonary hypertension. J Am Coll Cardiol. 2004;43 Suppl S:25S–32S. Review
4. Simonneau G, Gatzoulis MA, Adatia I, Celermajer D, Denton C, Ghofrani A, et al. Updated clinical classification of pulmonary hypertension. J Am Coll Cardiol. 2013;62(Suppl 25):D34–41. doi:10.1016/j.jacc.2013.10.029. Review
5. Guidelines for Treatment of Pulmonary Hypertension (JCS2006). Circ J. 2007;71, Suppl. IV.
6. Todorovich-Hunter L, Johnson DJ, Ranger P, Keeley FW, Rabinovitch M. Altered elastin and collagen sythesis associated with progressive pulmonary hypertension induced by monocrotaline: a biochemical and ultrastructural study. Lab Investig. 1988;58:184–95.

7. Yamaki S, Wagenvoort CA. Comparison of primary plexogenic arteriopathy in adults and children. A morphometric study in 40 patients. Br Heart J. 1985;54:428–34.
8. Dorfmüller P, Humbert M, Perros F, Sanchez O, Simonneau G, Müller KM, et al. Fibrous remodeling of the pulmonary venous system in pulmonary arterial hypertension associated with connective tissue diseases. Hum Pathol. 2007;38:893–902.
9. Klein-Weigel P, Opitz C, Riemekasten G. Systemic sclerosis – a systematic overview: part 1 – disease characteristics and classification, pathophysiologic concepts, and recommendations for diagnosis and surveillance. Vasa. 2011;40:6–19. doi:10.1024/0301-1526/a000065. Review
10. Launay D, Sitbon O, Hachulla E, Mouthon L, Gressin V, Rottat L, et al. Survival in systemic sclerosis-associated pulmonary arterial hypertension in the modern management era. Ann Rheum Dis. 2013;72:1940–6. doi:10.1136/annrheumdis-2012-202489.
11. Proudman SM, Stevens WM, Sahhar J, Celermajer D. Pulmonary arterial hypertension in systemic sclerosis: the need for early detection and treatment. Intern Med J. 2007;37:485–94. Review
12. Galiè N, Humbert M, JL V, Gibbs S, Lang I, Torbicki A, et al. 2015 ESC/ERS Guidelines for the diagnosis and treatment of pulmonary hypertension: The Joint Task Force for the Diagnosis and Treatment of Pulmonary Hypertension of the European Society of Cardiology (ESC) and the European Respiratory Society (ERS): Endorsed by: Association for European Paediatric and Congenital Cardiology (AEPC), International Society for Heart and Lung Transplantation (ISHLT). Eur Heart J. 2016;37:67–119. doi:10.1093/eurheartj/ehv317.
13. Khanna D, Gladue H, Channick R, Chung L, Distler O, Furst DE, et al. Recommendations for screening and detection of connective tissue disease-associated pulmonary arterial hypertension. Arthritis Rheum. 2013;65:3194–201. doi:10.1002/art.38172.
14. Yamaki S, Ishidoya T, Osuga Y, Arai S. Progressive pulmonary vascular disease after surgery in a case of patent ductus arteriosus with pulmonary hypertension. Tohoku J Exp Med. 1983;140:279–88.
15. Lantuéjoul S, Sheppard MN, Corrin B, Burke MM, Nicholson AG. Pulmonary veno-occlusive disease and pulmonary capillary hemangiomatosis – a clinicopathologic study of 35 cases. Am J Surg Pathol. 2006;30:850–7.
16. Montani D, Price LC, Dorfmuller P, Achouh L, Jaïs X, Yaïci A, et al. Pulmonary veno-occlusive disease. Eur Respir J. 2009;33:189–200. doi:10.1183/09031936.00090608. Review
17. Blauwet LA, Edwards WD, Tazelaar HD, McGregor CG. Surgical pathology of pulmonary thromboendarterectomy: a study of 54 cases from 1990 to 2001. Hum Pathol. 2003;34:1290–8.
18. Bernard J, Yi ES. Pulmonary thromboendarterectomy: a clinicopathologic study of 200 consecutive pulmonary thromboendarterectomy cases in one institution. Hum Pathol. 2007;38:871–7.
19. Hosokawa K, Ishibashi-Ueda H, Kishi T, Nakanishi N, Kyotani S, Ogino H. Histopathological multiple recanalized lesion is critical element of outcome after pulmonary thromboendarterectomy. Int Heart J. 2011;52:377–81.
20. Frazier AA, Galvin JR, Franks TJ, Rosado-De-Christenson ML. From the archives of the AFIP: pulmonary vasculature: hypertension and infarction. Radiographics. 2000;20:491–524.

Chapter 9
Pathophysiology and Genetics: BMPR2

Yoshihide Mitani

Abstract Recent advances in genomic research have provided us a deeper understanding of the pathogenesis of PAH. In the early 2000s, genetic linkage analysis using large families showed rare variants in the type II receptor for the bone morphogenetic protein (BMPR2), which is a member of the transforming growth factor-beta (TGF-β) cell signaling superfamily, are the first major genetic cause of PAH. In other linkage analyses and candidate gene approaches for TGF-β superfamily signaling pathway, ALK1, ENG, SMAD4, and SMAD9 were associated with the development of hereditary and other forms of PAH, which underscores the role of this pathway in the development of occlusive pulmonary vasculopathy. The whole genome sequencing in selected families and the analysis of common variation in large PAH population provided a wider view of the underlying genetic architecture of heritable and idiopathic PAH. Unmasking the biological link between BMPR2 mutations and occlusive pulmonary vascular pathology will identify new disease mechanisms and novel therapeutic targets in the future.

Keywords Pulmonary arterial hypertension • BMPR2 • Bone morphogenetic protein • ALK1 • Heritable PAH

9.1 Introduction

Pulmonary arterial hypertension (PAH) is a progressive and devastating disorder characterized by occlusive vasculopathy, including intimal hyperplasia and plexiform lesions in small pulmonary arteries [1]. These lesions, which comprised of proliferating endothelial cells, smooth muscle cells, and fibroblasts, ultimately lead to right ventricular failure and premature death [1]. Despite a recent advance in medical treatment, PAH still remains an incurable disease. It is therefore required to explore the pathophysiologic mechanisms involved in the development of novel

Y. Mitani (✉)
Mie University Graduate School of Medicine, Mie University, Tsu, Japan
e-mail: ymitani@clin.medic.mie-u.ac.jp

© Springer Science+Business Media Singapore 2017
Y. Fukumoto (ed.), *Diagnosis and Treatment of Pulmonary Hypertension*,
DOI 10.1007/978-981-287-840-3_9

therapeutics for this disease. Although the pathogenesis of PAH is still poorly understood, genetic and environmental risk factors may give us a clue to understanding mechanisms involved in this disorder.

Familial cases of PAH have been recognized for decades and are known to be inherited in an autosomal dominant manner with reduced penetration [2]. In the early 2000s, genetic linkage analysis using large families showed rare variants (mutations) in bone morphogenetic protein receptor type 2 (BMPR2) are the first major genetic cause of PAH [3, 4]. BMPR2 is the type II receptor for the bone morphogenetic protein, which is a member of the transforming growth factor-beta (TGF-β) cell signaling superfamily. Since 2000, mutations in other genes in the TGF-β superfamily signaling (i.e., ALK1, ENG, and SMAD9) have been discovered [5–7]. With the introduction of whole exome sequencing, rarer monogenic causes of PAH have been identified utilizing smaller families than required for linkage analysis. In addition to identifying rare causes of PAH, genome-wide association study (GWAS) has been applied to identify common variants predisposing to PAH in a large population.

Despite a remarkable progress in genetics, the biological mechanisms linking the mutation of BMPR2 and other genes to pathogenesis of disease remain poorly understood. This pathway appears to be critical in both cell differentiation and growth through transcriptional regulation of target genes for PAH. This review summarizes recent observations on the genetics and relevant pathobiology of PAH and potential future directions for the development of new therapeutics.

9.2 Genetics

9.2.1 Major Mutations

>300 independent BMPR2 mutations have been identified that account for approximately 75 % of patients with a family history of PAH and up to 25 % of sporadic cases [2]. Pathogenic mutations in the type I receptor ALK1 and the type III receptor endoglin cause PAH in patients associated with hereditary hemorrhagic telangiectasia (HHT) [5, 6]. These observations support a critical role for TGF-β superfamily members in the development of PAH. BMPR2 mutations comprise all major classes of loss of function mutations, including missense variants, nonsense mutations, frameshift defects, and splice site variation, as well as larger deletions or rearrangements affecting one or more exons or the entire gene which are not readily detectable by sequencing methods [8, 9]. These genetic findings suggest haploinsufficiency (HI) has been generally accepted as the predominant molecular mechanism by which a BMPR2 mutation predisposes to PAH [8, 9].

9.2.2 Other Rare Variants and Common Variants

In a candidate gene approach for TGF-β superfamily signaling pathway in patients without known mutations in PAH genes, rare variants in SMAD1, SMAD4, SMAD9, and the type I receptor BMPR1B were identified [7, 10, 11]. The association of BMPR2, ALK1, ENG, SMAD4, and SMAD9 with the development of hereditary and other forms of PAH underscores the pivotal role of this pathway in the development of occlusive pulmonary vasculopathy. In other candidate gene strategies, it has been reported that T-box transcription factor (TBX4) mutations are associated with pediatric PAH, although the prevalence of PAH in adult TBX4 mutation carriers is low [12]. Such parents with TBX4 mutations appeared to have previously unrecognized small patella syndrome, which is known to be caused by the TBX4 mutation. Mutations in the thrombospondin-1 (TSP1 gene), which regulate the activation of TGF-β and inhibit endothelial and smooth muscle cell proliferation, were found in three PAH families, implicating TSP1 as a modifier gene in familial PAH [13]. In whole exome sequencing to study a three-generation family with multiple family members with PAH but no identifiable PAH mutations, two frameshift mutations in caveolin-1 (CAV1) were identified in both familial cases and IPAH [14]. The expression of CAV1 is necessary for the formation of caveolae, which are plasma membrane invaginations and cytoplasmic vesicles presented in numerous cell types including endothelial and smooth muscle cells of the pulmonary vasculature. Caveolae are rich in cell surface receptors critical to initiation of a cellular signaling cascade such as the TGF-β superfamily, nitric oxide pathway, and G-protein-coupled receptors. Exome sequencing in another family with multiple affected family members without identifiable HPAH mutations was found to have a heterozygous novel missense variant in the potassium channel KCNK3 [15]. Exome sequencing revealed that EIF2AK4 (the eukaryotic translation initiation factor 2α kinase 4) mutations were found in idiopathic and familial cases of PCH/PVOD [16, 17].

Another approach for identifying genes predisposing for PAH is to perform GWAS of familial and idiopathic PAH patients without BMPR2 mutations. By adopting this approach, the cerebellin-2 precursor (CBLN2) gene was identified as an SNP [18]. CBLN2, which belongs to the cerebellin gene family encoding a group of secreted neuronal glycoproteins, is expressed in the lung, and its expression is higher in explanted lungs from individuals with PAH and in endothelial cells cultured from explanted PAH lungs. CBLN2 synthesized by endothelial cells can accelerate vascular SMC proliferation in a paracrine manner [18].

9.3   Clinical Phenotype

It has been known that 6 % of PAH patients reported a family history of PAH in the prospective National Institutes of Health registry [19]. However, in the 4th PH World Symposium (Dana Point, 2008) [9], the term familial PAH was replaced with HPAH, because 10–40 % of cases previously thought to be IPAH have BMPR2 mutations, and this may pose a hereditary risk to other family members [20]. These findings may be related to the fact a family history of PAH may be unrecognized in IPAH cases with BMPR2 mutations, as a consequence of either undiagnosed disease, incomplete penetrance, or de novo mutations. In patients with PAH associated with other conditions, approximately 20 % of ALK1 mutation carriers were found in anorexigen-induced PAH [21, 22]. However, BMPR2 mutations are not found in PAH patients associated with scleroderma or other connective tissue diseases, portal hypertension, or human immunodeficiency virus infection, except for some reports in CHDs [23]. Familial cases of pulmonary veno-occlusive diseases are rarely associated with a BMPR2 mutation [24].

Heritable PAH patients with BMPR2 mutations have an earlier age of onset and a more severe hemodynamic impairment at diagnosis. Patients with HPAH had higher mean pulmonary artery pressure, higher pulmonary vascular resistance, lower cardiac index, and worse survival, while such patients are more likely to be treated with parenteral epoprostenol or lung transplant [25, 26]. Both children and adults with PAH and BMPR2 mutations are less likely to respond to acute vasodilator testing and are unlikely to benefit from treatment with calcium channel blockade [27, 28]. Symptomatic HPAH patients with ALK1 mutations are associated with an earlier age of onset and more rapid disease progression than HPAH patients with BMPR2 mutations, although ALK1-positive patients had better hemodynamic status at diagnosis, but none responded to acute vasodilator challenge [29]. PAH patients carrying ALK1 mutations may develop both PAH and HHT. Since HHT has nearly complete penetrance at the age of 60 years, clinical symptom of HHT may be absent in ALK1 mutation carriers in the childhood or early adulthood.

Recent epidemiological data no longer support genetic anticipation in BMPR2-related familial PAH [30]. Analysis of families with sibships that have lived at least 57 years from first family diagnosis allows >85 % of mutation carriers to express disease. In these families, the apparent effect of lower age of onset in earlier generations disappears, because the time it takes for penetrance to occur in this illness can be up to 75 years of age in an apparently unaffected carrier. Furthermore, the usual genetic mechanisms for anticipation, trinucleotide repeat expansions, are not present in BMPR2 [30].

9.4 Penetrance and Risk Factors

HPAH is inherited in an autosomal dominant manner, but the average penetrance rate of BMPR2 mutations is estimated at 20 % [2, 9]. The reason for the incomplete penetrance of HPAH is poorly understood but may imply that additional genetic or environmental factors are required to cause disease phenotype. There is an influence of gender on the development of PAH. Female mutation carriers are about 2.5-fold more likely to develop FPAH than those of males [31]: The penetrance in female mutation carriers was approximately 42 %, and the penetrance of male was approximately 14 % [30]. A decrease in the ratio of the urinary estrogen metabolites 2-hydroxyestrogen and 16α-hydroxyestrone in affected females with a BMPR2 mutation was found, compared with non-affected females [32]. Significantly decreased levels of the estrogen-metabolizing gene CYP1B1 were found in affected females compared with unaffected females [33]. These findings suggest that altered estrogen metabolism could contribute to the penetrance of PAH in female BMPR2 mutation carriers and that CYP1B1 could be a sex-specific modifier gene. Unaffected mutation carrier-derived lymphocyte cell lines had higher levels of wide-type BMPR2 transcripts than familial PAH patient-derived lymphocyte cell lines, suggesting that the level of expression of wild-type BMPR2 allele transcripts is important in the pathogenesis of familial PAH caused by nonsense-mediated decay (NMD+) mutations [34]. BMPR2 has multiple alternative spliced variants, although the existence of a long and short isoform of BMPR2 has long been recognized. Patients had higher levels of isoform B compared with isoform A (B/A ratio) than carriers in cultured lymphocytes [35]. Alterations in BMPR2 isoform ratios may provide an explanation for the reduced penetrance among BMPR2 mutation carriers. An alternative idea of disease modification is a potential lung-specific alteration of protein function due to somatic mutation. The occurrence of somatic mutations of the BMPR2 gene within pulmonary vasculature cells could cause or aggravate BMPR2 haploinsufficiency, although previous work had failed to find this to be true among those with a germline BMPR2 mutation [36]. In contrast, a somatic SMAD9 gene mutation was found in the pulmonary vascular cells in BMPR2 mutation carriers with PAH, providing partial support for the "two-hit model" in BMPR2-PAH [37]. It is reported that BMPR2 mutation position may influence clinical phenotype. Specifically, PAH patients with a point mutation in the cytoplasmic tail of BMPR2 exhibited a later age of onset, lower pulmonary vascular resistance, and a higher proportion of acute vasodilator response, in contrast to patients with mutations outside of this domain [38]. There is a trend for more severe prognosis of the disease in males, particularly in male BMPR2 mutation carriers. This finding is consistent with the observation that PAH mortality is most closely associated with male gender [39].

9.5 Pediatric PAH

PAH in children has a broader spectrum of genetic causes than in adults. Pediatric PAH is associated with genetic syndromes with and without congenital heart disease or other anomalies [40]. PAH is an uncommon complication with all of these syndromes although more common in Down syndrome [40]. Genetic syndromes more commonly, but not necessarily, associated with CHD and PAH also include DiGeorge syndrome, VACTERL syndrome, CHARGE syndrome, Scimitar syndrome, and Noonan syndrome [40]. The mechanism for development of PH has not been definitely demonstrated for most genetic syndromes but could involve increased pulmonary blood flow with left-to-right shunts with CHD, pulmonary venous obstruction, or production of diffusible hepatic factors increasing the pulmonary pressures [40].

9.6   Pathophysiology and Pathobiology

Although current genetic epidemiology data support the association of BMPR2 mutations with heritable PAH, it is still poorly understood how such mutations cause the pathobiology in PAH. BMPR2 mutations have cell-specific variations in cell signaling within the pulmonary vasculature. Pulmonary vascular endothelial cells seem dysfunctional and more susceptible to apoptosis in the presence of a BMPR2 mutation [41]. However, pulmonary vascular smooth muscle cells with BMPR2 mutations have a failure of growth suppression. The proliferative pheno-type in PAH may be attributable to an increased release of growth factors that pro-mote exuberant smooth muscle cell proliferation by dysfunctional endothelial cells. Loss of BMPR2 in the endothelial layer of the pulmonary vasculature could lead to heightened susceptibility to inflammation. The enhanced transmigration of leuko-cytes observed in BMPR2-deficient endothelium after tumor necrosis factor α or transforming growth factor β1 stimulation was CXCR2 dependent [42]. BMPR2 acts to regulate the expression of CXCR2, which is related to leukocyte migration and extravasation on endothelial cells [43]. Alternatively, BMPR2-disrupted endo-thelial cells stimulated by tumor necrosis factor α exhibited heightened GM-CSF mRNA translation, increased inflammatory cell recruitment, and exacerbate PAH in hypoxic mice [44]. BMPR2 inhibits cytokine expression, activation of myocardin-related transcription factor A, and inhibition of NF-κB [45]. The increased TGF-β1 signaling in BMPR2-deficient cells is related to the induction of interleukin (IL)-6 and IL-8 expression through inappropriately altered NF-κB signaling [46].

9.7   Therapeutic Consideration

The pathophysiological relevance of BMPR2 mutations in PAH is supported by studies in mutant mice. Knockout models lacking exons 4 and 5 of BMPR2 develop mild-to-moderate disease phenotypes upon exposure to hypoxia and 5-lipoxygenase as previously described [8]. Conditional targeting of mutant alleles to pulmonary artery endothelial or smooth muscle cell layers has produced a PAH model [47, 48]. Most recently, a heterozygous knock-in mouse model of the p. R899* mutation has been shown to develop age-related disease [49]. Additionally, a rat model of PAH (BMPR2_140Ex1/+) has provided support to the hypothesis that endothelial-to-mesenchymal transition represents a pathophysiological process in PAH [50].

  Since decreased BMPR2 expression contributes to the development of experi-mental PAH, upregulating BMPR2 signaling is a rational approach for the treatment of PAH. On the basis of the findings that reduced BMPR2 expression also occurs in monocrotaline and chronic hypoxic rat models of PAH, delivery of BMPR2 by intravenous gene therapy attenuated the disease in these models [51, 52]. In the high-throughput screening of known chemicals to increase BMPR2 signaling and Id1 target gene expression, FK506 (tacrolimus) or BMP9 was demonstrated to reverse pulmonary vasculopathy in monocrotaline-treated rats and in rats treated with chronic hypoxia and VEGF receptor blockade [49, 53]. In the interaction of BMPR2 pathways with signaling pathways related to the conventional treatment, BMP7 increased ET-1 levels after BMPR2 knockdown, which was prevented by ALK2 knockdown [54]. Sildenafil enhanced canonical BMP signaling via cyclic GMP and cyclic GMP-dependent protein kinase I in vitro and in vivo and partly restored deficient BMP signaling in BMPR2 mutant PASMCs [55]. Prostacyclin analogs enhance inhibitor of DNA-binding protein 1 (Id1) expression in a cAMP-dependent manner in vitro and in vivo and restore deficient BMP signaling in BMPR2 mutant PASMCs [56].

9.8 Conclusions

Recent advances in genomic research have provided us a deeper understanding of the pathogenesis of PAH. Despite these advances, there remains uncertainty regarding the pathways that mediate mutations and the onset of disease and the generation of effective prevention or treatments based on such information. Comparisons between affected HPAH patients and their unaffected BMPR2 mutation carriers may confer further clues. Understanding what influences the onset of disease in BMPR2 mutation carriers may be critical for preventing this disorder. The whole genome sequencing in selected families and the analysis of common variation in large PAH population will provide a wider view of the underlying genetic architecture of heritable and idiopathic PAH and may explore the way to identify additional disease mechanisms and new therapeutic targets. Lastly, investigating the biological link between BMPR2 mutations and occlusive pulmonary vascular pathology per se would be required to bridge the gap between genetic mutations and the disease phenotype in human.

References

1. Tuder RM, Archer SL, Dorfmüller P, Erzurum SC, Guignabert C, Michelakis E, et al. Relevant issues in the pathology and pathobiology of pulmonary hypertension. J Am Coll Cardiol. 2013;62(25 Suppl):D4–12.
2. Soubrier F, Chung WK, Machado R, Grünig E, Aldred M, Geraci M, et al. Genetics and genomics of pulmonary arterial hypertension. J Am Coll Cardiol. 2013;62(25 Suppl):D13–21.
3. Deng Z, Morse JH, Slager SL, Cuervo N, Moore KJ, Venetos G, et al. Familial primary pulmonary hypertension (gene PPH1) is caused by mutations in the bone morphogenetic protein receptor-II gene. Am J Hum Genet. 2000;67(3):737–44.
4. International PPH Consortium, KB L, RD M, MW P, JR T, JA 3rd P, JE L, et al. Heterozygous germline mutations in BMPR2, encoding a TGF-beta receptor, cause familial primary pulmonary hypertension. Nat Genet. 2000;26(1):81–4.

5. Trembath RC, Thomson JR, Machado RD, Morgan NV, Atkinson C, Winship I, et al. Clinical and molecular genetic features of pulmonary hypertension in patients with hereditary hemorrhagic telangiectasia. N Engl J Med. 2001;345(5):325–34.

6. Chaouat A, Coulet F, Favre C, Simonneau G, Weitzenblum E, Soubrier F, et al. Endoglin germline mutation in a patient with hereditary haemorrhagic telangiectasia and dexfenfluramine associated pulmonary arterial hypertension. Thorax. 2004;59(5):446–8.

7. Shintani M, Yagi H, Nakayama T, Saji T, Matsuoka R. A new nonsense mutation of SMAD8 associated with pulmonary arterial hypertension. J Med Genet. 2009;46(5):331–7.

8. Machado RD, Aldred MA, James V, Harrison RE, Patel B, Schwalbe EC, et al. Mutations of the TGF-beta type II receptor BMPR2 in pulmonary arterial hypertension. Hum Mutat. 2006;27(2):121–32.

9. Machado RD, Eickelberg O, Elliott CG, Geraci MW, Hanaoka M, Loyd JE, et al. Genetics and genomics of pulmonary arterial hypertension. J Am Coll Cardiol. 2009;54(1 Suppl):S32–42.

10. Nasim MT, Ogo T, Ahmed M, Randall R, Chowdhury HM, Snape KM, et al. Molecular genetic characterization of SMAD signaling molecules in pulmonary arterial hypertension. Hum Mutat. 2011;32(12):1385–9.

11. Chida A, Shintani M, Nakayama T, Furutani Y, Hayama E, Inai K, et al. Missense mutations of the BMPR1B (ALK6) gene in childhood idiopathic pulmonary arterial hypertension. Circ J. 2012;76(6):1501–8.

12. Kerstjens-Frederikse WS, Bongers EM, Roofthooft MT, Leter EM, Douwes JM, Van Dijk A, et al. TBX4 mutations (small patella syndrome) are associated with childhood-onset pulmonary arterial hypertension. J Med Genet. 2013;50(8):500–6.

13. Broeckel U, Robbins IM, Wheeler LA, Cogan JD, Loyd JE. Loss-of-function thrombospondin-1 mutations in familial pulmonary hypertension. Am J Phys Lung Cell Mol Phys. 2012;302(6):L541–54.

14. Austin ED, Ma L, LeDuc C, Berman Rosenzweig E, Borczuk A, Phillips 3rd JA, et al. Whole exome sequencing to identify a novel gene (caveolin-1) associated with human pulmonary arterial hypertension. Circ Cardiovasc Genet. 2012;5(3):336–43.

15. Ma L, Roman-Campos D, Austin ED, Eyries M, Sampson KS, Soubrier F, et al. A novel channelopathy in pulmonary arterial hypertension. N Engl J Med. 2013;369(4):351–61.

16. Best DH, Sumner KL, Austin ED, Chung WK, Brown LM, Borczuk AC, et al. EIF2AK4 mutations in pulmonary capillary hemangiomatosis. Chest. 2014;145(2):231–6.

17. Eyries M, Montani D, Girerd B, Perret C, Leroy A, Lonjou C, et al. EIF2AK4 mutations cause pulmonary veno-occlusive disease, a recessive form of pulmonary hypertension. Nat Genet. 2014;46(1):65–9.

18. Germain M, Eyries M, Montani D, Poirier O, Girerd B, Dorfmüller P, et al. Genome-wide association analysis identifies a susceptibility locus for pulmonary arterial hypertension. Nat Genet. 2013;45(5):518–21.

19. Rich S, Dantzker DR, Ayres SM, Bergofsky EH, Brundage BH, Detre KM, et al. Primary pulmonary hypertension. A national prospective study. Ann Intern Med. 1987;107(2):216–23.

20. Thomson JR, Machado RD, Pauciulo MW, Morgan NV, Humbert M, Elliott GC, et al. Sporadic primary pulmonary hypertension is associated with germline mutations of the gene encoding BMPR-II, a receptor member of the TGF-beta family. J Med Genet. 2000;37(10):741–5.

21. Abdalla SA, Cymerman U, Rushlow D, Chen N, Stoeber GP, Lemire EG, et al. Novel mutations and polymorphisms in genes causing hereditary hemorrhagic telangiectasia. Hum Mutat. 2005;25(3):320–1.

22. Prigoda NL, Savas S, Abdalla SA, Piovesan B, Rushlow D, Vandezande K, et al. Hereditary haemorrhagic telangiectasia: mutation detection, test sensitivity and novel mutations. J Med Genet. 2006;43(9):722–8.

23. Roberts KE, McElroy JJ, Wong WP, Yen E, Widlitz A, Barst RJ, et al. BMPR2 mutations in pulmonary arterial hypertension with congenital heart disease. Eur Respir J. 2004;24(3):371–4.

24. Runo JR, Vnencak-Jones CL, Prince M, Loyd JE, Wheeler L, Robbins IM, et al. Pulmonary veno-occlusive disease caused by an inherited mutation in bone morphogenetic protein receptor II. Am J Respir Crit Care Med. 2003;167(6):889–94.
25. Sztrymf B, Coulet F, Girerd B, Yaici A, Jais X, Sitbon O, et al. Clinical outcomes of pulmonary arterial hypertension in carriers of BMPR2 mutation. Am J Respir Crit Care Med. 2008;177(12):1377–83.
26. Evans JD, Girerd B, Montani D, Wang XJ, Galiè N, Austin ED, et al. BMPR2 mutations and survival in pulmonary arterial hypertension: an individual participant data meta-analysis. Lancet Respir Med. 2016;4(2):129–37.
27. Elliott CG, Glissmeyer EW, Havlena GT, Carlquist J, McKinney JT, Rich S, et al. Relationship of BMPR2 mutations to vasoreactivity in pulmonary arterial hypertension. Circulation. 2006;113(21):2509–15.
28. Rosenzweig EB, Morse JH, Knowles JA, Chada KK, Khan AM, Roberts KE, et al. Clinical implications of determining BMPR2 mutation status in a large cohort of children and adults with pulmonary arterial hypertension. J Heart Lung Transplant. 2008;27(6):668–74.
29. Girerd B, Montani D, Coulet F, Sztrymf B, Yaici A, Jaïs X, et al. Clinical outcomes of pulmonary arterial hypertension in patients carrying an ACVRL1 (ALK1) mutation. Am J Respir Crit Care Med. 2010;181(8):851–61.
30. Larkin EK, Newman JH, Austin ED, Hemnes AR, Wheeler L, Robbins IM, et al. Longitudinal analysis casts doubt on the presence of genetic anticipation in heritable pulmonary arterial hypertension. Am J Respir Crit Care Med. 2012;186(9):892–6.
31. Loyd JE. Genetics and gene expression in pulmonary hypertension. Chest. 2002;121(3 Suppl):46S–50S.
32. Austin ED, Cogan JD, West JD, Hedges LK, Hamid R, Dawson EP, et al. Alterations in oestrogen metabolism: implications for higher penetrance of familial pulmonary arterial hypertension in females. Eur Respir J. 2009;34(5):1093–9.
33. West J, Cogan J, Geraci M, Robinson L, Newman J, Phillips JA, et al. Gene expression in BMPR2 mutation carriers with and without evidence of pulmonary arterial hypertension suggests pathways relevant to disease penetrance. BMC Med Genet. 2008;1:45.
34. Hamid R, Cogan JD, Hedges LK, Austin E, Phillips 3rd JA, Newman JH, et al. Penetrance of pulmonary arterial hypertension is modulated by the expression of normal BMPR2 allele. Hum Mutat. 2009;30(4):649–54.
35. Cogan J, Austin E, Hedges L, Womack B, West J, Loyd J, et al. Role of BMPR2 alternative splicing in heritable pulmonary arterial hypertension penetrance. Circulation. 2012;126(15):1907–16.
36. Machado RD, James V, Southwood M, Harrison RE, Atkinson C, Stewart S, et al. Investigation of second genetic hits at the BMPR2 locus as a modulator of disease progression in familial pulmonary arterial hypertension. Circulation. 2005;111(5):607–13.
37. Aldred MA, Comhair SA, Varella-Garcia M, Asosingh K, Xu W, Noon GP, et al. Somatic chromosome abnormalities in the lungs of patients with pulmonary arterial hypertension. Am J Respir Crit Care Med. 2010;182(9):1153–60.
38. Girerd B, Coulet F, Jaïs X, Eyries M, Van Der Bruggen C, De Man F, et al. Characteristics of pulmonary arterial hypertension in affected carriers of a mutation located in the cytoplasmic tail of bone morphogenetic protein receptor type 2. Chest. 2015;147(5):1385–94.
39. Humbert M, Sitbon O, Chaouat A, Bertocchi M, Habib G, Gressin V, et al. Survival in patients with idiopathic, familial, and anorexigen-associated pulmonary arterial hypertension in the modern management era. Circulation. 2010;122:156–63.
40. Ma L, Chung WK. The genetic basis of pulmonary arterial hypertension. Hum Genet. 2014;133(5):471–9.
41. Teichert-Kuliszewska K, Kutryk MJ, Kuliszewski MA, Karoubi G, Courtman DW, et al. Bone morphogenetic protein receptor-2 signaling promotes pulmonary arterial endothelial cell survival: implications for loss-of-function mutations in the pathogenesis of pulmonary hypertension. Circ Res. 2006;98(2):209–17.

42. Burton VJ, Ciuclan LI, Holmes AM, Rodman DM, Walker C, Budd DC. Bone morphogenetic protein receptor II regulates pulmonary artery endothelial cell barrier function. Blood. 2011;117(1):333–41.

43. Burton VJ, Holmes AM, Ciuclan LI, Robinson A, Roger JS, Jarai G, et al. Attenuation of leukocyte recruitment via CXCR1/2 inhibition stops the progression of PAH in mice with genetic ablation of endothelial BMPR-II. Blood. 2011;118(17):4750–8.

44. Sawada H, Saito T, Nickel NP, Alastalo TP, Glotzbach JP, Chan R, Haghighat L, Fuchs G, Januszyk M, Cao A, Lai YJ, Perez Vde J, Kim YM, Wang L, et al. Reduced BMPR2 expression induces GM-CSF translation and macrophage recruitment in humans and mice to exacerbate pulmonary hypertension. J Exp Med. 2014;211(2):263–80.

45. Wang D, Prakash J, Nguyen P, Davis-Dusenbery BN, Hill NS, Layne MD, et al. Bone morphogenetic protein signaling in vascular disease: anti-inflammatory action through myocardin-related transcription factor A. J Biol Chem. 2012;287(33):28067–77.

46. Davies RJ, Holmes AM, Deighton J, Long L, Yang X, Barker L, et al. BMP type II receptor deficiency confers resistance to growth inhibition by TGF-β in pulmonary artery smooth muscle cells: role of proinflammatory cytokines. Am J Phys Lung Cell Mol Phys. 2012;302(6):L604–15.

47. West J, Fagan K, Steudel W, Fouty B, Lane K, Harral J, et al. Pulmonary hypertension in transgenic mice expressing a dominant-negative BMPRII gene in smooth muscle. Circ Res. 2004;94(8):1109–14.

48. Hong KH, Lee YJ, Lee E, Park SO, Han C, Beppu H, et al. Genetic ablation of the BMPR2 gene in pulmonary endothelium is sufficient to predispose to pulmonary arterial hypertension. Circulation. 2008;118(7):722–30.

49. Long L, Ormiston ML, Yang X, Southwood M, Gräf S, Machado RD, et al. Selective enhancement of endothelial BMPR-II with BMP9 reverses pulmonary arterial hypertension. Nat Med. 2015;21(7):777–85.

50. Ranchoux B, Antigny F, Rucker-Martin C, Hautefort A, Péchoux C, Bogaard HJ, et al. Endothelial-to-mesenchymal transition in pulmonary hypertension. Circulation. 2015;131(11):1006–18.

51. Reynolds AM, Holmes MD, Danilov SM, Reynolds PN. Targeted gene delivery of BMPR2 attenuates pulmonary hypertension. Eur Respir J. 2012;39(2):329–43.

52. Reynolds AM, Xia W, Holmes MD, Hodge SJ, Danilov S, Curiel DT, et al. Bone morphogenetic protein type 2 receptor gene therapy attenuates hypoxic pulmonary hypertension. Am J Phys Lung Cell Mol Phys. 2007;292(5):L1182–92.

53. Spiekerkoetter E, Tian X, Cai J, Hopper RK, Sudheendra D, Sawada H, et al. FK506 activates BMPR2, rescues endothelial dysfunction, and reverses pulmonary hypertension. J Clin Invest. 2013;123(8):3600–13.

54. Star GP, Giovinazzo M, Langleben D. ALK2 and BMPR2 knockdown and endothelin-1 production by pulmonary microvascular endothelial cells. Microvasc Res. 2013;85:46–53.

55. Yang J, Li X, Al-Lamki RS, Wu C, Weiss A, Berk J, et al. Sildenafil potentiates bone morphogenetic protein signaling in pulmonary arterial smooth muscle cells and in experimental pulmonary hypertension. Arterioscler Thromb Vasc Biol. 2013;33(1):34–42.

56. Yang J, Li X, Al-Lamki RS, Southwood M, Zhao J, Lever AM, et al. Smad-dependent and smad-independent induction of id1 by prostacyclin analogues inhibits proliferation of pulmonary artery smooth muscle cells in vitro and in vivo. Circ Res. 2010;107(2):252–62.

Part III
Treatment of Pulmonary Arterial Hypertension (PAH)

Chapter 10
Prostacyclin

Satoshi Akagi

Abstract A decrease of prostacyclin plays an important role in the pathogenesis of pulmonary arterial hypertension (PAH). Prostacyclin replacement therapy using prostacyclin and prostacyclin analogues has been developed for treatment of PAH. Prostacyclin has not only potent vasodilatory effects but also antiproliferative and pro-apoptotic effects on pulmonary artery smooth muscle cells, which lead to the potential for reverse remodeling of pulmonary arteries. Prostacyclin analogues, iloprost and treprostinil, improve exercise capacity, symptoms, and hemodynamics. Prostacyclin, epoprostenol, improves exercise capacity, symptoms, and hemodynamics and is the only treatment shown to reduce long-term mortality in patients with idiopathic PAH. Furthermore, high-dose intravenous epoprostenol therapy has a potential for remarkable improvement of hemodynamics and exercise capacity. Intravenous delivery of epoprostenol requires a central catheter, which sometimes causes catheter-related troubles. Catheter-related infection is the most serious complication and causes aggravation of PAH. Use of a closed-hub system could prevent bacterial invasion from the catheter hub in patients treated with intravenous epoprostenol. Prostacyclin is a key factor in pathogenesis and treatment of PAH.

Keywords Prostacyclin • Antiproliferative effect • Pro-apoptotic effect • Reverse remodeling • Catheter-related infection

10.1 Properties of Prostacyclin

In 1935, Ulf Svante von Euler discovered and isolated a new chemical from the prostate glands of a sheep and a human that contracted smooth muscles of various organs. He named the material "prostaglandin." In 1960–1970, Sune Bergstrom, Bengt Samuelsson, and John Vane discovered various prostaglandins and their

S. Akagi (✉)
Department of Cardiovascular Medicine, Okayama University Graduate School of Medicine, Dentistry and Pharmaceutical Sciences, Okayama University,
2-5-1 shikata-cho Kitaku, Okayama 700-8558, Japan
e-mail: akagi-s@cc.okayama-u.ac.jp

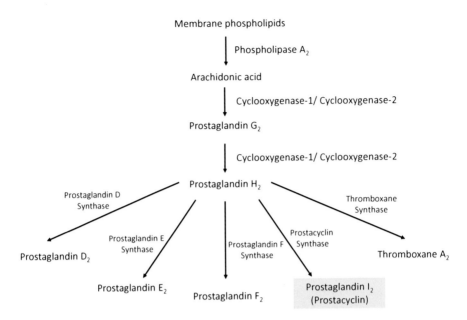

Fig. 10.1 Arachidonic acid cascade

cascades and determined their chemical structures [1–4]. They were awarded the Nobel Prize in Physiology or Medicine in 1982 after isolating and elucidating the chemical structures of prostaglandins.

Prostacyclin is formed by cyclooxygenase from arachidonic acid (Fig. 10.1). Arachidonic acid is released from membrane phospholipids by phospholipase A_2. Cyclooxygenase (COX-1 or COX-2) converts arachidonic acid to prostaglandin H_2. Prostaglandin H_2 is isomerized to either prostacyclin by prostaglandin I synthase or to thromboxane A_2 by thromboxane A synthase. Prostacyclin released from endothelial cells acts on a specific cell-surface receptor (IP receptor) on vascular smooth muscle cells and platelets. Prostacyclin has properties of vasodilatation and platelet aggregation. The binding of prostacyclin to IP receptors on vascular smooth muscle cells triggers the activation of adenylate cyclase and increases intracellular cyclic AMP, which induces vasodilatation.

10.2 Deficiency of Prostacyclin in Pulmonary Arterial Hypertension

An imbalance between the release of prostacyclin and that of thromboxane A_2 is found in pulmonary arterial hypertension (PAH) since prostacyclin I synthase is downregulated [5]. Increase of thromboxane A_2 and decrease of prostacyclin lead to excess vasoconstriction, which elevates pulmonary artery pressure. Thus, prostacyclin replacement therapy using prostacyclin and prostacyclin analogues has been developed for treatment of PAH. Prostacyclin and its analogues act on pulmonary artery smooth muscle cells (PASMCs) and induce pulmonary artery vasodilatation.

10.3 Characteristics of Prostacyclin Analogues and Prostacyclin

10.3.1 Prostacyclin Analogues

Iloprost, treprostinil, and beraprost are prostacyclin analogues used for treatment of PAH. These prostacyclin analogues are chemically stable in solution, and their plasma half-lives are longer than that of prostacyclin: ~30 min for iloprost and beraprost and <4.5 h for treprostinil. Iloprost is provided by inhalation. Treprostinil is provided by continuous subcutaneous infusion or intravenous infusion. A micro-infusion pump and a small subcutaneous catheter are used for subcutaneous administration of treprostinil. Treprostinil is stable at room temperature for only 48 h. Patients prepare and change medications once every 2 days. Beraprost is provided as an oral preparation.

10.3.2 Prostacyclin

Epoprostenol, like endogenous prostacyclin, is available for treatment of PAH. It is a chemically unstable compound and its plasma half-life is about 6 min. After mixing epoprostenol with a solvent, the compound is degraded spontaneously. Epoprostenol is stable at room temperature for only 8 h or at cooling for 24 h. Recently, a thermostable formulation of epoprostenol that does not require cooling packs has been approved in many countries. Epoprostenol is continuously delivered intravenously via a central venous catheter with an infusion pump. Patients are daily required to prepare and to change medications.

10.4 Additional Effects of Prostacyclin Analogues and Prostacyclin

10.4.1 Antiproliferative Effects on PASMCs

Platelet-derived growth factor stimulation caused excess proliferation of PASMCs obtained from patients with PAH [6–8]. Iloprost and treprostinil inhibited the proliferation of PASMCs [9, 10]. The antiproliferative effects of prostacyclin analogues are preserved despite IP receptor downregulation. Peroxisome proliferator-activated receptor γ may be related to the inhibition of PASMC proliferation in patients with PAH. Thus, these prostacyclin analogues have antiproliferative effects on PASMCs.

10.4.2   Pro-apoptotic Effect on PASMCs

Gene microarray studies showed that lungs from patients with PAH had a decreased pro-apoptotic/antiapoptotic gene expression ratio [11]. Bone morphogenetic protein (BMP)-2 and BMP-7 increased apoptosis of normal PASMCs. However, apoptosis induced by BMP-2 or BMP-7 was inhibited in PAH-PASMCs [12]. These results indicated that PAH-PASMCs have a property of resistance to apoptosis. Basic research revealed that epoprostenol induced apoptosis via a Fas ligand, an apoptosis-inducing member of the TNF cytokine family, in PAH-PASMCs (Fig. 10.2) [13, 14]. Thus, epoprostenol has a potential effect to induce apoptosis of PAH-PASMCs.

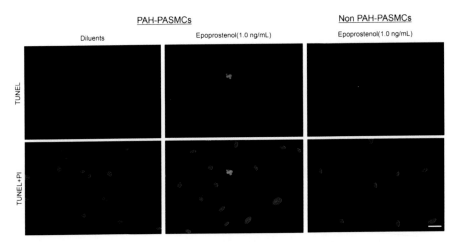

Fig. 10.2   Representative images reflecting findings of induction of apoptosis. For PAH experiments, pulmonary artery samples were obtained from patients with idiopathic PAH at lung transplantation. For non-PAH experiments, non-PAH-PASMCs were obtained from patients with lung cancer at lung lobectomy. Epoprostenol or its diluents using the flow circuit for 24 h were administered in PAH-PASMCs and non-PAH-PASMCs. A TUNEL assay was performed using an ApopTag Fluorescein In Situ Apoptosis Detection Kit (Chemicon International Inc.) to assess apoptosis of PASMCs. Nuclear morphology was examined by labeling with prodium iodium (*PI*). *Green* is TUNEL positive. *Red* is PI. PAH-PASMCs treated with epoprostenol at a high concentration showed TUNEL-positive nuclei. TUNEL-positive nuclei were not observed in PAH-PASMCs treated with only diluents and non-PAH-PASMCs treated with epoprostenol. Bar=20 μm

10.4.3   Reverse Remodeling Effects on Pulmonary Arteries

Prostacyclin analogues and prostacyclin have antiproliferative and pro-apoptotic effects on PASMCs. These effects have a potential for causing reverse remodeling of pulmonary arteries. Recently, pathological features of PAH patients treated with currently available medications have been reported [15]. No significant difference was found in medial thickness between patients with IPAH and controls. It has been reported that less medial hypertrophy was observed in a patient whose hemodynamics improved after receiving high-dose epoprostenol therapy [16]. Thus, high-dose epoprostenol has a potential effect to reverse pulmonary arteries remodeling.

10.5   Prostacyclin Therapy for Patients with PAH

The table shows a summary of results of treatment with prostacyclin analogues and prostacyclin in clinical trials (Table 10.1).

10.5.1   Iloprost

The effects of inhaled iloprost in patients with PAH were evaluated in a randomized control study [17]. The patients received daily repetitive iloprost inhalation (6–9 times, 2.5–5 µg/inhalation, median dose of 30 µg daily). Inhaled iloprost improved exercise capacity, symptoms, and hemodynamics. The addition of inhaled iloprost for patients who had already been treated with bosentan was also evaluated [18, 19]. One study showed an increase in exercise capacity and good tolerance with the addition of inhaled iloprost compared with a placebo, but the other study showed no improvement of exercise capacity. On the basis of these results, inhaled iloprost is recommended for PAH patients by the World Health Organization functional class (WHO-FC) III (class I, evidence level B) [20].

The inhalation technique allows for more intrapulmonary selectivity. Iloprost is thought to be deposited on terminal bronchioles and then penetrates the airway and directly diffuses into the walls of small pulmonary arteries [21]. Although all prostacyclin analogues induce systemic vasodilatation along with pulmonary vasodilatation, which causes headache, flashing, and hypotension, inhaled iloprost is thought to directly act on pulmonary arteries and thus to have less systemic side effects. Furthermore, the dose for significant effects is much smaller with inhalation than with oral, subcutaneous or intravenous administration. However, iloprost has to be inhaled 6–9 times per day to achieve good clinical effects, and inhalation is thus a burden for patients.

Table 10.1 Summary of clinical trials with pulmonary arterial hypertension with regard to prostacyclin and prostacyclin analogues

Drug	Administration	Dose	Study design	Disease	Patient no.	Background therapy	Duration	WHO-FC	Primary outcome	PAP change (mmHg)	Ref
Iloprost	Inha	30 µg/day	DB.RCT	IPAH.SS	203	–	3 months	III or IV	6MWD, improve	−4.6	[17]
		27 µg/day	DB.RCT	IPAH.APAH	67	bosentan	3 months	III or IV	6MWD, improve	−6.0	[18]
		30 µg/day	OL.RCT	IPAH	40	bosentan	3 months	III	6MWD, not improve	–	[19]
Treprostinil	s.c.	9.3 ng/kg/min	DB.RCT	IPAH.APAH	470	–	3 months	II–IV	6MWD, improve	−2.3	[22]
	i.v.	41 ng/kg/min	OL	IPAH.APAH	16	–	3 months	III or IV	6MWD, improve	−4.2	[23]
Beraprost	oral	80 µg/day	DB.RCT	IPAH.APAH	130	–	3 months	II or III	6MWD, improve	−1.0	[25]
		120 µg/day	DB.RCT	IPAH.APAH	116	–	12 months	II or III	6MWD, not improve	+1.0	[26]
		120–360 µg/day	OL	IPAH.APAH	46	–	3 months	I–III	6MWD, improve	−2.8	[27]

Epoprostenol	i.v.	7.9 ng/kg/min	OL.RCT	IPAH	24	–	8 weeks	II–IV	PVR, improve	–9.3	[28]
		9.2 ng/kg/min	OL.RCT	IPAH	81	–	3 months	III or IV	6MWD, improve	–2.4	[29]
		11.2 ng/kg/min	OL.RCT	APAH	111	–	3 months	II–IV	6MWD, improve	–5.0	[30]
		14 ng/kg/min	Obser	IPAH	178	–	26 months	III or IV	Survival, improve	–8.0	[31]
		21–57 ng/kg/min	Obser	IPAH	162	–	36 months	III or IV	Survival, improve	–8.0	[32]
		40 ng/kg/min	Obser	IPAH	27	–	16 months	III or IV	PVR, improve	–15	[34]
		107 ng/kg/min	Obser	IPAH	16	–	45 months	III or IV	PAP, improve	–19	[35]

Inha inhalation, *s.c.* subcutaneous, *i.v.* intravenous, *DB* double blind, *OL* open label, *RCT* randomized control trial, *obser* observational study, *IPAH* idiopathic pulmonary arterial hypertension, *APAH* associated pulmonary arterial hypertension, *WHO-FC* World Health Organization functional class, *6MWD* 6-min-walk distance, *PVR* pulmonary vascular resistance, *PAP* pulmonary artery pressure

10.5.2   Treprostinil

The effect of subcutaneously administered treprostinil for patients with PAH was evaluated in a randomized control study [22]. Subcutaneous treprostinil (mean dose: 9.3 ng/kg/min) improved exercise capacity, symptoms, and hemodynamics. Higher doses of treprostinil (mean dose: >13.8 ng/kg/min) resulted in more significant improvement. The effects of intravenously administered treprostinil for patients with PAH were evaluated in a small, open-label, uncontrolled study [23]. Intravenous treprostinil improved exercise capacity and symptoms in patients with PAH. On the basis of these results, subcutaneous treprostinil is recommended for PAH patients by WHO-FC III (class I, evidence level B), and intravenous treprostinil is recommended for PAH patients by WHO-FC III (class IIa, evidence level C) [20].

Treatment with treprostinil is initiated at a dose of 1–2 ng/kg/min, and the dose is increased gradually to the maximal tolerated dose based on clinical symptoms and side effects in each case. The optimal dose range is thought to be between 20 and 80 ng/kg/min. The dose of intravenous treprostinil is two to three times higher than the dose of intravenous epoprostenol [24].

The use of a permanent central venous catheter can be avoided with subcutaneous treprostinil therapy. However, infusion site pain is a common adverse side effect that leads to discontinuation of subcutaneous treprostinil therapy. The pain does not appear to be dose related. Less change of the infusion needle might improve infusion site pain. Thrombocytopenia is rare in patients treated with treprostinil unlike in patients treated with epoprostenol.

10.5.3   Beraprost

The effects of beraprost for patients with PAH were evaluated in two randomized control studies [25, 26]. Oral beraprost improved exercise capacity in the short term but did not improve hemodynamics and long-term survival. Long-acting beraprost is available in Japan. Treatment with long-acting beraprost improved exercise capacity and hemodynamics in the short term [27]. On the basis of these results, beraprost is not recommended for PAH patients (class IIb, evidence level C) [20].

10.5.4   Epoprostenol

The efficacy of continuous intravenous administration of epoprostenol was examined in three randomized control studies for PAH patients with WHO-FC III and IV [28–30]. Epoprostenol improved symptoms, exercise capacity, and hemodynamics. Furthermore, intravenous epoprostenol is the only treatment shown to reduce long-term mortality in patients with idiopathic PAH [31–34]. On the basis of these results, intravenous epoprostenol is recommended for PAH patients with WHO-FC III and IV (class I, evidence level A) [20].

Treatment with epoprostenol is initiated at a dose of 1–2 ng/kg/min. The dose of epoprostenol is increased by 1–2 ng/kg/min daily, weekly or monthly, to the maximal tolerated dose based on clinical symptoms and side effects in each case. The appropriate dose range is thought to be 25–40 ng/kg/min based on the results of previous studies [31, 32]. Although the efficacy of treatment with epoprostenol at doses greater than 40 ng/kg/min is not known, the efficacy of high-dose epoprostenol has been reported in patients with idiopathic PAH [35]. The hemodynamics and exercise capacity of 14 idiopathic PAH patients treated with epoprostenol at doses greater than 40 ng/kg/min (mean dose: 107±40 ng/kg/min) were analyzed. Significant decreases from baseline values were seen in mean pulmonary artery pressure (from 66±16 to 47±12 mmHg, P<0.001) and pulmonary vascular resistance (from 21.6±8.3 to 6.9±2.9 Wood units, P<0.001). Compared with the baseline state, high-dose epoprostenol therapy reduced mean pulmonary artery pressure by 30 % and pulmonary vascular resistance by 68 %. BNP and 6-min-walk distances were significantly improved. High-dose epoprostenol therapy has a potential for remarkable improvements in hemodynamics and exercise capacity.

Intravenous epoprostenol therapy has several side effects. Epoprostenol has a potent vasodilatory effect on not only pulmonary arteries but also systemic arteries. The most frequent adverse events caused by systemic vasodilatation are headache, flushing, and jaw pain. Elevation of cyclic AMP caused by epoprostenol leads to the secretion of chloride ions and water in the gastrointestinal tract, which causes diarrhea. Thrombocytopenia develops in some PAH patients treated with epoprostenol [36]. There was a negative correlation between the dose of epoprostenol and platelet count. The platelet count increased in PAH patients who transitioned from epoprostenol to treprostinil [37], although the reason remains unknown. Abnormal thyroid function was found in some PAH patients treated with epoprostenol, though the relation to epoprostenol is still unknown. Epoprostenol often affects the systemic vascular bed more than it does the pulmonary vascular bed. Initiation of epoprostenol therapy can cause severe systemic hypotension, which leads to hemodynamic collapse in vulnerable patients with WHO-FC IV [38]. Thus, preventing hemodynamic instability is important to initiate epoprostenol therapy. Temporary use of catecholamine is safe for hemodynamic support at the initiation of epoprostenol therapy and does not affect short-term or long-term mortality in patients with PAH [39].

Intravenous epoprostenol has several complications related to the central catheter such as catheter-related infection, thrombosis, and temporary interruption of infusion due to malfunction of the pump. Catheter-related infection is the most important and serious complication. Catheter infection rate was reported to be 0.26 per 1000 catheter days in PAH patients treated with epoprostenol [40]. Catheter-related infections were categorized according to infection routes into catheter-related bloodstream infection (CRSBI) and tunnel infection. CRBSI could be caused by bacterial invasion through the catheter connection. Tunnel infection could be caused by direct bacterial invasion through the catheter insertion site. Since the catheter hub was the most important source of CRBSI, use of a closed-hub system could prevent bacterial invasion from the catheter hub. Actually, the incidence of CRBSI significantly decreased with the use of a closed-hub system in PAH patients treated with intravenous epoprostenol [41].

10.6   Perspective on Prostacyclin Therapy

Inhaled iloprost, subcutaneous treprostinil, and intravenous epoprostenol are beneficial treatment of PAH. Recently, the efficacy and safety of selexipag, an orally available, selective prostacyclin receptor agonist, has been examined in patients with PAH. We would be able to use the various therapeutic options of prostacyclin in the near future.

References

1. Moncada S, Gryglewski R, Bunting S, Vane JR. An enzyme isolated from arteries transforms prostaglandin endoperoxides to an unstable substance that inhibits platelet aggregation. Nature. 1976;263(5579):663–5.
2. Bunting S, Gryglewski R, Moncada S, Vane JR. Arterial walls generate from prostaglandin endoperoxides a substance (prostaglandin X) which relaxes strips of mesenteric and coeliac arteries and inhibits platelet aggregation. Prostaglandins. 1976;12(6):897–913.
3. Gryglewski RJ, Bunting S, Moncada S, Flower RJ, Vane JR. Arterial walls are protected against deposition of platelet thrombi by a substance (prostaglandin X) which they make from prostaglandin endoperoxides. Prostaglandins. 1976;12(5):685–713.
4. Moncada S, Gryglewski RJ, Bunting S, Vane JR. A lipid peroxide inhibits the enzyme in blood vessel microsomes that generates from prostaglandin endoperoxides the substance (prostaglandin X) which prevents platelet aggregation. Prostaglandins. 1976;12(5):715–37.
5. Tuder RM, Cool CD, Geraci MW, Wang J, Abman SH, Wright L, et al. Prostacyclin synthase expression is decreased in lungs from patients with severe pulmonary hypertension. Am J Respir Crit Care Med. 1999;159(6):1925–32.
6. Nakamura K, Akagi S, Ogawa A, Kusano KF, Matsubara H, Miura D, et al. Pro-apoptotic effects of imatinib on PDGF-stimulated pulmonary artery smooth muscle cells from patients with idiopathic pulmonary arterial hypertension. Int J Cardiol. 2012;159(2):100–6.
7. Fujio H, Nakamura K, Matsubara H, Kusano KF, Miyaji K, Nagase S, et al. Carvedilol inhibits proliferation of cultured pulmonary artery smooth muscle cells of patients with idiopathic pulmonary arterial hypertension. J Cardiovasc Pharmacol. 2006;47(2):250–5.
8. Ogawa A, Nakamura K, Matsubara H, Fujio H, Ikeda T, Kobayashi K, et al. Prednisolone inhibits proliferation of cultured pulmonary artery smooth muscle cells of patients with idiopathic pulmonary arterial hypertension. Circulation. 2005;112(12):1806–12.
9. Falcetti E, Hall SM, Phillips PG, Patel J, Morrell NW, Haworth SG, et al. Smooth muscle proliferation and role of the prostacyclin (IP) receptor in idiopathic pulmonary arterial hypertension. Am J Respir Crit Care Med. 2010;182(9):1161–70.
10. Clapp LH, Finney P, Turcato S, Tran S, Rubin LJ, Tinker A. Differential effects of stable prostacyclin analogs on smooth muscle proliferation and cyclic AMP generation in human pulmonary artery. Am J Respir Cell Mol Biol. 2002;26(2):194–201.

11. Geraci MW, Moore M, Gesell T, Yeager ME, Alger L, Golpon H, et al. Gene expression patterns in the lungs of patients with primary pulmonary hypertension: a gene microarray analysis. Circ Res. 2001;88(6):555–62.

12. Zhang S, Fantozzi I, Tigno DD, Yi ES, Platoshyn O, Thistlethwaite PA, et al. Bone morphogenetic proteins induce apoptosis in human pulmonary vascular smooth muscle cells. Am J Phys Lung Cell Mol Phys. 2003;285(3):L740–54.

13. Akagi S, Nakamura K, Matsubara H, Kusano KF, Kataoka N, Oto T, et al. Prostaglandin I2 induces apoptosis via upregulation of Fas ligand in pulmonary artery smooth muscle cells from patients with idiopathic pulmonary arterial hypertension. Int J Cardiol. 2013;165(3):499–505.

14. Akagi S, Nakamura K, Matsubara H, Ogawa A, Sarashina T, Ejiri K, et al. Epoprostenol therapy for pulmonary arterial hypertension. Acta Med Okayama. 2015;69(3):129–36.

15. Stacher E, Graham BB, Hunt JM, Gandjeva A, Groshong SD, McLaughlin VV, et al. Modern age pathology of pulmonary arterial hypertension. Am J Respir Crit Care Med. 2012;186(3):261–72.

16. Akagi S, Nakamura K, Matsubara H, Ohta-Ogo K, Yutani C, Miyaji K, et al. Reverse remodeling of pulmonary arteries by high-dose prostaglandin I2 therapy: a case report. J Cardiol Cases. 2014;9(5):173–6.

17. Olschewski H, Simonneau G, Galie N, Higenbottam T, Naeije R, Rubin LJ, et al. Inhaled iloprost for severe pulmonary hypertension. N Engl J Med. 2002;347(5):322–9.

18. McLaughlin VV, Oudiz RJ, Frost A, Tapson VF, Murali S, Channick RN, et al. Randomized study of adding inhaled iloprost to existing bosentan in pulmonary arterial hypertension. Am J Respir Crit Care Med. 2006;174(11):1257–63.

19. Hoeper MM, Leuchte H, Halank M, Wilkens H, Meyer FJ, Seyfarth HJ, et al. Combining inhaled iloprost with bosentan in patients with idiopathic pulmonary arterial hypertension. Eur Respir J. 2006;28(4):691–4.

20. Galie N, Corris PA, Frost A, Girgis RE, Granton J, Jing ZC, et al. Updated treatment algorithm of pulmonary arterial hypertension. J Am Coll Cardiol. 2013;62(25 Suppl):D60–72.

21. Gomberg-Maitland M, Olschewski H. Prostacyclin therapies for the treatment of pulmonary arterial hypertension. Eur Respir J. 2008;31(4):891–901.

22. Simonneau G, Barst RJ, Galie N, Naeije R, Rich S, Bourge RC, et al. Continuous subcutaneous infusion of treprostinil, a prostacyclin analogue, in patients with pulmonary arterial hypertension: a double-blind, randomized, placebo-controlled trial. Am J Respir Crit Care Med. 2002;165(6):800–4.

23. Tapson VF, Gomberg-Maitland M, McLaughlin VV, Benza RL, Widlitz AC, Krichman A, et al. Safety and efficacy of IV treprostinil for pulmonary arterial hypertension: a prospective, multicenter, open-label, 12-week trial. Chest. 2006;129(3):683–8.

24. Sitbon O, Manes A, Jais X, Pallazini M, Humbert M, Presotto L, et al. Rapid switch from intravenous epoprostenol to intravenous treprostinil in patients with pulmonary arterial hypertension. J Cardiovasc Pharmacol. 2007;49(1):1–5.

25. Galie N, Humbert M, Vachiery JL, Vizza CD, Kneussl M, Manes A, et al. Effects of beraprost sodium, an oral prostacyclin analogue, in patients with pulmonary arterial hypertension: a randomized, double-blind, placebo-controlled trial. J Am Coll Cardiol. 2002;39(9):1496–502.

26. Barst RJ, McGoon M, McLaughlin V, Tapson V, Rich S, Rubin L, et al. Beraprost therapy for pulmonary arterial hypertension. J Am Coll Cardiol. 2003;41(12):2119–25.

27. Kunieda T, Nakanishi N, Matsubara H, Ohe T, Okano Y, Kondo H, et al. Effects of long-acting beraprost sodium (TRK-100STP) in Japanese patients with pulmonary arterial hypertension. Int Heart J. 2009;50(4):513–29.

28. Rubin LJ, Mendoza J, Hood M, McGoon M, Barst R, Williams WB, et al. Treatment of primary pulmonary hypertension with continuous intravenous prostacyclin (epoprostenol). Results of a randomized trial. Ann Intern Med. 1990;112(7):485–91.

29. Barst RJ, Rubin LJ, Long WA, McGoon MD, Rich S, Badesch DB, et al. A comparison of continuous intravenous epoprostenol (prostacyclin) with conventional therapy for primary pulmonary hypertension. N Engl J Med. 1996;334(5):296–301.
30. Badesch DB, Tapson VF, McGoon MD, Brundage BH, Rubin LJ, Wigley FM, et al. Continuous intravenous epoprostenol for pulmonary hypertension due to the scleroderma spectrum of disease. A randomized, controlled trial. Ann Intern Med. 2000;132(6):425–34.
31. Sitbon O, Humbert M, Nunes H, Parent F, Garcia G, Herve P, et al. Long-term intravenous epoprostenol infusion in primary pulmonary hypertension: prognostic factors and survival. J Am Coll Cardiol. 2002;40(4):780–8.
32. McLaughlin VV, Shillington A, Rich S. Survival in primary pulmonary hypertension: the impact of epoprostenol therapy. Circulation. 2002;106(12):1477–82.
33. Shapiro SM, Oudiz RJ, Cao T, Romano MA, Beckmann XJ, Georgiou D, et al. Primary pulmonary hypertension: improved long-term effects and survival with continuous intravenous epoprostenol infusion. J Am Coll Cardiol. 1997;30(2):343–9.
34. McLaughlin VV, Genthner DE, Panella MM, Rich S. Reduction in pulmonary vascular resistance with long-term epoprostenol (prostacyclin) therapy in primary pulmonary hypertension. N Engl J Med. 1998;338(5):273–7.
35. Akagi S, Nakamura K, Miyaji K, Ogawa A, Kusano KF, Ito H, et al. Marked hemodynamic improvements by high-dose epoprostenol therapy in patients with idiopathic pulmonary arterial hypertension. Circ J. 2010;74(10):2200–5.
36. Chin KM, Channick RN, de Lemos JA, Kim NH, Torres F, Rubin LJ. Hemodynamics and epoprostenol use are associated with thrombocytopenia in pulmonary arterial hypertension. Chest. 2009;135(1):130–6.
37. Gomberg-Maitland M, Tapson VF, Benza RL, McLaughlin VV, Krichman A, Widlitz AC, et al. Transition from intravenous epoprostenol to intravenous treprostinil in pulmonary hypertension. Am J Respir Crit Care Med. 2005;172(12):1586–9.
38. Davies S, McKenna F, Turney J, Wright V. Severe hypotension due to epoprostenol. Lancet. 1984;2(8416):1401–2.
39. Akagi S, Ogawa A, Miyaji K, Kusano K, Ito H, Matsubara H. Catecholamine support at the initiation of epoprostenol therapy in pulmonary arterial hypertension. Ann Am Thorac Soc. 2014;11(5):719–27.
40. Oudiz RJ, Widlitz A, Beckmann XJ, Camanga D, Alfie J, Brundage BH, et al. Micrococcus-associated central venous catheter infection in patients with pulmonary arterial hypertension. Chest. 2004;126(1):90–4.
41. Akagi S, Matsubara H, Ogawa A, Kawai Y, Hisamatsu K, Miyaji K, et al. Prevention of catheter-related infections using a closed hub system in patients with pulmonary arterial hypertension. Circ J. 2007;71(4):559–64.

Chapter 11
Targeting the NO-sGC-cGMP Pathway in Pulmonary Arterial Hypertension

Hiroshi Watanabe and Quang-Kim Tran

Abstract Pulmonary arterial hypertension (PAH) is characterized by an increase of more than 25 mmHg in pulmonary arterial blood pressure and a pulmonary capillary wedge pressure ≤ 15 mmHg. If left untreated, PAH is fatal, with only 34 % survival rate after 5 years (D'Alonzo GE, Barst RJ, Ayres SM, Bergofsky EH, Brundage BH, Detre KM, Fishman AP, Goldring RM, Groves BM, Kernis JT et al. Ann Intern Med 115, 343–9, (1991)). Pathologically, PAH is characterized by changes in the pulmonary arterial vascular wall leading to occlusion, increased pressure, right ventricular heart failure, and death. Current therapies for PAH include increasing the nitric oxide (NO)-soluble guanylate cyclase (sGC)-cyclic guanosine monophosphate (cGMP) axis, improving the prostacyclin pathway, or inhibiting the endothelin pathway. The NO-sGC-cGMP axis is a critical signaling cascade in PAH. Nitric oxide activates sGC, resulting in the synthesis of cGMP, a key mediator of pulmonary arterial vasodilatation that may also inhibit vascular smooth muscle proliferation and platelet aggregation. Dysregulation of the NO-sGC-cGMP axis results in pulmonary vascular inflammation, thrombosis, and constriction and ultimately leads to death from right heart failure. In this chapter, we will briefly discuss the role of the NO-sGC-cGMP pathway in PAH, potential and established treatment modalities to target this pathway, and their clinical applications.

Keywords Nitric oxide (NO) • Soluble guanylate cyclase (sGC) • Cyclic guanosine monophosphate (cGMP) • sGC stimulator • Phosphodiesterase Type 5 (PDE5) inhibitor

H. Watanabe (✉)
Department of Clinical Pharmacology and Therapeutics, Hamamatsu University School of Medicine, Handayama 1-20-1, Higashi-ku, Hamamatsu 431-3192, Japan
e-mail: hwat@hama-med.ac.jp

Q.-K. Tran
Department of Physiology and Pharmacology, Des Moines University College of Osteopathic Medicine, 3200 Grand Avenue, Des Moines, IA 50312, USA

© Springer Science+Business Media Singapore 2017
Y. Fukumoto (ed.), *Diagnosis and Treatment of Pulmonary Hypertension*,
DOI 10.1007/978-981-287-840-3_11

11.1 Targeting Nitric Oxide Production and Availability in PAH

Numerous studies have demonstrated decreases in NO availability in the lungs of PAH patients. NO measured directly via gas sampling or indirectly via NO products from PAH lungs is lower than in normal individuals [2]. The degree of reduction in NO production also appears to be correlated with the severity of PAH [3]. Investigations over the years have dissected various components of the NO signaling pathway in PAH. Changes in some components are clear and have been exploited therapeutically.

11.1.1 Endothelial Nitric Oxide Synthase (eNOS)

Physiologically, NO is produced in response to chemical stimuli such as bradykinin, acetylcholine, and histamine and physical stimuli such as shear stress and mechanical stretch. The production of nitric oxide is catalyzed in the vascular endothelium by eNOS. Endothelial NOS exists as a dimer, in which each monomer contains two domains that function as a reductase and an oxygenase. The C-terminal reductase domain of one monomer binds nicotinamide adenine dinucleotide phosphate (NADPH), flavin mononucleotide (FMN), and flavin adenine dinucleotide (FAD) and is connected to the N-terminal oxygenase domain of the other monomer. The oxygenase domain contains a heme group and binds tetrahydrobiopterin, oxygen, and L-arginine. NOS activation is initiated by flavin-mediated electron transfer from NADPH bound on the reductase domain to the heme in the oxygenase domain [4]. This electron transfer process is controlled by Ca^{2+}/calmodulin (CaM) binding to a sequence that links the reductase to the oxygenase domain. Endothelial NOS has an absolute dependence on Ca^{2+}/CaM and binds Ca^{2+}-saturated CaM with picomolar dissociation constant [5, 6]. Regulation of Ca^{2+} and CaM signals in the endothelium therefore is important for the physiological production of NO [6–9]. In an experimental model of hypoxic pulmonary hypertension, the acute decrease in eNOS activity was suggested to be due to abnormality in intracellular Ca^{2+} homeostasis, whereas chronic hypoxic pulmonary hypertension was due more to reduction in other cofactors for eNOS [10]. Additionally, eNOS contains multiple phosphorylation sites, whose individual or combined phosphorylation contributes significantly to the function of the enzyme [11–15]. Activation of eNOS also depends on the availability of other cofactors and substrates such as tetrahydrobiopterin and zinc [16].

11.1.2 Alterations in eNOS Expression in PAH

In 1995, Giad and Saleh reported that eNOS expression is substantially reduced in patients with primary pulmonary hypertension [17]. The reduction in eNOS expression level was linearly correlated with the development of plexiform lesions in patients with the clinical diagnosis of primary pulmonary hypertension. The reduction in eNOS expression in this group of patients was more pronounced in small pulmonary arteries compared to medium or large pulmonary arteries. These findings were corroborated by studies showing that targeted disruption of eNOS gene in the pulmonary vasculature led to pulmonary vasoconstriction and hypertension [18]. Consistently, cell-based transferring eNOS gene to the pulmonary vasculature in experimentally induced pulmonary hypertension reduced right ventricular pressure [19]. Most recently, the eNOS gene-enhanced progenitor cell therapy for pulmonary arterial hypertension – the PHACeT trial – was carried out as a phase 1 trial testing the tolerability of culture-derived endothelial progenitor cells transfected with eNOS in seven PAH patients unresponsive to PAH-specific therapies [20]. Only transient hemodynamic improvements were observed, but there were significant improvements in the 6-min walk distance at 1, 3, and 6 months of therapy.

11.1.3   Alterations in eNOS Regulatory Inputs

Overall, studies of eNOS in PAH have been focusing on examination of changes in eNOS expression; whether changes in other regulatory inputs of eNOS activity play a role in PAH is currently not known. Regardless of eNOS expression, these regulatory inputs are essential in controlling NO production and availability. For example, interaction with Ca^{2+}-saturated CaM is a prerequisite for eNOS activity. CaM binding per se is dependent on phosphorylation status of a number of residues, including Thr-495 [15], Ser-615 [12], Ser1177, and a combination thereof [13]. Phosphorylation at Thr495 substantially reduced eNOS-CaM interaction, while combined phosphorylation at Ser615 and 1177 increases the Ca^{2+} sensitivity for eNOS interaction with CaM, eNOS activation, and NO production [13]. Hypoxia has been shown to substantially decrease store-operated Ca^{2+} entry, eNOS phosphorylation at Ser1177, and interaction between the synthase and its other regulatory proteins [21]. These are essential factors controlling eNOS functions and affect NO production independently of eNOS expression levels. In line with this finding, statin treatment protects eNOS activity in hypoxia-induced pulmonary hypertension by increasing eNOS phosphorylation at Ser1177, promoting eNOS dissociation from inhibitory protein such as caveolin-1 and Hsp90 [22].

11.1.4   Arginase

In addition to eNOS expression and regulation, endothelial NO production depends on the amount of L-arginine, which is converted by arginase in the urea cycle to ornithine [23]. It was intuitive that increased arginase expression and activity might play a role in the reduction in NO availability seen in PAH patients. Xu et al. observed that eNOS expression was not reduced in PAH patients, but serum arginase activity was doubled. This increase was linearly correlated with the increases in right ventricular pressure [24]. It was also shown that pulmonary vascular smooth muscle cell proliferation is induced by hypoxia via the induction of arginase [25]. Arginase expression was also increased in experimental pulmonary arterial embolism [26]. Cell-based studies suggested that increasing cAMP by activating adenylyl cyclase or inhibiting phosphodiesterase 3 prevents hypoxia-induced increases in arginase mRNA and proliferation of pulmonary arterial smooth muscle cells [27]. These studies are consistent with the well-known antiproliferative role of nitric oxide. However, to date, no clinical studies have explored an approach to downregulate arginase in patients with PAH.

11.1.5   Nitric Oxide and Nitric Oxide Donors in PAH

NO is a potent vasodilator that is rapidly inactivated by binding to hemoglobin. Due to its very short half-life and selective for the pulmonary vasculature when used via inhalation, exogenous NO offers several benefits for patients with PAH. A particular advantage of inhaled NO over systemic vasodilators is that it exerts its vasodilatory effects in well-ventilated areas of the lungs, thereby distributing blood flow from less ventilated areas to better ventilated areas for ideal ventilation-perfusion matching [28]. With its potent vasodilator effect, nitric oxide has long been used for a number of respiratory diseases, including respiratory distress syndrome [29, 30], pulmonary hypertension due to heart failure [31], chronic obstructive lung diseases [32], or pulmonary arterial hypertension [33]. It is a very effective therapy for neonates born with persistent pulmonary hypertension, improving systemic oxygenation in 53 % subjects in comparison to 7 % treated with conventional method [34]. Inhaled nitric oxide also reduces the use of extracorporeal membrane oxygenation in these subjects, despite an unclear effect on mortality in critically ill infants with hypoxic respiratory failure [35]. However, a number of disadvantages limit the use of NO and nitrates in PAH. First, NO has to be delivered continuously due to its very short half-life. Second, withdrawal of inhaled NO may be associated with dangerous rebound pulmonary hypertension [36]. Additionally, the efficacy of nitrates is limited by the development of tolerance. Resistance to NO and nitrates can be developed as a result of changes in the redox state of the heme in sGC, resulting in reduced binding affinity of heme to sGC and as such eliminating the effect of NO [37].

11.2   Targeting Soluble Guanylyl Cyclase (sGC) in PAH

Soluble guanylyl cyclase functions to catalyze the conversion of GTP to cGMP. The enzyme exists as a heterodimer, consisting of a larger α-subunit and a smaller heme-binding β-subunit. In the resting state, the β-subunit contains a ferrous heme iron

(Fe^{2+}) that binds NO with picomolar affinity, which enhances sGC activity by several hundredfold [38, 39]. Other circulating peptides such as natriuretic peptide can activate particulate (pGC) guanylyl cyclase to convert GTP to cGMP. Overall, cGMP accumulation leads to vasodilatation, inhibits vascular smooth muscle proliferation and fibrosis, and exerts antithrombotic and anti-inflammatory effects. These effects are controlled by cGMP-dependent protein kinases, cGMP-dependent ion channels, and phosphodiesterases [40]. Activation of cyclic GMP-dependent protein kinase I (cGKI) decreases cytosolic Ca^{2+} concentration indirectly via activation of membrane K^+ channels leading to hyperpolarization of vascular smooth muscle cell membrane. Additionally, cGKI phosphorylates vasodilator-stimulated phosphoprotein (VASP), an actin-binding protein whose phosphorylation status is related to the proliferation of vascular smooth muscle cells [41]. These effects lead to relaxation of smooth muscle cells. Increases in sGC expression level have been described in hypoxia-induced PAH models as well as in patients with PAH [42, 43]; however, sGC oxidation and the related loss of sGC's heme group have also been reported [44]. Oxidation of the heme iron to the ferric state (Fe^{3+}) dramatically reduces the affinity of sGC for NO [45]. Given the limitations of NO and NO donors, direct stimulators or activators of sGC have been developed. Stimulators of sGC act by directly stimulating sGC and increasing the NO sensitivity of ferrous-iron heme sGC, thereby motivating sGC activity in the presence of low NO availability. Activators of sGC, on the contrary, substitute for the heme-NO complex and activate oxidized (ferric-iron heme) or heme-free sGC independently of NO [46–49]. Only sGC stimulators are now approved for PAH; sGC activators are currently still being tested.

11.2.1   Stimulation of sGC with Riociguat

Riociguat is the first approved medication from the novel class of sGC stimulators and the only agent approved for treating both chronic thromboembolic hypertension (CTEPH) and PAH. Riociguat is able to restore the homeostatic effects of NO that are diminished as a result of phenotypic alterations associated with PAH. In a 12-week randomized, double-blind, placebo-controlled trial in 443 patients, riociguat brought significant improvements in pulmonary vascular resistance ($P<0.001$), NT-proBNP levels ($P<0.001$), WHO functional class ($P=0.003$), time to clinical worsening ($P=0.005$), and Borg dyspnea score ($P=0.002$) [50]. The symptomatic benefit appeared to be similar in patients who continued to take the endothelin receptor inhibitors or prostanoids and in those who were not taking a vasodilator other than riociguat. In a 16-week, double-blind trial in 261 patients with chronic thromboembolic pulmonary hypertension in whom surgery was not feasible or had failed, riociguat was more effective than placebo on symptoms; there was improvement in functional class in, respectively, 33 % and 15 % of patients [51]. Improvements in 6-min walk distance (6MWD) in patients with PAH during the phase 3 PATENT-1 trial were comparable to other oral agents approved for the treatment of PAH. Improvements in 6MWD in patients with CTEPH during the phase 3 CHEST-1 trial were greater than those previously observed with other oral PAH-directed therapies [50, 51]. Hypotension is the dose-limiting adverse effect of riociguat, and dose titration needs to be performed to avoid substantial decreases in blood pressure.

11.3 Targeting Phosphodiesterase Type 5 (PDE5) in PAH

11.3.1 Increasing cGMP

Cyclic GMP signaling is terminated by cGMP-hydrolyzing phosphodiesterase enzymes. PDE5 has the effect of inactivating cGMP by catabolizing it to 5'GMP. In PAH, the expression and the activity of PDE5 are enhanced in smooth muscle cells and the right ventricular myocardium [52–54]. Reduced NO bioavailability and the enhancement of PDE5 activity both lead to lower cGMP concentration and result in vasoconstriction and smooth muscle cell proliferation and promote the resistance against apoptosis (Fig. 11.1). The PDE5A subtype selectively hydrolyzes cGMP. Sildenafil and tadalafil, inhibitors of PDE5A, block the breakdown of cGMP, increase cGMP concentration, relax smooth muscle cells, and finally cause vasorelaxation. In addition, PDE5 inhibitors possess antiproliferative and proapoptotic effects and are expected to reverse the remodeling process taking place in pulmonary arteries in PAH [55]. PDE5 is mainly distributed in smooth muscles of the corpus cavernosum in penile tissue and the lung blood vessels. Although PDE5 expression in isolated myocytes has been reported, PDE5 activity is rather low

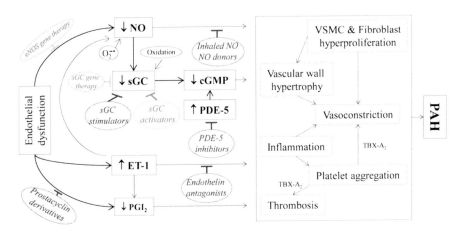

Fig. 11.1 Pathophysiology and therapy of PAH. *Red* approved drug classes, *green* contemplated therapies, therapies being tested. *PAH* pulmonary arterial hypertension, *NO* nitric oxide, *sGC* soluble guanylyl cyclase, *cGMP* cyclic guanylyl monophosphate, *PDE5* phosphodiesterase type 5, *ET-1* endothelin-1, *PGI2* prostacyclin, *TBX-A2* thromboxane A2 (Modified from [58])

compared to that in lung tissue [56]. The main sites of action of PDE5 inhibitors are thus limited in these organs, and the selectivity of these agents for lung tissue is maintained, even when given by systemic oral administration.

11.3.2 Ameliorating Ventricular Function

PDE5 inhibition exerts little influence on baseline cardiac function [57]. However, increased cGMP by PDE5 inhibitors or sGC stimulators could inhibit the PDE3 subtype, which in turn leads to increased levels of cAMP, resulting in a positive inotropic effect [58]. Furthermore, PKG activation following the rise of cGMP by PDE5 inhibition causes opening of the mitochondrial K_{ATP} channels in cardiac cells [59, 60]. Because the regulation of mitochondrial volume and electron transport are the preeminent mechanisms in maintaining mitochondrial function in the intact myocardium, opening of the mitochondrial K_{ATP} channels could bring cardioprotective effects [61, 62]. A direct effect on cardiac cells by PDE5 inhibitors has been suggested in patients with diabetic dilated cardiomyopathy after a 3-month administration of sildenafil (100 mg/day) along with the improvement of myocardial morphology and function, reduction of circulating MCP-1, and reduction of TGF-β [63]. Additionally, cGMP-PKG is involved in the regulation of titin, which influences the myocardial cell flexibility and passive rigidity [64]. In vitro studies suggest that phosphorylation of titin reduces myocyte/myofiber stiffness. Thus, titin can be phosphorylated by cGMP-activated protein kinase (PKG). Intracellular cGMP production is stimulated by B-type natriuretic peptide (BNP) and degraded by PDE5A. In animal studies, acute cGMP-enhancing treatment with sildenafil and BNP improves LV diastolic distensibility in vivo, in part, by phosphorylating titin [65].

11.3.3 Sildenafil

Sildenafil is selective and potent inhibitor of cGMP PDE5. Inhibition of PDE5 increases the cellular levels of cGMP by blocking its degradation to 5'GMP, leading to vascular smooth muscle relaxation. Sildenafil is widely used to dilate penile arteries in patients with erectile dysfunction (ED). Because PDE5 is abundant in the lung as well as penile tissues, it has been hypothesized that the drug can also be used to dilate pulmonary arteries in patients with PAH as well as the patients with ED. In animal models, sildenafil induced pulmonary vasodilation by a NO-dependent mechanism without decreasing systemic artery pressure [66, 67]. Following several case reports suggesting that oral sildenafil may be beneficial as a selective pulmonary vasodilator in patients with PAH [68, 69], SUPER, a double-blind, placebo-controlled, randomized study, demonstrated that sildenafil improved exercise capacity, WHO functional class, and hemodynamics in patients with symptomatic

PAH [70]. In the SUPER study, 278 patients with symptomatic PAH were randomly assigned to placebo or sildenafil (20, 40, or 80 mg) orally three times daily for 12 weeks. The primary end point was the change from baseline to week 12 in the distance walked in 6 min, which increased from baseline in all sildenafil groups; the mean placebo-corrected treatment effects were 45 m (+13.0 %), 46 m (+13.3 %), and 50 m (+14.7 %) for 20, 40, and 80 mg of sildenafil, respectively ($P<0.001$ for all comparisons). All sildenafil doses reduced the mean pulmonary artery pressure ($P=0.04$, $P=0.01$, and $P<0.001$, respectively), pulmonary vascular resistance (-171 dyn·s·cm^{-5}, -192 dyn·s·cm^{-5}, -310 dyn·s·cm^{-5}, respectively), and improved the WHO functional class ($P=0.003$, $P<0.001$, and $P<0.001$, respectively). Flushing, dyspepsia, and diarrhea were observed as side effects [70]. Following the SUPER study, the long-term safety and tolerability of sildenafil treatment of PAH were assessed in SUPER-2, an open-label uncontrolled extension study that continued until the last patient completed 3 years of sildenafil treatment [71]. Patients titrated to sildenafil 80 mg tid; one dose reduction for tolerability was allowed during the titration phase. At 3 years post-SUPER-1 baseline, the majority of patients (60 %) improved or maintained their functional status, and 46 % maintained or improved 6MWD. Data from SUPER-2 also suggest that the patients assigned to sildenafil treatment in SUPER-1 had better prognosis than the placebo group. This strongly suggests that earlier treatment with sildenafil could bring better outcome in the treatment for PAH.

11.3.4 Tadalafil

Tadalafil is also a phosphodiesterase type 5 inhibitor like sildenafil, yet with more prolonged half-life. The pulmonary arterial hypertension and response to tadalafil (PHIRST) study, a 16-week, double-blind, placebo-controlled study, randomized 405 patients with PAH to placebo or tadalafil 2.5, 10, 20, or 40 mg orally once daily [72]. Tadalafil increased the distance walked in 6 min, the primary end point, in a dose-dependent manner. Overall, the mean placebo-corrected treatment effect was 33 m (95 % confidence interval, 15 to 50 m). In the bosentan-naive group, the treatment effect was 44 m (95 % confidence interval, 20 to 69 m) compared with 23 m (95 % confidence interval, -2 to 48 m) in patients on background bosentan therapy. Tadalafil 40 mg improved the time to clinical worsening ($P=0.041$), incidence of clinical worsening (68 % relative risk reduction; $P=0.038$), and health-related quality of life. Patients completing the 16-week study could enter a long-term extension study (PHIRST-2), which showed that long-term treatment with tadalafil was well tolerated in patients with pulmonary arterial hypertension. In patients receiving either T20 mg or T40 mg, the improvements in 6MWD demonstrated in the 16-week PHIRST study appeared sustained for up to 52 additional weeks of treatment in PHIRST-2 [73].

11.4   Concluding Remarks

The NO-cGMP-PKG axis is an essential axis in the pathophysiology and treatment of PAH. Multiple classes of agents are now approved for the treatment of PAH that act on one or more components of this axis (Fig. 11.1). Additionally, certain gene therapies targeting eNOS and sGC have been contemplated. A desirable pharmacological agent for PAH should have little effect on the systemic circulation, selectively decrease pulmonary vascular resistance, and increase inotropic function of the right ventricle. The phosphodiesterase type 5 inhibitors and the sGC stimulator riociguat, with careful dose titration, can satisfy these requirements.

References

1. D'Alonzo GE, Barst RJ, Ayres SM, Bergofsky EH, Brundage BH, Detre KM, Fishman AP, Goldring RM, Groves BM, Kernis JT, et al. Survival in patients with primary pulmonary hypertension. Results from a national prospective registry. Ann Intern Med. 1991;115:343–9.
2. Kaneko FT, Arroliga AC, Dweik RA, Comhair SA, Laskowski D, Oppedisano R, Thomassen MJ, Erzurum SC. Biochemical reaction products of nitric oxide as quantitative markers of primary pulmonary hypertension. Am J Respir Crit Care Med. 1998;158:917–23.
3. Archer SL, Djaballah K, Humbert M, Weir KE, Fartoukh M, Dall'ava-Santucci J, Mercier JC, Simonneau G, Dinh-Xuan AT. Nitric oxide deficiency in fenfluramine- and dexfenfluramine-induced pulmonary hypertension. Am J Respir Crit Care Med. 1998;158:1061–7.
4. Dudzinski DM, Igarashi J, Greif D, Michel T. The regulation and pharmacology of endothelial nitric oxide synthase. Annu Rev Pharmacol Toxicol. 2006;46:235–76.
5. Bredt DS, Snyder SH. Isolation of nitric oxide synthetase, a calmodulin-requiring enzyme. Proc Natl Acad Sci U S A. 1990;87:682–5.
6. Tran QK, Black DJ, Persechini A. Dominant affectors in the calmodulin network shape the time courses of target responses in the cell. Cell Calcium. 2005;37:541–53.
7. Tran QK, Watanabe H. Calcium signalling in the endothelium. Handb Exp Pharmacol, 2006;145–87.
8. Tran QK, VerMeer M, Burgard MA, Hassan AB, Giles J. Hetero-oligomeric complex between the G protein-coupled estrogen receptor 1 and the plasma membrane Ca2+−ATPase 4b. J Biol Chem. 2015;290:13293–307.
9. Tran, Q. K., Firkins, R., Giles, J., Francis, S., Matnishian, V., Tran, P., VerMeer, M., Jasurda, J., Burgard, M. A., and Gebert-Oberle, B. Estrogen enhances linkage in the vascular endothelial calmodulin network via a feedforward mechanism at the G protein-coupled estrogen receptor 1. J Biol Chem, 2016;pii: jbc.M115.697334.
10. Shaul PW, Wells LB, Horning KM. Acute and prolonged hypoxia attenuate endothelial nitric oxide production in rat pulmonary arteries by different mechanisms. J Cardiovasc Pharmacol. 1993;22:819–27.
11. Mount PF, Kemp BE, Power DA. Regulation of endothelial and myocardial NO synthesis by multi-site eNOS phosphorylation. J Mol Cell Cardiol. 2007;42:271–9.
12. Tran QK, Leonard J, Black DJ, Persechini A. Phosphorylation within an autoinhibitory domain in endothelial nitric oxide synthase reduces the Ca(2+) concentrations required for calmodulin to bind and activate the enzyme. Biochemistry. 2008;47:7557–66.
13. Tran QK, Leonard J, Black DJ, Nadeau OW, Boulatnikov IG, Persechini A. Effects of combined phosphorylation at Ser-617 and Ser-1179 in endothelial nitric-oxide synthase on

EC50(Ca2+) values for calmodulin binding and enzyme activation. J Biol Chem. 2009;284:11892–9.

14. Boo YC, Jo H. Flow-dependent regulation of endothelial nitric oxide synthase: role of protein kinases. Am J Phys Cell Physiol. 2003;285:C499–508.

15. Fleming I, Fisslthaler B, Dimmeler S, Kemp BE, Busse R. Phosphorylation of Thr(495) regulates Ca(2+)/calmodulin-dependent endothelial nitric oxide synthase activity. Circ Res. 2001;88:E68–75.

16. Forstermann U, Munzel T. Endothelial nitric oxide synthase in vascular disease: from marvel to menace. Circulation. 2006;113:1708–14.

17. Giaid A, Saleh D. Reduced expression of endothelial nitric oxide synthase in the lungs of patients with pulmonary hypertension. N Engl J Med. 1995;333:214–21.

18. Steudel W, Ichinose F, Huang PL, Hurford WE, Jones RC, Bevan JA, Fishman MC, Zapol WM. Pulmonary vasoconstriction and hypertension in mice with targeted disruption of the endothelial nitric oxide synthase (NOS 3) gene. Circ Res. 1997;81:34–41.

19. Campbell AI, Kuliszewski MA, Stewart DJ. Cell-based gene transfer to the pulmonary vasculature: Endothelial nitric oxide synthase overexpression inhibits monocrotaline-induced pulmonary hypertension. Am J Respir Cell Mol Biol. 1999;21:567–75.

20. Granton J, Langleben D, Kutryk MB, Camack N, Galipeau J, Courtman DW, Stewart DJ. Endothelial NO-synthase gene-enhanced progenitor cell therapy for pulmonary arterial hypertension: the PHACeT trial. Circ Res. 2015;117:645–54.

21. Murata T, Sato K, Hori M, Ozaki H, Karaki H. Decreased endothelial nitric-oxide synthase (eNOS) activity resulting from abnormal interaction between eNOS and its regulatory proteins in hypoxia-induced pulmonary hypertension. J Biol Chem. 2002;277:44085–92.

22. Murata T, Kinoshita K, Hori M, Kuwahara M, Tsubone H, Karaki H, Ozaki H. Statin protects endothelial nitric oxide synthase activity in hypoxia-induced pulmonary hypertension. Arterioscler Thromb Vasc Biol. 2005;25:2335–42.

23. Durante W. Role of arginase in vessel wall remodeling. Front Immunol. 2013;4:111.

24. Xu W, Kaneko FT, Zheng S, Comhair SA, Janocha AJ, Goggans T, Thunnissen FB, Farver C, Hazen SL, Jennings C, Dweik RA, Arroliga AC, Erzurum SC. Increased arginase II and decreased NO synthesis in endothelial cells of patients with pulmonary arterial hypertension. FASEB J. 2004;18:1746–8.

25. Chen B, Calvert AE, Cui H, Nelin LD. Hypoxia promotes human pulmonary artery smooth muscle cell proliferation through induction of arginase. Am J Phys Lung Cell Mol Phys. 2009;297:L1151–9.

26. Watts JA, Marchick MR, Gellar MA, Kline JA. Up-regulation of arginase II contributes to pulmonary vascular endothelial cell dysfunction during experimental pulmonary embolism. Pulm Pharmacol Ther. 2011;24:407–13.

27. Chen B, Calvert AE, Meng X, Nelin LD. Pharmacologic agents elevating cAMP prevent arginase II expression and proliferation of pulmonary artery smooth muscle cells. Am J Respir Cell Mol Biol. 2012;47:218–26.

28. Frostell C, Fratacci MD, Wain JC, Jones R, Zapol WM. Inhaled nitric oxide. A selective pulmonary vasodilator reversing hypoxic pulmonary vasoconstriction. Circulation. 1991;83:2038–47.

29. Rossaint R, Falke KJ, Lopez F, Slama K, Pison U, Zapol WM. Inhaled nitric oxide for the adult respiratory distress syndrome. N Engl J Med. 1993;328:399–405.

30. Fierobe L, Brunet F, Dhainaut JF, Monchi M, Belghith M, Mira JP, Dall'ava-Santucci J, Dinh-Xuan AT. Effect of inhaled nitric oxide on right ventricular function in adult respiratory distress syndrome. Am J Respir Crit Care Med. 1995;151:1414–9.

31. Journois D, Pouard P, Mauriat P, Malhere T, Vouhe P, Safran D. Inhaled nitric oxide as a therapy for pulmonary hypertension after operations for congenital heart defects. J Thorac Cardiovasc Surg. 1994;107:1129–35.

32. Moinard J, Manier G, Pillet O, Castaing Y. Effect of inhaled nitric oxide on hemodynamics and VA/Q inequalities in patients with chronic obstructive pulmonary disease. Am J Respir Crit Care Med. 1994;149:1482–7.

33. Williamson DJ, Hayward C, Rogers P, Wallman LL, Sturgess AD, Penny R, Macdonald PS. Acute hemodynamic responses to inhaled nitric oxide in patients with limited scleroderma and isolated pulmonary hypertension. Circulation. 1996;94:477–82.

34. Roberts Jr JD, Fineman JR, Morin 3rd FC, Shaul PW, Rimar S, Schreiber MD, Polin RA, Zwass MS, Zayek MM, Gross I, Heymann MA, Zapol WM. Inhaled nitric oxide and persistent pulmonary hypertension of the newborn. The Inhaled Nitric Oxide Study Group. N Engl J Med. 1997;336:605–10.

35. Neonatal Inhaled Nitric Oxide Study, G. Inhaled nitric oxide in full-term and nearly full-term infants with hypoxic respiratory failure. N Engl J Med. 1997;336:597–604.

36. Miller OI, Tang SF, Keech A, Celermajer DS. Rebound pulmonary hypertension on withdrawal from inhaled nitric oxide. Lancet. 1995;346:51–2.

37. Fernhoff NB, Derbyshire ER, Underbakke ES, Marletta MA. Heme-assisted S-nitrosation desensitizes ferric soluble guanylate cyclase to nitric oxide. J Biol Chem. 2012;287:43053–62.

38. Zhao Y, Brandish PE, Ballou DP, Marletta MA. A molecular basis for nitric oxide sensing by soluble guanylate cyclase. Proc Natl Acad Sci U S A. 1999;96:14753–8.

39. Stone JR, Marletta MA. Spectral and kinetic studies on the activation of soluble guanylate cyclase by nitric oxide. Biochemistry. 1996;35:1093–9.

40. Hofmann F, Feil R, Kleppisch T, Schlossmann J. Function of cGMP-dependent protein kinases as revealed by gene deletion. Physiol Rev. 2006;86:1–23.

41. Chen L, Daum G, Chitaley K, Coats SA, Bowen-Pope DF, Eigenthaler M, Thumati NR, Walter U, Clowes AW. Vasodilator-stimulated phosphoprotein regulates proliferation and growth inhibition by nitric oxide in vascular smooth muscle cells. Arterioscler Thromb Vasc Biol. 2004;24:1403–8.

42. Li D, Zhou N, Johns RA. Soluble guanylate cyclase gene expression and localization in rat lung after exposure to hypoxia. Am J Phys. 1999;277:L841–7.

43. Schermuly RT, Stasch JP, Pullamsetti SS, Middendorff R, Muller D, Schluter KD, Dingendorf A, Hackemack S, Kolosionek E, Kaulen C, Dumitrascu R, Weissmann N, Mittendorf J, Klepetko W, Seeger W, Ghofrani HA, Grimminger F. Expression and function of soluble guanylate cyclase in pulmonary arterial hypertension. Eur Respir J. 2008;32:881–91.

44. Wolin MS, Gupte SA, Mingone CJ, Neo BH, Gao Q, Ahmad M. Redox regulation of responses to hypoxia and NO-cGMP signaling in pulmonary vascular pathophysiology. Ann N Y Acad Sci. 2010;1203:126–32.

45. Hoshino, M. L., L.; Ford, P.C. (1999) Nitric oxide complexes of metalloporphyrins. An overview of some mechanistic studies. Coord Chem Rev 187, 75-102

46. Dasgupta A, Bowman L, D'Arsigny CL, Archer SL. Soluble guanylate cyclase: a new therapeutic target for pulmonary arterial hypertension and chronic thromboembolic pulmonary hypertension. Clin Pharmacol Ther. 2015;97:88–102.

47. Stasch JP, Pacher P, Evgenov OV. Soluble guanylate cyclase as an emerging therapeutic target in cardiopulmonary disease. Circulation. 2011;123:2263–73.

48. Evgenov OV, Pacher P, Schmidt PM, Hasko G, Schmidt HH, Stasch JP. NO-independent stimulators and activators of soluble guanylate cyclase: discovery and therapeutic potential. Nat Rev Drug Discov. 2006;5:755 68.

49. Stasch JP, Evgenov OV. Soluble guanylate cyclase stimulators in pulmonary hypertension. Handb Exp Pharmacol. 2013;218:279–313.

50. Ghofrani HA, Galiè N, Grimminger F, Grünig E, Humbert M, Jing ZC, Keogh AM, Langleben D, Kilama MO, Fritsch A, Neuser D, Rubin LJ; PATENT-1 Study Group. Riociguat for the treatment of pulmonary arterial hypertension. N Engl J Med, 2013, 25;369(4):330–340

51. Ghofrani HA, D'Armini AM, Grimminger F, et al. Riociguat for the treatment of chronic thromboembolic pulmonary hypertension. N Engl J Med. 2013;369(4):319–29.

52. Black SM, Sanchez LS, Mata-Greenwood E, et al. sGC and PDE5 are elevated in lambs with increased pulmonary blood flow and pulmonary hypertension. Am J Phys Lung Cell Mol Phys. 2001;281:L1051–7.

53. Murray F, MacLean MR, Pyne NJ. Increased expression of the cGMP-inhibited camp-specific (PDE3) and cGMP binding cGMP-specific (PDE5) phosphodiesterases in models of pulmonary hypertension. Br J Pharmacol. 2002;137:1187–94.

54. Nagendran J, Archer SL, Soliman D, et al. Phosphodiesterase type 5 is highly expressed in the hypertrophied human right ventricle, and acute inhibition of phosphodiesterase type 5 improves contractility. Circulation. 2007;116:238–48.

55. Wharton J, Strange JW, Møller GM, et al. Antiproliferative effects of phosphodiesterase type 5 inhibition in human pulmonary artery cells. Am J Respir Crit Care Med. 2005;172:105–13.

56. Guazzi M. Clinical use of phosphodiesterase-5 inhibitors in chronic heart failure. Circ Heart Fail. 2008;1:272–80.

57. Corbin J, Rannels S, Neal D, Chang P, Grimes K, Beasley A, Francis S. Sildenafil citrate does not affect cardiac contractility in human or dog heart. Curr Med Res Opin. 2003;19:747–52.

58. Tran QK, Watanabe H. Novel oral prostacyclin analog with thromboxane synthase inhibitory activity for management of pulmonary arterial hypertension. Circ J. 2013;77:1994–5.

59. Ockaili R, Salloum F, Hawkins J, Kukreja RC. (2002) Sildenafil (Viagra) induces powerful cardioprotective effect via opening of mitochondrial KATP channels in rabbits. *Am J Physiol Heart Circ Physiol* 283: H1263–H1269.

60. Salloum FN, Ockaili RA, Wittkamp M, Marwaka VR, Kukreja RC. Vardenafil: a novel type 5 phosphodiesterase inhibitor reduces myocardial infarct size following ischemia/reperfusion injury via opening of mitochondrial KATP channels in rabbits. J Mol Cell Cardiol. 2006;40:405–11.

61. Garlid KD, Paucek P, Yarov-Yarovoy V, et al. Cardioprotective effect of diazoxide and its interaction with mitochondrial ATP-sensitive K channels: possible mechanism of cardioprotection. Circ Res. 1997;81:1072–82.

62. Dos Santos P, Kowaltowski AJ, Laclau MN, et al. (2002) Mechanisms by which opening the mitochondrial ATP-sensitive K channel protects the ischemic heart. A*m J Physiol Heart Circ Physiol* 283:H284–H295.

63. Giannetta E, Isidori AM, Galea N, Carbone I, Mandosi E, Vizza CD, Naro F, Morano S, Fedele F, Lenzi A. Chronic Inhibition of cGMP phosphodiesterase 5A improves diabetic cardiomyopathy: a randomized, controlled clinical trial using magnetic resonance imaging with myocardial tagging. Circulation. 2012;125(19):2323–33.

64. Krüger M, Kötter S, Grützner A, Lang P, Andresen C, Redfield MM, Butt E, dos Remedios CG, Linke WA. Protein kinase G modulates human myocardial passive stiffness by phosphorylation of the titin springs. Circ Res. 2009;104(1):87–94.

65. Bishu K, Hamdani N, Mohammed SF, Kruger M, Ohtani T, Ogut O, Brozovich FV, Burnett Jr JC, Linke WA, Redfield MM. Sildenafil and B-type natriuretic peptide acutely phosphorylate titin and improve diastolic distensibility in vivo. Circulation. 2011;124(25):2882–91.

66. Weimann J, Ullrich R, Hromi J, Fujino Y, Clark MW, Bloch KD, Zapol WM. Sildenafil is a pulmonary vasodilator in awake lambs with acute pulmonary hypertension. Anesthesiology. 2000;92(6):1702–12.

67. Ichinose F, Erana-Garcia J, Hromi J, Raveh Y, Jones R, Krim L, MW C, JD W, KD B, WM Z. Nebulized sildenafil is a selective pulmonary vasodilator in lambs with acute pulmonary hypertension. Crit Care Med. 2001;29(5):1000–5.

68. Prasad S, Wilkinson J, Gatzoulis MA. Sildenafil in primary pulmonary hypertension. N Engl J Med. 2000;343(18):1342.

69. Watanabe H, Ohashi K, Takeuchi K, Yamashita K, Yokoyama T, Tran QK, Satoh H, Terada H, Ohashi H, Hayashi H. Sildenafil for primary and secondary pulmonary hypertension. Clin Pharmacol Ther. 2002;71(5):398–402.

70. Galiè N, Ghofrani HA, Torbicki A, Barst RJ, Rubin LJ, Badesch D, Fleming T, Parpia T, Burgess G, Branzi A, Grimminger F, Kurzyna M, Simonneau G, Sildenafil Use in Pulmonary

Arterial Hypertension (SUPER) Study Group. Sildenafil citrate therapy for pulmonary arterial hypertension. N Engl J Med. 2005;353(20):2148–57.

71. Rubin LJ, Badesch DB, Fleming TR, Galiè N, Simonneau G, Ghofrani HA, Oakes M, Layton G, Serdarevic-Pehar M, McLaughlin VV, Barst RJ, SUPER-2 Study Group. Long-term treatment with sildenafil citrate in pulmonary arterial hypertension: the SUPER-2 study. Chest. 2011;140(5):1274–83.

72. Galiè N, Brundage BH, Ghofrani HA, Oudiz RJ, Simonneau G, Safdar Z, Shapiro S, White RJ, Chan M, Beardsworth A, Frumkin L, Barst RJ; Pulmonary Arterial Hypertension and Response to Tadalafil (PHIRST) Study Group. Tadalafil therapy for pulmonary arterial hypertension. Circulation. 2009, 119(22):2894-2903.

73. Oudiz RJ, Brundage BH, Galiè N, Ghofrani HA, Simonneau G, Botros FT, Chan M, Beardsworth A, Barst RJ, PHIRST Study Group. Tadalafil for the treatment of pulmonary arterial hypertension: a double-blind 52-week uncontrolled extension study. J Am Coll Cardiol. 2012;60(8):768–74.

Chapter 12
Endothelin Receptor Antagonist

Noriaki Emoto

Abstract Endothelin (ET)-1, a peptide mainly produced by vascular endothelial cells, has potent and long-lasting vasoconstrictive effect. In addition, ET-1 has been shown to induce a variety of biological effects including cell proliferation, inflammation, and fibrosis. Thus, ET-1 has attracted considerable attention as a potential therapeutic target for cardiovascular diseases and has shown the greatest clinical potential in the treatment of pulmonary arterial hypertension (PAH). In recent years, ET receptor antagonists (ERAs) have become a well-established class of therapeutic agents with obvious effects in the management of PAH. This chapter outlines the current knowledge and understanding of the physiological and pathogenic roles of the ET system as well as the clinical pharmacology of the ERAs used in the treatment of PAH.

Keywords Endothelin • Endothelin receptor antagonist • Bosentan • Ambrisentan • Macitentan

12.1 Endothelin (ET) System

Endothelin (ET)-1, a 21-amino acid peptide with two disulfide bonds, was identified in the supernatant of cultured porcine aortic endothelial cells as a potent vasoconstrictive agent [1]. Shortly after the discovery of ET-1, two structurally related isopeptides, named ET-2 and ET-3, were isolated [2]. ET-1 is the predominant

N. Emoto (✉)
Clinical Pharmacy, Kobe Pharmaceutical University,
4-19-1 Motoyama-kitamachi, Higashinada-ku, Kobe, Hyogo 658-8558, Japan

Division of Cardiovascular Medicine, Kobe University Graduate School of Medicine,
7-5-1 Kusunoki, Chuo-ku, Kobe, Hyogo 650-0017, Japan
e-mail: emoto@kobepharma-u.ac.jp; emoto@med.kobe-u.ac.jp

© Springer Science+Business Media Singapore 2017
Y. Fukumoto (ed.), *Diagnosis and Treatment of Pulmonary Hypertension*,
DOI 10.1007/978-981-287-840-3_12

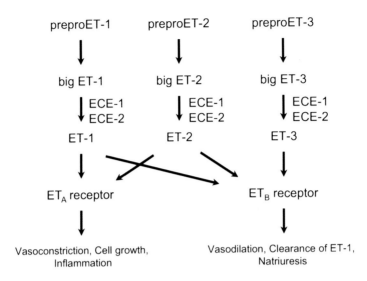

Fig. 12.1 Components of the endothelin pathway. The endothelins (ETs) are a family of 21-residue peptides consisting of three structurally related isoforms, namely, ET-1, ET-2, and ET-3. The corresponding preproendothelins are processed by furin-like enzymes into biologically inactive intermediates called big ETs. ET-converting enzymes, ECE-1 and ECE-2, proteolytically activate big ETs via cleavage at the common Trp21 residue. ETs act on two types of G protein-coupled receptors, ET_A and ET_B receptors, to mediate a variety of biological actions

isopeptide mainly involved in regulating the cardiovascular system, and vascular endothelial cells are the most abundant source of ET-1 [3]. In addition to endothelial cells, ET-1 is expressed in a wide variety of cells including vascular smooth muscle cells, cardiomyocytes, fibroblasts, macrophages, bronchial epithelial cells, and neurons [4].

The ETs are produced from their corresponding approximately 200-residue pre-propolypeptides that are encoded by three distinct genes (Fig. 12.1). These peptides are converted to inactive 38- or 39-amino acid intermediates called big ETs by furin-like endopeptidase. The big ETs are then proteolytically activated via a cleavage at Trp^{21}-Val^{22} by the ET-converting enzymes (ECEs), ECE-1 and ECE-2 [5, 6].

ETs act on two pharmacologically and molecularly distinct subtypes of G-protein-coupled receptors termed ET_A and ET_B receptors [7, 8]. Both receptors are expressed in a wide range of cell types with distinct but partially overlapping tissue distributions. In the vasculature, both ET_A and ET_B receptors on smooth muscle cells mediate the direct vasoconstrictor actions of ET-1, whereas endothelial ET_B receptors induce vasodilation via the ET-induced release of prostacyclin (PGI_2) and nitric oxide (NO) (Fig. 12.2). ET_B receptors mediate the clearance of circulating ET-1, particularly in the vascular beds of the lungs and kidneys [9, 10].

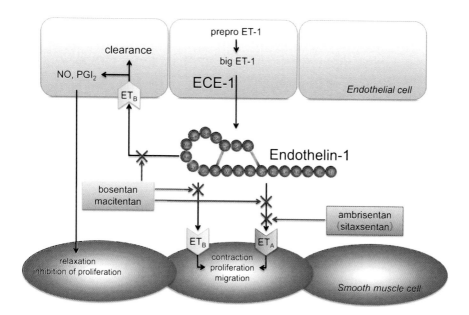

Fig. 12.2 Vascular endothelin system and representative endothelin receptor antagonists.
Endothelin (ET)-1 is produced by endothelial cells and acts on ET_A and ET_B receptors located on
the vascular smooth muscle cells to induce contraction, proliferation, and migration. ET-1 acts on
ET_B receptor in endothelial cells to produce nitric oxide (NO) and prostacyclin (PGI_2), which leads
to relaxation and inhibition of smooth muscle cell proliferation

12.2 Physiology and Pathophysiology of ET System

12.2.1 ETs in Development

A series of gene knockout experiments in mice have revealed the importance of the
ET system in the development of neural crest-derived cells (Fig. 12.3). ET-1- or
ET_A-deficient animals have craniofacial and cardiovascular abnormalities, which
results in embryonic lethality or death shortly after birth [11, 12]. Furthermore,
ET-3- or ET_B-deficient animals exhibit aganglionic megacolon and coat color spot-
ting and die at 3–6 weeks of age [13, 14]. *ECE-1* gene-deficient mice show the
additive phenotypes of animals lacking ET-1/ET_A and ET-3/ET_B pathways [15].

12.2.2 ETs in Pulmonary Arterial Hypertension (PAH)

Preclinical studies in animal models of PAH and clinical studies in patients with
PAH have shown a striking upregulation of ET-1 in the pulmonary arterial vasculature in diseased but not normal pulmonary arteries [16, 17]. These observations led

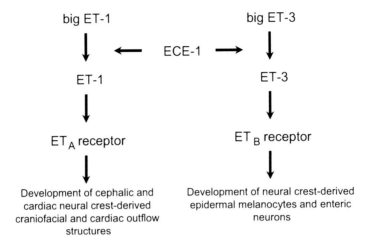

Fig. 12.3 Role of endothelin (ET) system in developmental stage of gene knockout mice.
Gene knockout experiments in mice have unexpectedly defined the importance of the ET system
in development. ET-1–ECE-1–ET_A axis is important for the development of embryonic cephalic
and cardiac neural crest-derived craniofacial and cardiac outflow structures. ET-3–ECE-1–ET_B
axis is responsible for the development of neural crest-derived epidermal melanocytes and enteric
neurons

to the hypothesis that ET-1 might be implicated in the pathogenesis of PAH and
could be a novel therapeutic target for PAH. This was further supported by evidence
that the plasma and lung levels of ET-1 increase in patients with PAH and correlate
with disease severity and prognosis [18–22]. Moreover, in preclinical models of
PAH, pharmacological blockade of the ET system improves the hemodynamics,
right ventricular hypertrophy, and survival [23].

12.2.3 Pathophysiological Roles of ET System in genetically Modified PAH Mice

The embryonic lethality or juvenile death of mice with genetically modified
ET-related genes hindered the analysis of the pathophysiological roles of the ET
system in adult animals. Therefore, mice with a conditional knockout of ET-1 exclusively in endothelial cells were generated and characterized [24]. These mice were
born without developmental abnormalities and survived to adulthood. The generation and characterization of several disease models using this mouse strain revealed
that ET-1 plays an essential role not only in the maintenance of blood pressure but
also in the induction of inflammation and fibrosis [25–27]. In addition, ET-1 has an
anti-apoptotic function in cardiomyocytes [28]. These observations suggest pathological roles for ET-1 in PAH including the abnormal proliferation of endothelial

and smooth muscle cells, inflammation, and fibrosis in addition to excessive vaso-constriction of the pulmonary vasculature (Fig. 12.4) [29, 30].

12.3   ERAs

There are currently three ERAs available on the market for the treatment of PAH, bosentan, ambrisentan, and macitentan (Table 12.1) [31]. Bosentan and macitentan are dual ET receptor blockers with similar affinity for the ET_A and ET_B receptors (Fig. 12.2), while ambrisentan is a relatively selective ET_A receptor antagonist.

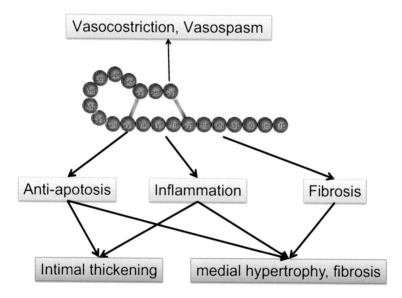

Fig. 12.4 Pathological roles of endothelin (ET)-1 in etiology of pulmonary arterial hypertension (PAH). Experimental observations of conditional knockout mice suggest that ET-1 is involved in the pathogenesis of PAH via multiple biological actions including vasoconstriction, vasospasm, antiapoptosis, inflammation, and fibrosis

Table 12.1 Pharmacological and pharmacokinetic properties of endothelin receptor antagonists

	Bosentan	Ambrisentan	Macitentan
FDA approval	2001	2007	2013
Mechanism of action	Dual ET_A/ET_B antagonism	Selective ET_A antagonism	Dual ET_A/ET_B antagonism
Selectivity ET_A:ET_B	30:1	4000:1	50:1
Half-life	5.4 h	15 h	17.5 h
Dosing range	62.5–125 mg	5–10 mg	10 mg
Dosing frequency	Twice daily	Once daily	Once daily

Sitaxsentan, another ET_A-selective antagonist, was previously available in Europe, Australia, and Canada, but was withdrawn from the market in 2010 owing to several fatalities attributed to acute liver failure [32, 33].

12.3.1 Structure, Specificity, Pharmacokinetics, and Drug Interactions of ERAs

12.3.1.1 Bosentan

Bosentan, a non-peptide pyrimidine derivative, is a specific and competitive antagonist of both ET_A and ET_B receptors [34, 35]. The usual dosage of bosentan is 125 mg twice a day after a 4-week titration period (62.5 mg twice a day). Bosentan has multiple drug interactions due to its enzymatic induction of cytochrome P450 (CYP) 2C9 and CYP3A4. The co-administration of bosentan and warfarin has been reported to reduce plasma warfarin concentrations and consequently decrease the international normalized ratio (INR) levels. Monitoring the prothrombin time (PT)-INR is advised when the dosage of bosentan is changed; however, significant clinical effects from co-administration of bosentan and warfarin are very rare in clinical practice, and the modification of the oral anticoagulant is seldom necessary.

Ketoconazole approximately doubles the exposure to bosentan because of the inhibition of CYP3A4. Furthermore, concomitant treatment with cyclosporine A increases the initial bosentan trough concentration, presumably by inhibiting the hepatic uptake transporter system. Therefore, the combined use of bosentan and cyclosporine A is contraindicated. In addition, the co-administration of glibenclamide and bosentan increases the incidence of elevated aminotransferase levels. Finally, co-administration of bosentan and sildenafil in PAH decrease the sildenafil level while that of bosentan is increased. However, current prescribing information does not recommend any dose adjustments for these combination therapies [36].

12.3.1.2 Ambrisentan

Ambrisentan, a carboxylic ERA, is the only selective antagonist of the ET_A receptor currently available for the treatment of PAH at an approved dosage of 5 or 10 mg once daily [37–39]. Food does not affect the bioavailability of ambrisentan, which is metabolized primarily by glucuronidation and to a lesser extent by CYP3A4, CYP3A5, and CYP2C19. Ambrisentan has a low propensity for drug-drug interactions because it only slightly induces and inhibits hepatic CYP450 [40]. Therefore, it can be safely administered with sildenafil or warfarin without any dose adjustment [41]. A significant interaction has only been reported with cyclosporine A, which caused a twofold increase in the ambrisentan concentration [42]. Therefore, for co-administration with cyclosporine A, ambrisentan has a fixed dose adjustment of 5 mg daily.

12.3.1.3   Macitentan

Macitentan is a new oral, dual ERA with a 50-fold higher affinity for ET_A than for ET_B receptors [43]. Macitentan belongs to the new chemical class of sulfamides, and its development led to an increased tissue penetration and more sustained receptor blockade than that obtained with other ERAs. Macitentan has been approved for the treatment of PAH at a dose of 10 mg once daily [44].

In vivo, macitentan is metabolized to its major pharmacologically active metabolite, ACT-132577, which is produced by oxidative depropylation by CYP3A4. While ACT-132577 is fivefold less potent than macitentan is, it achieves plasma levels that are four to five times higher because of its long half-life (approximately 48 h) [45]. Although macitentan metabolism is affected by the inhibition of CYP3A4, the changes are not considered clinically relevant, and no dose adjustment is required when it is combined with CYP3A4 inhibitors [46]. Furthermore, the concomitant administration of cyclosporine A had no clinically significant effect on the macitentan level or that of its metabolites at steady state [45]. Regarding drug interactions with warfarin or sildenafil, concomitant treatment with macitentan did not lead to a clinically relevant modification of the pharmacokinetics of each drug. Therefore, macitentan can be co-administered with warfarin or sildenafil without requiring a dose adjustment [47, 48].

12.3.2   Efficacy of ERAs in PAH

12.3.2.1   Bosentan

Bosentan was the first ERA approved for use in patients with PAH. Its availability represents a major advance in the management of PAH by improving the functional class, exercise capacity, and hemodynamic parameters, as well as delaying the clinical worsening of the disease [49]. The first double-blind, placebo-controlled study, BREATHE-1, which included 213 patients with idiopathic PAH (IPAH) or connective tissue-associated PAH, showed an improved exercise capacity (assessed using the 6-minute walking distance) and functional class at both 125 and 250 mg daily doses of bosentan [50]. The risk of clinical disease progression was reduced by bosentan compared with the placebo. A later study, EARLY, showed improved pulmonary vascular resistance (PVR) levels and a significantly delayed time to clinical progression in treated patients compared to that in patients with mildly symptomatic PAH treated with placebo [51]. Moreover, bosentan significantly improved the quality of life in patients with IPAH or PAH associated with connective tissue disease [52]. Bosentan therapy was also evaluated in a multicenter, double-blind, randomized, and placebo-controlled study in patients with functional class III Eisenmenger syndrome [53]. Bosentan did not worsen oxygen saturation, and compared to the placebo it reduced the PVR index and mean pulmonary arterial pressure, while it increased the exercise capacity. In addition, bosentan was proven to improve the hemodynamics of patients with human immunodeficiency virus (HIV)-related PAH or portopulmonary hypertension [54, 55]. Table 12.2 summarizes the randomized controlled trials (RCTs) performed with bosentan and other ERAs.

12.3.2.2 Ambrisentan

Ambrisentan has been studied in two pivotal phase-III multicenter, randomized, placebo-controlled trials, ARIES-1 and ARIES-2 [56]. The 6-min walking distance increased in all ambrisentan-treated groups. Improvements in time to clinical worsening, functional class, quality of life, Borg dyspnea score, and brain natriuretic peptide (BNP) were also observed. Furthermore, the 2-year extension study confirmed the improvements in the exercise capacity and good tolerability profile were persistent [57]. Ambrisentan was generally well tolerated and had a low risk of inducing liver dysfunction over the study period [58]. Recently, the randomized, double-blinded, multicenter, AMBITION study showed that initial combination therapy with ambrisentan/tadalafil in naïve PAH patients demonstrated a significantly lower risk of clinical failure-related events than monotherapy with ambrisentan or tadalafil did [59]. This result supports its rationale use for treating patients with PAH as part of an initial combination therapy to improve clinical outcomes.

12.3.2.3 Macitentan

Macitentan was studied in a multicenter, double-blind, placebo-controlled, long-term, event-driven, randomized study (SERAPHIN) [60]. This study was the first to use a morbidity-mortality composite endpoint. Furthermore, the study was designed to evaluate the efficacy and safety of macitentan using a primary endpoint of time from initiation of treatment to the first occurrence of a composite endpoint of death, atrial septostomy, lung transplantation, initiation of treatment with parenteral prostanoids, or worsening PAH in 742 patients with symptomatic PAH and treated for up to 3.5 years. The patients were randomized to receive either the placebo or macitentan 3 or 10 mg daily. There were 30 and 45 % risk reductions in the primary endpoint with the 3- and 10-mg doses, respectively. Interestingly, macitentan 10 mg significantly reduced the risk of the primary endpoint event versus the placebo in both treatment-naïve patients and those receiving background PAH-specific therapies (such as sildenafil) at the study entry. Treatment with macitentan in the SERAPHIN study was well tolerated and the more frequently reported adverse events were nasopharyngitis, headache, and anemia. The incidence of peripheral edema and elevation of liver aminotransferases were similar in the placebo and macitentan groups.

Table 12.2 Characteristics of the main clinical trials of endothelin receptor antagonists in patients with pulmonary hypertension

Drugs	Study	Type	No. of patients	Etiology	Length of study	Primary endpoint
Ambrisentan	ARIES-1 [56]	Randomized, double-blind, placebo-controlled, multicenter	202	IPAH, APAH	12 weeks	6MWD
	ARIES-2 [56]	Randomized, double-blind, placebo-controlled, multicenter	192	IPAH, APAH	12 weeks	6MWD
	ARIES-E [57]	Randomized, open label, multicenter, extension study	383	IPAH, APAH	2 years	6MWD
	AMBITION [59]	Randomized, double-blind, placebo-controlled, multicenter	500	IPAH, APAH	Event driven (73.9 weeks)	Time to clinical failure

(continued)

Table 12.2 (continued)

Drugs	Study	Type	No. of patients	Etiology	Length of study	Primary endpoint
Bosentan	Study-351 [49]	Randomized, double-blind, placebo-controlled, multicenter	32	IPAH, APAH-SSc	12 weeks	6MWD
	BREATHE-1 [50]	Randomized, double-blind, placebo-controlled, multicenter	213	IPAH, APAH-CTD	16 weeks	6MWD
	BREATHE-2 [70]	Randomized, double-blind, placebo-controlled, multicenter	33	IPAH, APAH-CTD	16 weeks	TPR
	BREATHE-5 [53]	Randomized, double-blind, placebo-controlled, multicenter	54	E:senmenger syndrome	16 weeks	SpO_2, PVR
	McLaughlin et al. [71]	Randomized, open label, multicenter, extension study	169	IPAH	2.1 years	NA
	EARLY [51]	Randomized, double-blind, placebo-controlled, multicenter	185	IPAH, APAH	6 months	6MWD
Macitentan	SERAPHIN [60]	Randomized, double-blind, placebo-controlled, multicenter	742	IPAH, APAH	Event driven (115 weeks)	Time to clinical worsening

IPAH idiopathic pulmonary arterial hypertension, *APAH* associated pulmonary arterial hypertension, *SSc* systemic sclerosis, *CTD* connective tissue disease, *6MWD* 6-minute walk distance, *TPR* total pulmonary resistance, *SpO₂* finger oxygen saturation, *PVR* pulmonary vascular resistance, *NA* not applicable

12.3.3 Safety of ERAs

12.3.3.1 General Side Effects

Treatment with ERAs is generally well tolerated, and their associated dose-dependent side effects, which are caused by vasodilatory properties, include peripheral edema, headache, nasal congestion, flushing, or nausea. Hypotension and palpitation have also been reported for treatment with ERAs. Among the ERAs currently available for PAH treatment, macitentan appears to be the best tolerated regarding liver dysfunction and peripheral edema [61].

12.3.3.2 Liver Dysfunction

Liver dysfunction is the main adverse effect observed with ERAs and bosentan is known to be associated with reversible, dose-dependent, and in most cases asymptomatic, elevation of aminotransferases [62]. The increase in liver enzymes usually occurs during the first 6 months of treatment with bosentan but could also appear later on. To prevent this adverse event, a gradual dose increase is recommended (62 mg twice daily for the first month and 125 mg twice daily after that). Furthermore, aminotransferase elevation could normalize after the bosentan dosage is decreased or treatment is interrupted. The reported annual rate of aminotransferases level elevation was approximately 10 %. Therefore, liver function testing should be performed monthly in patients receiving bosentan. Similarly, monitoring is recommended in the case of dosage modification or possible drug-drug interaction.

Ambrisentan has not been shown to increase the risk of liver enzyme elevation over placebo [63, 64]. Ambrisentan belongs to the group of carboxylic ERAs, which unlike sulfonamide ERAs such as bosentan and sitaxsentan are devoid of hepatotoxicity. Ambrisentan is a safe alternative when bosentan has to be discontinued because of increased liver aminotransferase levels.

Macitentan does not inhibit canalicular bile acid transport in rats, which could indicate a better liver safety profile than that of bosentan [65]. In the SERAPHIN study, no difference in the proportion of liver enzyme abnormalities was observed between the placebo and macitentan groups [60].

12.3.3.3 Edema

Peripheral edema is a notable side effect of the ERA, and its mechanism is currently unclear. One possible mechanism is that the edema may be mediated by primary effects on sodium and water retention by the nephrons [66]. Another explanation could be the activation of the myocardial ET system in heart failure in patients with PAH, which could be a compensatory mechanism to preserve cardiac contractility

[28, 67]. ERAs might potentially deteriorate cardiac function, which explains some of the peripheral edema observed clinically with these agents. Moreover, a higher incidence of peripheral edema is observed in PAH patients treated with ambrisentan than in those treated with dual ERAs [68]. This observation may support the hypothesis that the peripheral edema is mediated by circulating ET-1 and its activation of the ET_B receptor. Nevertheless, in numerous cases, peripheral edema may be managed by the using an appropriate class and amount of the combined diuretic.

12.3.3.4   Anemia

Decreased hemoglobin levels and anemia are other side effects observed during ERA treatment and the mechanism underlying the decrease in hemoglobin level has not been fully elucidated. This decrease could be explained by the hemodilution induced by vasodilatation and intravascular fluid retention. Anemia may aggravate the symptoms (such as dyspnea and palpitation) and, hence, increase the risk of heart failure. Therefore, monitoring the hemoglobin level is recommended in patients treated with ERAs.

12.3.3.5   Teratogenicity

The teratogenic effects reported in animals treated with bosentan and developmental abnormalities observed in genetically modified mice with altered ET-related genes have led to its official contraindication in pregnancy [69]. Similar to bosentan, ambrisentan and macitentan are considered teratogens, which could cause early developmental fetal defects. In childbearing women, ERAs could be prescribed if contraception is proved, along with a negative pregnancy test performed before initiation of the treatment and, after that, monthly. In particular, bosentan may decrease plasma concentrations of estroprogestative oral contraceptives, and additional or alternative contraceptive methods are required when treatment with bosentan is proposed in women of childbearing potential. Nevertheless, pregnancy is formally contraindicated in PAH treatment since it could be an aggravating factor in the prognosis of the disease.

12.4   Place of ERAs in PAH Treatment Algorithm

ERAs have been proven efficacious in PAH treatment with relatively few adverse effects, becoming an indispensable monotherapy or combination therapy with drugs targeting alternate pathways. Three ERAs are currently recommended as first-line therapy for patients with FC II and III PAH [31]. The current clinical data suggests that selective and dual ERAs are similarly efficacious in improving the clinical outcome in patients with PAH, although they exhibit different safety profiles. The advantage that ambrisentan and macitentan have over bosentan is their once daily oral dose, which improves the quality of life and adherence of patients with PAH to treatment regimens. Moreover, the adverse events and drug-drug interactions appear to be a clinical consideration for the choice of drug. Regarding the general safety profile, macitentan appears to be safer and has a lower potential for drug-drug interactions than the other agents do.

12.5 Conclusions

The ERAs were the first oral therapy for PAH and remain a critical component of the therapeutic algorithm for this highly symptomatic, progressive, and life-threatening disease. ERAs have demonstrated improvements in exercise capacity, functional status, pulmonary hemodynamics, and clinical outcome in several randomized placebo-controlled trials, thereby representing a pivotal therapy for PAH. However, it is important to note that treatment with ERAs is not a curative approach. Even without the aggravation of symptom or exercise capacity with ERA treatment, periodical monitoring of hemodynamics is mandatory, and the therapeutic strategy should be reconsidered if and when needed.

References

1. Yanagisawa M, Kurihara H, Kimura S, Tomobe Y, Kobayashi M, Mitsui Y, et al. A novel potent vasoconstrictor peptide produced by vascular endothelial cells. Nature. 1988;332(6163):411–5. doi:10.1038/332411a0.
2. Inoue A, Yanagisawa M, Kimura S, Kasuya Y, Miyauchi T, Goto K, et al. The human endothelin family: three structurally and pharmacologically distinct isopeptides predicted by three separate genes. Proc Natl Acad Sci U S A. 1989;86(8):2863–7.
3. Vignon-Zellweger N, Heiden S, Miyauchi T, Emoto N. Endothelin and endothelin receptors in the renal and cardiovascular systems. Life Sci. 2012;91(13–14):490–500. doi:10.1016/j.lfs.2012.03.026.
4. Kedzierski RM, Yanagisawa M. Endothelin system: the double-edged sword in health and disease. Annu Rev Pharmacol Toxicol. 2001;41:851–76. doi:10.1146/annurev.pharmtox.41.1.851.
5. Xu D, Emoto N, Giaid A, Slaughter C, Kaw S, deWit D et al. ECE-1: a membrane-bound metalloprotease that catalyzes the proteolytic activation of big endothelin-1. Cell 1994;78(3):473-485. doi:10.1016/0092-8674(94)90425-1 [pii].
6. Emoto N, Yanagisawa M. Endothelin-converting enzyme-2 is a membrane-bound, phosphoramidon-sensitive metalloprotease with acidic pH optimum. J Biol Chem. 1995;270(25):15262–8.
7. Arai H, Hori S, Aramori I, Ohkubo H, Nakanishi S. Cloning and expression of a cDNA encoding an endothelin receptor. Nature. 1990;348(6303):730–2. doi:10.1038/348730a0.
8. Sakurai T, Yanagisawa M, Takuwa Y, Miyazaki H, Kimura S, Goto K, et al. Cloning of a cDNA encoding a non-isopeptide-selective subtype of the endothelin receptor. Nature. 1990;348(6303):732–5. doi:10.1038/348732a0.

9. Dupuis J, Stewart DJ, Cernacek P, Gosselin G. Human pulmonary circulation is an important site for both clearance and production of endothelin-1. Circulation. 1996;94(7):1578–84.

10. Fukuroda T, Fujikawa T, Ozaki S, Ishikawa K, Yano M, Nishikibe M. Clearance of circulating endothelin-1 by ETB receptors in rats. Biochem Biophys Res Commun. 1994;199(3):1461–5. doi:10.1006/bbrc.1994.1395.

11. Kurihara Y, Kurihara H, Suzuki H, Kodama T, Maemura K, Nagai R, et al. Elevated blood pressure and craniofacial abnormalities in mice deficient in endothelin-1. Nature. 1994;368(6473):703–10. doi:10.1038/368703a0.

12. Clouthier DE, Hosoda K, Richardson JA, Williams SC, Yanagisawa H, Kuwaki T, et al. Cranial and cardiac neural crest defects in endothelin-A receptor-deficient mice. Development. 1998;125(5):813–24.

13. Baynash AG, Hosoda K, Giaid A, Richardson JA, Emoto N, Hammer RE, et al. Interaction of endothelin-3 with endothelin-B receptor is essential for development of epidermal melano-cytes and enteric neurons. Cell. 1994;79(7):1277–85.

14. Hosoda K, Hammer RE, Richardson JA, Baynash AG, Cheung JC, Giaid A, et al. Targeted and natural (piebald-lethal) mutations of endothelin-B receptor gene produce megacolon associated with spotted coat color in mice. Cell. 1994;79(7):1267–76.

15. Yanagisawa H, Yanagisawa M, Kapur RP, Richardson JA, Williams SC, Clouthier DE, et al. Dual genetic pathways of endothelin-mediated intercellular signaling revealed by targeted disruption of endothelin converting enzyme-1 gene. Development. 1998;125(5):825–36.

16. Miyagawa K, Emoto N. Current state of endothelin receptor antagonism in hypertension and pulmonary hypertension. Ther Adv Cardiovasc Dis. 2014;8(5):202–16. doi:10.1177/1753944714541511.

17. Barton M, Yanagisawa M. Endothelin: 20 years from discovery to therapy. Can J Physiol Pharmacol. 2008;86(8):485–98. doi:10.1139/Y08-059.

18. Stewart DJ, Levy RD, Cernacek P, Langleben D. Increased plasma endothelin-1 in pulmonary hypertension: marker or mediator of disease? Ann Intern Med. 1991;114(6):464–9.

19. Giaid A, Yanagisawa M, Langleben D, Michel RP, Levy R, Shennib H, et al. Expression of endothelin-1 in the lungs of patients with pulmonary hypertension. N Engl J Med. 1993;328(24):1732–9. doi:10.1056/NEJM199306173282402.

20. Silva Marques J, Martins SR, Calisto C, Goncalves S, Almeida AG, de Sousa JC, et al. An exploratory panel of biomarkers for risk prediction in pulmonary hypertension: emerging role of CT-proET-1. J Heart Lung Transplant. 2013;32(12):1214–21. doi:10.1016/j.healun.2013.06.020.

21. Montani D, Souza R, Binkert C, Fischli W, Simonneau G, Clozel M, et al. Endothelin-1/endothelin-3 ratio: a potential prognostic factor of pulmonary arterial hypertension. Chest. 2007;131(1):101–8. doi:10.1378/chest.06-0682.

22. Rubens C, Ewert R, Halank M, Wensel R, Orzechowski HD, Schultheiss HP, et al. Big endothelin-1 and endothelin-1 plasma levels are correlated with the severity of primary pulmonary hypertension. Chest. 2001;120(5):1562–9.

23. Dupuis J, Hoeper MM. Endothelin receptor antagonists in pulmonary arterial hypertension. Eur Respir J. 2008;31(2):407–15. doi:10.1183/09031936.00078207.

24. Kisanuki YY, Emoto N, Ohuchi T, Widyantoro B, Yagi K, Nakayama K, et al. Low blood pressure in endothelial cell-specific endothelin 1 knockout mice. Hypertension. 2010;56(1):121–8. doi:10.1161/HYPERTENSIONAHA.109.138701.

25. Anggrahini DW, Emoto N, Nakayama K, Widyantoro B, Adiarto S, Iwasa N, et al. Vascular endothelial cell-derived endothelin-1 mediates vascular inflammation and neointima formation following blood flow cessation. Cardiovasc Res. 2009;82(1):143–51. doi:10.1093/cvr/cvp026.

26. Adiarto S, Emoto N, Iwasa N, Yokoyama M. Obesity-induced upregulation of myocardial endothelin-1 expression is mediated by leptin. Biochem Biophys Res Commun. 2007;353(3):623–7. doi:10.1016/j.bbrc.2006.12.066.

27. Hartopo AB, Emoto N, Vignon-Zellweger N, Suzuki Y, Yagi K, Nakayama K, et al. Endothelin-converting enzyme-1 gene ablation attenuates pulmonary fibrosis via CGRP-cAMP/EPAC1 pathway. Am J Respir Cell Mol Biol. 2013;48(4):465–76. doi:10.1165/rcmb.2012-0354OC.

28. Heiden S, Vignon-Zellweger N, Masuda S, Yagi K, Nakayama K, Yanagisawa M, et al. Vascular endothelium derived endothelin-1 is required for normal heart function after chronic pressure overload in mice. PLoS One. 2014;9(2):e88730. doi:10.1371/journal.pone.0088730.

29. Van Hung T, Emoto N, Vignon-Zellweger N, Nakayama K, Yagi K, Suzuki Y, et al. Inhibition of vascular endothelial growth factor receptor under hypoxia causes severe, human-like pulmonary arterial hypertension in mice: potential roles of interleukin-6 and endothelin. Life Sci. 2014;118(2):313–28. doi:10.1016/j.lfs.2013.12.215.

30. Satwiko MG, Ikeda K, Nakayama K, Yagi K, Hocher B, Hirata K, et al. Targeted activation of endothelin-1 exacerbates hypoxia-induced pulmonary hypertension. Biochem Biophys Res Commun. 2015;465(3):356–62. doi:10.1016/j.bbrc.2015.08.002.

31. Galie N, Humbert M, JL Vachiery, Gibbs S, Lang I, Torbicki A et al. 2015 ESC/ERS Guidelines for the diagnosis and treatment of pulmonary hypertension: The Joint Task Force for the Diagnosis and Treatment of Pulmonary Hypertension of the European Society of Cardiology (ESC) and the European Respiratory Society (ERS): Endorsed by: Association for European Paediatric and Congenital Cardiology (AEPC), International Society for Heart and Lung Transplantation (ISHLT). Eur Respir J. 2015;46(4):903–75. doi:10.1183/13993003.01032-2015.

32. Lavelle A, Sugrue R, Lawler G, Mulligan N, Kelleher B, Murphy DM, et al. Sitaxentan-induced hepatic failure in two patients with pulmonary arterial hypertension. Eur Respir J. 2009;34(3):770–1. doi:10.1183/09031936.00058409.

33. Lee WT, Kirkham N, Johnson MK, Lordan JL, Fisher AJ, Peacock AJ. Sitaxentan-related acute liver failure in a patient with pulmonary arterial hypertension. Eur Respir J. 2011;37(2):472–4. doi:10.1183/09031936.00091610.

34. Clozel M, Breu V, Burri K, Cassal JM, Fischli W, Gray GA, et al. Pathophysiological role of endothelin revealed by the first orally active endothelin receptor antagonist. Nature. 1993;365(6448):759–61. doi:10.1038/365759a0.

35. Clozel M, Breu V, Gray GA, Kalina B, Loffler BM, Burri K, et al. Pharmacological characterization of bosentan, a new potent orally active nonpeptide endothelin receptor antagonist. J Pharmacol Exp Ther. 1994;270(1):228–35.

36. Burgess G, Hoogkamer H, Collings L, Dingemanse J. Mutual pharmacokinetic interactions between steady-state bosentan and sildenafil. Eur J Clin Pharmacol. 2008;64(1):43–50. doi:10.1007/s00228-007-0408-z.

37. Riechers H, Albrecht HP, Amberg W, Baumann E, Bernard H, Bohm HJ, et al. Discovery and optimization of a novel class of orally active nonpeptidic endothelin-A receptor antagonists. J Med Chem. 1996;39(11):2123–8. doi:10.1021/jm960274q.

38. Casserly B, Klinger JR. Ambrisentan for the treatment of pulmonary arterial hypertension. Drug Design Dev Therapy. 2009;2:265–80.

39. Galie N, Badesch D, Oudiz R, Simonneau G, McGoon MD, Keogh AM, et al. Ambrisentan therapy for pulmonary arterial hypertension. J Am Coll Cardiol. 2005;46(3):529–35. doi:10.1016/j.jacc.2005.04.050.

40. Frampton JE. Ambrisentan. Am J Cardiovasc Drugs. 2011;11(4):215–26. doi:10.2165/11207340-000000000-00000.

41. D'Alto M. An update on the use of ambrisentan in pulmonary arterial hypertension. Ther Adv Respir Dis. 2012;6(6):331–43. doi:10.1177/1753465812458014.

42. Venitz J, Zack J, Gillies H, Allard M, Regnault J, Dufton C. Clinical pharmacokinetics and drug-drug interactions of endothelin receptor antagonists in pulmonary arterial hypertension. J Clin Pharmacol. 2012;52(12):1784–805. doi:10.1177/0091270011423662.

43. Iglarz M, Binkert C, Morrison K, Fischli W, Gatfield J, Treiber A, et al. Pharmacology of macitentan, an orally active tissue-targeting dual endothelin receptor antagonist. J Pharmacol Exp Ther. 2008;327(3):736–45. doi:10.1124/jpet.108.142976.

44. Sidharta PN, van Giersbergen PL, Dingemanse J. Safety, tolerability, pharmacokinetics, and pharmacodynamics of macitentan, an endothelin receptor antagonist, in an ascending multiple-dose study in healthy subjects. J Clin Pharmacol. 2013;53(11):1131–8. doi:10.1002/jcph.152.

45. Bruderer S, Aanismaa P, Homery MC, Hausler S, Landskroner K, Sidharta PN, et al. Effect of cyclosporine and rifampin on the pharmacokinetics of macitentan, a tissue-targeting dual endothelin receptor antagonist. AAPS J. 2012;14(1):68–78. doi:10.1208/s12248-011-9316-3.

46. Atsmon J, Dingemanse J, Shaikevich D, Volokhov I, Sidharta PN. Investigation of the effects of ketoconazole on the pharmacokinetics of macitentan, a novel dual endothelin receptor antagonist, in healthy subjects. Clin Pharmacokinet. 2013;52(8):685–92. doi:10.1007/s40262-013-0063-8.

47. Sidharta PN, Dietrich H, Dingemanse J. Investigation of the effect of macitentan on the pharmacokinetics and pharmacodynamics of warfarin in healthy male subjects. Clinic Drug Investig. 2014;34(8):545–52. doi:10.1007/s40261-014-0207-0.

48. Sidharta PN, van Giersbergen PL, Wolzt M, Dingemanse J. Investigation of mutual pharmacokinetic interactions between macitentan, a novel endothelin receptor antagonist, and sildenafil in healthy subjects. Br J Clin Pharmacol. 2014;78(5):1035–42. doi:10.1111/bcp.12447.

49. Channick RN, Simonneau G, Sitbon O, Robbins IM, Frost A, Tapson VF, et al. Effects of the dual endothelin-receptor antagonist bosentan in patients with pulmonary hypertension: a randomised placebo-controlled study. Lancet. 2001;358(9288):1119–23. doi:10.1016/S0140-6736(01)06250-X.

50. Rubin LJ, Badesch DB, Barst RJ, Galie N, Black CM, Keogh A, et al. Bosentan therapy for pulmonary arterial hypertension. N Engl J Med. 2002;346(12):896–903. doi:10.1056/NEJMoa012212.

51. Galie N, Rubin L, Hoeper M, Jansa P, Al-Hiti H, Meyer G, et al. Treatment of patients with mildly symptomatic pulmonary arterial hypertension with bosentan (EARLY study): a double-blind, randomised controlled trial. Lancet. 2008;371(9630):2093–100. doi:10.1016/S0140-6736(08)60919-8.

52. Keogh AM, McNeil KD, Wlodarczyk J, Gabbay E, Williams TJ. Quality of life in pulmonary arterial hypertension: improvement and maintenance with bosentan. J Heart Lung Transplant. 2007;26(2):181–7. doi:10.1016/j.healun.2006.11.009.

53. Galie N, Beghetti M, Gatzoulis MA, Granton J, Berger RM, Lauer A, et al. Bosentan therapy in patients with Eisenmenger syndrome: a multicenter, double-blind, randomized, placebo-controlled study. Circulation. 2006;114(1):48–54. doi:10.1161/CIRCULATIONAHA.106.630715.

54. Sitbon O, Gressin V, Speich R, Macdonald PS, Opravil M, Cooper DA, et al. Bosentan for the treatment of human immunodeficiency virus-associated pulmonary arterial hypertension. Am J Respir Crit Care Med. 2004;170(11):1212–7. doi:10.1164/rccm.200404-445OC.

55. Savale L, Magnier R, Le Pavec J, Jais X, Montani D, O'Callaghan DS, et al. Efficacy, safety and pharmacokinetics of bosentan in portopulmonary hypertension. Eur Respir J. 2013;41(1):96–103. doi:10.1183/09031936.00117511.

56. Galie N, Olschewski H, Oudiz RJ, Torres F, Frost A, Ghofrani HA, et al. Ambrisentan for the treatment of pulmonary arterial hypertension: results of the ambrisentan in pulmonary arterial hypertension, randomized, double-blind, placebo-controlled, multicenter, efficacy (ARIES) study 1 and 2. Circulation. 2008;117(23):3010–9. doi:10.1161/CIRCULATIONAHA.107.742510.

57. Oudiz RJ, Galie N, Olschewski H, Torres F, Frost A, Ghofrani HA, et al. Long-term ambrisentan therapy for the treatment of pulmonary arterial hypertension. J Am Coll Cardiol. 2009;54(21):1971–81. doi:10.1016/j.jacc.2009.07.033.

58. Klinger JR, Oudiz RJ, Spence R, Despain D, Dufton C. Long-term pulmonary hemodynamic effects of ambrisentan in pulmonary arterial hypertension. Am J Cardiol. 2011;108(2):302–7. doi:10.1016/j.amjcard.2011.03.037.

59. Galie N, Barbera JA, Frost AE, Ghofrani HA, Hoeper MM, McLaughlin VV, et al. Initial use of Ambrisentan plus Tadalafil in pulmonary arterial hypertension. N Engl J Med. 2015;373(9):834–44. doi:10.1056/NEJMoa1413687.
60. Pulido T, Adzerikho I, Channick RN, Delcroix M, Galie N, Ghofrani HA, et al. Macitentan and morbidity and mortality in pulmonary arterial hypertension. N Engl J Med. 2013;369(9):809–18. doi:10.1056/NEJMoa1213917.
61. Sidharta PN, van Giersbergen PL, Halabi A, Dingemanse J. Macitentan: entry-into-humans study with a new endothelin receptor antagonist. Eur J Clin Pharmacol. 2011;67(10):977–84. doi:10.1007/s00228-011-1043-2.
62. Benedict N, Seybert A, Mathier MA. Evidence-based pharmacologic management of pulmonary arterial hypertension. Clin Ther. 2007;29(10):2134–53. doi:10.1016/j.clinthera.2007.10.009.
63. McGoon MD, Frost AE, Oudiz RJ, Badesch DB, Galie N, Olschewski H, et al. Ambrisentan therapy in patients with pulmonary arterial hypertension who discontinued bosentan or sitaxsentan due to liver function test abnormalities. Chest. 2009;135(1):122–9. doi:10.1378/chest.08-1028.
64. Ben-Yehuda O, Pizzuti D, Brown A, Littman M, Gillies H, Henig N, et al. Long-term hepatic safety of ambrisentan in patients with pulmonary arterial hypertension. J Am Coll Cardiol. 2012;60(1):80–1. doi:10.1016/j.jacc.2012.03.025.
65. Bolli MH, Boss C, Binkert C, Buchmann S, Bur D, Hess P, et al. The discovery of N-[5-(4-bromophenyl)-6-[2-[(5-bromo-2-pyrimidinyl)oxy]ethoxy]-4-pyrimidinyl]-N′-p ropylsulfamide (Macitentan), an orally active, potent dual endothelin receptor antagonist. J Med Chem. 2012;55(17):7849–61. doi:10.1021/jm3009103.
66. Vignon-Zellweger N, Heiden S, Emoto N. Renal function and blood pressure: molecular insights into the biology of endothelin-1. Contrib Nephrol. 2011;172:18–34. doi:10.1159/000328164.
67. Nagendran J, Sutendra G, Paterson I, Champion HC, Webster L, Chiu B, et al. Endothelin axis is upregulated in human and rat right ventricular hypertrophy. Circ Res. 2013;112(2):347–54. doi:10.1161/CIRCRESAHA.111.300448.
68. Trow TK, Taichman DB. Endothelin receptor blockade in the management of pulmonary arterial hypertension: selective and dual antagonism. Respir Med. 2009;103(7):951–62. doi:10.1016/j.rmed.2009.02.016.
69. Dhillon S, Keating GM. Bosentan: a review of its use in the management of mildly symptomatic pulmonary arterial hypertension. Am J Cardiovasc Drugs. 2009;9(5):331–50. doi:10.2165/11202270-000000000-00000.
70. Humbert M, Barst RJ, Robbins IM, Channick RN, Galie N, Boonstra A, et al. Combination of bosentan with epoprostenol in pulmonary arterial hypertension: BREATHE-2. Eur Resp J. 2004;24(3):353–9. doi:10.1183/09031936.04.00028404.
71. McLaughlin VV, Sitbon O, Badesch DB, Barst RJ, Black C, Galie N, et al. Survival with first-line bosentan in patients with primary pulmonary hypertension. Eur Respir J. 2005;25(2):244–9. doi:10.1183/09031936.05.00054804.

Chapter 13
Lung Transplantation

Hiroshi Date

Abstract Bilateral cadaveric lung transplantation (CLT) is the most common procedure for pulmonary arterial hypertension (PAH) according to the report from International Society for Heart and Lung Transplantation. The 5-year survival after CLT is approximately 50 %, and pulmonary hypertension (PH) is known to be a significant risk factor of early death after lung transplantation.

Because of severe shortage of cadaveric lungs in Japan, living-donor lobar lung transplantation (LDLLT) is often the only realistic option for very sick PAH patients especially for children.

Between 1998 and 2015, lung transplantation has been performed in 464 patients at nine lung transplant centers in Japan. Among these, the author and his colleagues have performed 184 lung transplants including 111 LDLLTs and 73 CLTs. Thirty-five of them (19 %) were diagnosed with PH. Twenty-four patients received LDLLT and 11 patients received CLT. The 5-year survival rate was 81.2 % for PH patients ($n = 35$) and was 72.2 % for non-PH patients ($n = 149$).

Lung transplantation is a viable treatment in patients with PAH who failed to respond medical treatment.

Keywords Pulmonary arterial hypertension • Pulmonary hypertension • Cadaveric lung transplantation • Living-donor lobar lung transplantation

13.1 History

The first successful heart-lung transplantation (HLT) was performed in 1981 in a patient with pulmonary arterial hypertension (PAH) at Stanford University by Dr. Bruce A Reitz [1]. It was believed that not only the lung but also the heart had to be replaced for a patient with severe PAH because of associated right heart failure.

H. Date, M.D. (✉)
Department of Thoracic Surgery, Kyoto University Graduate School of Medicine,
54 Kawahara-cho, Shogoin, Sakyo-ku, Kyoto 606-8507, Japan
e-mail: hdate@kuhp.kyoto-u.ac.jp

© Springer Science+Business Media Singapore 2017
Y. Fukumoto (ed.), *Diagnosis and Treatment of Pulmonary Hypertension*,
DOI 10.1007/978-981-287-840-3_13

In 1983, Dr. Joel D Cooper performed the first successful single lung transplantation (SLT) for a patient with idiopathic pulmonary fibrosis at Toronto University [2]. The first application of SLT for pulmonary hypertension was reported by Dr. G Alexander Patterson in a patient with Eisenmenger's syndrome due to patient ductus arteriosus [3]. The recovery of right heart failure was demonstrated by the reduction of pulmonary arterial pressure. However, the following experience of SLT for PAH was not satisfactory because it was associated with high incidence of reperfusion lung edema. It is for this reason that bilateral lung transplantation (BLT) has become the standard transplant procedure for PAH.

Bilateral living-donor lobar lung transplantation (LDLLT) was clinically developed at the University of Southern California as a procedure for patients considered too ill to await cadaveric transplantation [4]. It was originally applied almost exclusively to patients with cystic fibrosis. We and others have expanded the indications for LDLLT to include both pediatric [4, 5] and adult [6, 7] IPAH patients. Although LDLLT was initially performed in the USA, its use has decreased there because of the recent change by the Organ Procurement and Transplantation Network to an urgency/benefit allocation system for cadaveric donor lungs. For the past several years, reports on LDLLT almost exclusively have been from Japan [8–10], where the average waiting time for a cadaveric lung is still more than 2 years.

13.2 Indication for Lung Transplantation

13.2.1 Recipient Selection

13.2.1.1 Cadaveric Lung Transplantation

Lung transplantation is indicated for patients with end-stage lung disease who are failing maximal medical therapy and whose life expectancy is limited. Because of the severe cadaveric donor shortage, upper age limit is set in Japan. Candidates should be less than 55 years old for bilateral lung transplantation, and they should be less than 60 years old for single lung transplantation at the time of registration on Japanese Organ Transplant Network (JOTN) waiting list.

Because of the remarkable improvements in medical treatment for PAH during the past decade, determining the indications and timing for transplantation as a PAH treatment is a difficult challenge. The US Registry to Evaluate Early and Long-Term PAH Disease Management (REVEAL) [11] reported the following factors to be associated with increased mortality: NYHA functional class IV, male gender with age >60 years old, pulmonary vascular resistance (PVR) >30 Wood units, PAH associated with portal hypertension, or a family history of PAH. NYHA functional class III, increased mean right atrial pressure, decreased resting systolic blood pressure or an elevated heart rate, decreased 6-min walk distance, increased brain natriuretic peptide, renal insufficiency, PAH associated with connective tissue diseases, decreased DLCO, and the presence of pericardial effusion were also associated with increased mortality.

Table 13.1 Selection of lung transplant candidates for patients with pulmonary vascular diseases

Timing for referal
NYHA functional class III or IV symptoms during escalating therapy
Rapidly progressive disease
Use of parenteral targeted pulmonary arterial hypertension therapy regardless of symptoms or NYHA functional class
Known or suspected pulmonary veno-occlusive disease or pulmonary capillary hemangiomatosis
Timing of transplant listing
NYHA functional class III or IV despite a trial of at least 3 months of combination therapy incuding prostanoids
Cardiac index of less than 2 liters/min/m2
Mean right atrial pressure > 15 mmHg
6-minute walk test < 350 m
Development of significant hemoptysis, pericardial effusion, or signs of progressive right heart failure

J Heart Lung Transplantation 2015 [12]

Table 13.2 Indication of living-donor lobar lung transplantation for patients with pulmonary arterial hypertension

Patients who fulfill the guidelines of cadaveric lung transplantation (Table 13.1)
Critically ill patients who fail in maximal medical treatment including epoprostenol therapy
Patients who would die or become unsuitable recipients before cadaveric lungs become available

The Pulmonary Scientific Council of the International Society for Heart and Lung Transplantation updated a consensus document for the selection of lung transplant candidates in the guidelines for referral and transplantation in 2014 (Table 13.1) [12].

13.2.1.2   Living-Donor Lobar Lung Transplantation

Patients being considered for LDLLT should meet the criteria for conventional bilateral CLT except that age should be less than 65 years old. Because LDLLT subjects healthy donors to a lower lobectomy procedure associated with potentially serious complications, hospitalization, discomfort and loss of work, as well as the irreversible reduction in lung function, we have accepted only critically ill PAH patients who failed maximal medical treatment including epoprostenol therapy (Table 13.2). Although knowledge of the predictors of survival in patients with PAH is helpful, ultimately the timetable must be set by the unique situation of each patient. In our LDLLT experience, most of PAH patients were on high-dose intravenous epoprostenol with inotropic support and were bed bound.

13.2.2   Donor Selection

13.2.2.1   Cadaveric Lung Transplantation

The Japanese transplant law finally became effective in October 1997 and cadaveric lung transplantation (CLT) was officially approved. However, it was somewhat a very strict law resulting in very small practice of CLTs for the next decade. In 2010, the Japanese Organ Transplant Law was amended so that the family of the brain-dead donors can make a decision for organ donation. The revision of the law significantly increased the number of organ donations from brain-dead donors, and CLT has become a more realistic option for adult Japanese patients since then.

Ideal brain-dead donor should have clear chest X-ray, good blood gas (PaO2 > 300 mmHg with 100% oxygen), and age less than 60 years old. Use of marginal donors is one of the strategies for organ shortage. A medical consult system has been established in Japan to maintain various organ conditions suitable for the subsequent donation. The utility ratio of the lungs of brain-dead donors in Japan is indeed over 60%, and it is much higher than that reported in the United States (approximately 20%).

13.2.2.2   Living-Donor Lobar Lung Transplantation

Eligibility criteria for living lobar lung donation at Kyoto University are summarized in Table 13.3. Potential donors should be mentally competent, willing to donate free of coercion, medically and psychosocially suitable, fully informed of the risks and benefits as a donor, and fully informed of risks, benefits, and alternative treatment available to the recipient. In our institutions, potential donors are interviewed by three physicians with an observer to safeguard against coercion and to ensure donor comprehension of the procedure. The interview is performed at least three times to provide potential donors multiple opportunities to question, reconsider, or withdraw as a donor.

Appropriate size matching between donor and recipient is important in LDLLT. It is often inevitable that small grafts are implanted in LDLLT, in which only two lobes are implanted. Excessively small grafts may cause high pulmonary artery pressure, resulting in lung edema. A pleural space problem may increase the risk of empyema. Overexpansion of the donor lobes may contribute to obstructive physiology by early closure of small airways. We have previously proposed a formula to estimate the graft forced vital capacity (FVC) based on the donor's measured FVC and the number of pulmonary segments implanted. Given that the right lower lobe consists of five segments, the left lower lobe four segments, and the whole lung 19 segments, total forced vital capacity (FVC) of the two grafts is estimated by the following equation [8]:

Total FVC of the 2 grafts = Measeured FVC of the right donor × 5/19 + Measured FVC of the left donor × 4/19

This "functional size matching" has been used to determine the lower threshold of undersized grafts. When the total FVC of the two grafts is more than 45 % of the

Table 13.3 The eligibility
criteria for living lung
donation (Kyoto University)

Medical criteria
Age 20–60 years
ABO blood type compatible with recipient
Relatives within the third degree or a spouse
No significant past medical history
No recent viral infection
No significant abnormalities on echocardiogram and electrocardiogram
No significant ipsilateral pulmonary pathology on computed tomography
Arterial oxygen tension $\geq$ 80 mmHg (room air)
Forced vital capacity, forced expiratory volume in one second $\geq$ 85 % of predicted
No previous ipsilateral thoracic surgery
No active tobacco smoking
Social and ethical criteria
No significant mental disorders proved by a psychiatrist
No ethical issues or concerns about donor motivation

predicted FVC of the recipient (calculated from a knowledge of height, age, and sex), we accept the size disparity. For PH patients, the ratio should be more than 50%.

For "anatomical size matching," three-dimensional (3D) computed tomography (CT) volumetric images are now in practice (Fig. 13.1). The upper and lower thresholds of anatomical size matching have not been determined at the present time. We have accepted a wide range of volume ratios between the donor's lower lobe graft and the corresponding recipient's chest cavity [13].

13.3   Recipient Operation

13.3.1   Bilateral Cadaveric Lung Transplantation

Patients are anesthetized and intubated with a single-lumen endotracheal tube in children and with a left-sided double-lumen endotracheal tube in adults. When the patient's hemodynamic instability is remarkable, partial cardiopulmonary bypass is initiated using the femoral vessels under local anesthesia. Then, the recipient is anesthetized and intubated. A Swan-Ganz catheter is placed. Intraoperative transesophageal echocardiography is employed routinely. The "clamshell" incision is used and the sternum is transected. The sternum is notched at the level of transection by aiming the sternal saw at a 45° angle and cutting toward the midpoint to facilitate postoperative sternal adaptation. Pleural and hilar dissection is carried out before

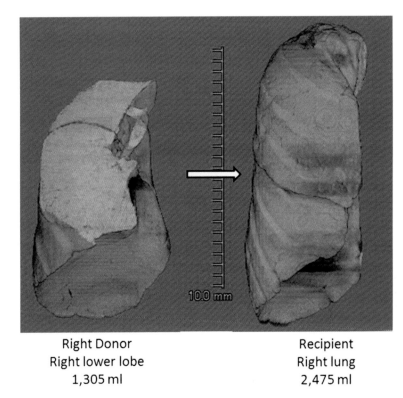

Right Donor   **Recipient**
Right lower lobe   **Right lung**
1,305 ml   **2,475 ml**

Fig. 13.1 Anatomical size matching using three-dimensional volumetry in living-donor lobar lung transplantation. The recipient was an adult female with bronchiolitis obliterans whose right hemithorax was 2475 ml. The right donor was her son whose right lower lobe was 1305 ml. Chest X-ray showed no detectable dead space after transplantation

heparinization to reduce blood loss. The ascending aorta and the right atrium are cannulated after heparinization, and patients are placed on standard cardiopulmonary bypass. We have utilized extracorporeal membrane oxygenation (ECMO) instead of conventional cardiopulmonary bypass (CPB) in most LDLLT procedures since 2012. Activated clotting time is maintained between 180 and 200 s. Use of ECMO with relatively low activated clotting time significantly reduces intraoperative bleeding.

After right pneumonectomy, the right donor lung implantation is performed. The anastomosis sequence of the recipient is the bronchus, left atrium, and pulmonary artery. The bronchial anastomosis is begun with a running 4–0 polydioxanone suture for the membranous portion and completed with simple interrupted sutures or figure of eight suture for the cartilaginous portion. Bronchial wrapping is not employed. The left atrial anastomosis is performed using a running 5–0 Prolene suture. Finally, the pulmonary artery anastomosis is performed in an end-to-end fashion using a running Prolene suture. In pulmonary hypertension patients, pulmonary artery anastomosis is often challenging due to marked size discrepancy. To compensate the

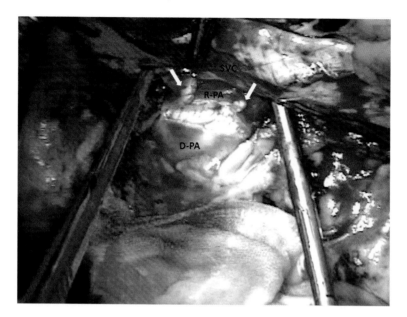

Fig. 13.2 Right pulmonary artery anastomosis during cadaveric bilateral lung transplantation. In patients with pulmonary hypertension, the pulmonary artery is markedly dilated. A vascular clamp is placed behind the superior vena cava (SVC). The right pulmonary artery is transected proximal to the first branch. Leaving long pulmonary artery might increase the risk of arterial kinking after reperfusion. Note the huge size discrepancy between the recipient pulmonary artery (R-PA) and the donor lobar pulmonary artery (D-PA). To compensate the huge size discrepancy, two tack stitches (*white arrows*) were placed on the recipient pulmonary artery in this case

huge size discrepancy, one to four tack stitches are placed on the recipient pulmonary artery (Fig. 13.2). Just before reperfusion, 500 mg of methylprednisolone is given intravenously, and nitric oxide inhalation is initiated at 10–20 ppm. Following right lung implantation, left pneumonectomy and left donor lung implantation is performed in the same manner.

A left atrial line is placed through the left appendage to monitor left atrial pressure. Cardiopulmonary bypass is gradually weaned and then stopped. Heparin is reversed by protamine and careful hemostasis is performed. Two chest tubes are placed in each chest cavity, and the chest is closed in the standard fashion.

13.3.2 Living-Donor Lobar Lung Transplantation

The technique of living-donor lobar lung transplantation is quite similar to that of bilateral cadaveric lung transplantation. The venous anastomosis is placed between the donor's inferior pulmonary vein and the recipient's upper pulmonary vein. Native upper lobes may be preserved when two lower lobe grafts are too small [14].

13.4   Postoperative Management

The patient is kept intubated at a positive end-expiratory pressure of 5 cm H_2O for at least 2 days. Weaning from the ventilator is intentionally slow, and a tracheostomy is performed when patients show any signs of sputum retention. Suction of the chest drainage tubes starts at 10 cm H_2O and gradually decreases to water seal in a couple of days. Fiber-optic bronchoscopy is performed every 12 h while the patient is intubated to assess donor airway viability and to suction any retained secretions. Postoperative immunosuppression is a triple drug therapy consisting of cyclosporine (CSA) or tacrolimus (FK), mycophenolate mofetil (MMF), and corticosteroids. In CLT, transbronchial lung biopsy offers a safe and accurate means of diagnosis of acute rejection and has emerged as the procedure of choice. However, the risk of pneumothorax and bleeding from transbronchial lung biopsy may be higher in LDLLT because the small grafts are receiving high blood flow. It is for this reason that we judge acute rejection on the basis of radiographic and clinical findings. Early acute rejection episodes are characterized by dyspnea, low-grade fever, leukocytosis, hypoxemia, and diffuse interstitial infiltrate on chest radiographs. Because two lobes are donated by different donors, acute rejection is usually seen unilaterally. A trial bolus dose of methylprednisolone 500 mg is administered, and various clinical signs are carefully observed. If acute rejection is indeed the problem, two additional daily bolus doses of methylprednisolone are given.

Because graft ischemic time is short in LDLLT, primary graft dysfunction is infrequently encountered as compared with CLT in general. However, we have encountered severe lung edema associated with left ventricular dysfunction in the early postoperative period both in LDLLT and CLT for patients with pulmonary hypertension. Some patients required ECMO support (Fig. 13.3). Contrary to the early right ventricular function recovery, the impaired left ventricular function persists at 2 months despite findings that left ventricular geometry is restored earlier after reversal of pulmonary hypertension [15]. Chronic preoperative preload reduction may adversely affect left ventricular compliance and muscle stiffness. Most of the patients developing lung edema respond to therapy including steroid pulse, inotropic drugs, afterload reduction with vasodilators, and nitric oxide inhalation. We recommend that patients to be kept on a ventilator for at least 5 days and weaned from the ventilator very slowly along with inotropic support.

13.5   Outcome and Prognosis

According to the registry of International Society for Heart and Lung Transplantation (ISHLT), the 5-year survival after lung transplantation is approximately 50 % [16]. Pulmonary hypertension is known to be a significant risk factor of early death after lung transplantation.

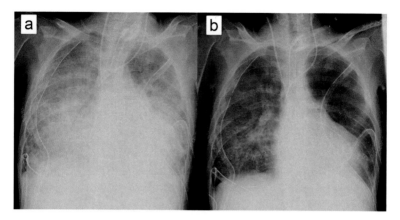

Fig. 13.3 **Severe lung edema after cadaveric bilateral lung transplantation in an adult male patient with idiopathic pulmonary arterial hypertension.** (**a**) On day 7, extracorporeal membrane oxygenation (ECMO) was placed due to severe lung edema. (**b**) On day 10, chest X-ray showed marked improvement and ECMO could be removed

Between 1998 and 2015, lung transplantation has been performed in 464 patients at nine lung transplant centers in Japan. Among these, the author and his colleagues have performed 184 lung transplants including 111 LDLLTs and 73 CLTs.

Thirty-five of them (19 %) were diagnosed with pulmonary hypertension. Twenty-four patients received LDLLT and 11 patients received CLT. Final pathologic diagnoses of the excised lungs were idiopathic pulmonary arterial hypertension (IPAH) in 23 patients, pulmonary veno-occlusive disease (PVOD) in three patients, Eisenmenger syndrome in three patients, pulmonary hypertension associated with connective tissue diseases in two patients, pulmonary capillary hemagiomatosis (PCH) in one patient, and others in three patients.

There were 25 females and 10 males with ages ranging from 6 to 63 years (average 26.4 years). Nine of the patients were children and 26 were adults. Chest X-rays showed dramatic improvement of cardiomegaly both in CLT and LDLLT (Fig. 13.4). Mean pulmonary artery pressure is normalized by the time of discharge and pulmonary hemodynamics continued to be excellent at 3 years (Fig. 13.5) posttransplant. The 5-year survival rate was 81.2 % for pulmonary hypertension (PH) patients (n = 35) and was 72.2 % for non-PH patients (n = 149) (Fig. 13.6).

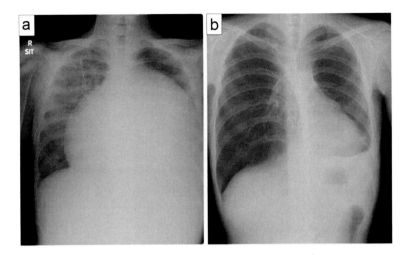

Fig. 13.4 Dramatic improvement of cardiomegaly in a 14-year-old male with idiopathic pulmonary arterial hypertension receiving LDLLT. (**a**) Pretransplant. (**b**) Six months after receiving living-donor lobar lung transplantation (LDLLT)

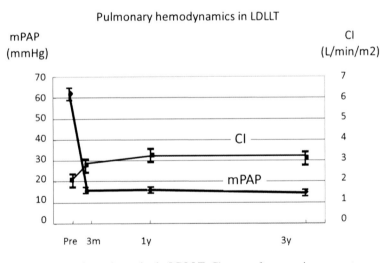

Fig. 13.5 Pulmonary hemodynamics in LDLLT. Changes of mean pulmonary artery pressure (mPAP) and cardiac index (CI) before and after living-donor lobar lung transplantation (LDLLT)

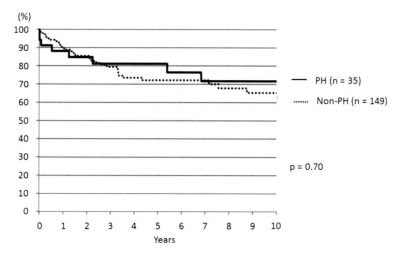

Fig. 13.6 Survival after lung transplantation (*n* = **184**). The 5-year survival rate was 81.2 % for pulmonary hypertension (PH) patients (*n* = 35) and was 72.2 % for non-PH patients (*n* = 149)

13.6   Summary

Lung transplantation is a viable treatment in patients with PAH who failed to respond medical treatment. Because of severe shortage of cadaveric lungs in Japan, living-donor lobar lung transplantation is often the only realistic option for very sick PAH patients especially for children.

References

1. Reitz BA, Wallwork JL, Hunt SA, et al. Heart-lung transplantation: successful therapy for patients with pulmonary vascular disease. N Engl J Med. 1982;306:557–64.
2. The Toronto Lung Transplant Group. Unilateral lung transplantation for pulmonary fibrosis. N Engl J Med. 1986;314:1140–5.
3. Fremes SE, Patterson GA, Williams WG, et al. Single lung transplantation and closure of patent ductus arteriosus for Eisenmenger's syndrome. Toronto Lung Transplant Group. J Thorac Cardiovasc Surg. 1990;100:1–5.
4. Starnes VA, Bowdish ME, Woo MS, et al. A decade of living lobar lung transplantation. Recipient outcomes. J Thorac Cardiovasc Surg. 2004;127:114–22.
5. Date H, Sano Y, Aoe M, Matsubara H, Kusano K, Goto K, Tedoriya T, Shimizu N. Living-donor single lobe lung transplantation for primary pulmonary hypertension in a child. J Thorac Cardiovasc Surg. 2002;123:1211–3.
6. Date H, Nagahiro I, Aoe M, Matsubara H, Kusano K, Goto K, Shimizu N. Living-donor lobar lung transplantation for primary pulmonary hypertension in an adult. J Thorac Cardiovasc Surg. 2001;122:817–8.

7. Date H, Kusano KF, Matsubara H, et al. Living-donor lobar lung transplantation for pulmonary arterial hypertension after failure of epoprostenol therapy. J Am Coll Cardiol. 2007;50:523–7.

8. Date H, Aoe M, Nagahiro I, et al. Living-donor lobar lung transplantation for various lung diseases. J Thorac Cardiovasc Surg. 2003;126:476–81.

9. Date H, Aoe M, Sano Y, et al. Improved survival after living-donor lobar lung transplantation. J Thorac Cardiovasc Surg. 2004;128:933–40.

10. Date H, Sato M, Aoyama A, et al. Living-donor lobar lung transplantation provides similar survival to cadaveric lung transplantation even for very ill patients. Eur J Cardiothorac Surg. 2015;47:967–72.

11. Benza RL, Miller DP, Gomberg-Maitland M, et al. Predicting survival in pulmonary arterial hypertension: insights from the Registry to Evaluate Early and Long-Term Pulmonary Arterial Hypertension Disease Management (REVEAL). Circulation. 2010;122:164–72.

12. Weill D, Benden C, Corris PA, et al. A consensus document for the selection of lung transplant candidates: 2014 – an update from the pulmonary transplantation council of the International Society for Heart and Lung Transplantation. J Heart Lung Transplant. 2015;34:1–15.

13. Chen F, Kubo T, Yamada T, et al. Adaptation over a wide range of donor graft lung size discrepancies in living-donor lobar lung transplantation. Am J Transplant. 2013;13:1336–42.

14. Aoyama A, Chen F, Minakata K, et al. Sparing native upper lobes in living-donor lobar lung transplantation: Five cases from a single center. Am J Transplant. 2015;15:3202–7.

15. Toyooka S, Kusano KF, Goto K, et al. Right but left ventricular function recovers early after living-donor lobar lung transplantation in patients with pulmonary arterial hypertension. J Thorac Cardiovasc Surg. 2009;138:222–6.

16. Yusen RD, Edwards LB, Kucheryavaya AY, et al. The registry of the International Society for Heart Lung Transplantation: Thirty-second official adult lung and heart-lung transplantation report – 2015; focus theme: early graft failure. J Heart Lung Transplant. 2015;34:1264–77.

Part IV
Treatment of Chronic Thromboembolic Pulmonary Hypertension (CTEPH)

Chapter 14
Medical Therapy for Chronic Thromboembolic Pulmonary Hypertension

Toru Satoh

Abstract Prior to the development of pulmonary endarterectomy (PEA), a surgical removal of organized chronic thrombi, there had long been no efficacious treatment to improve the prognosis of patients with chronic thromboembolic pulmonary hypertension (CTEPH). Anticoagulants are initiated when CTEPH is diagnosed to prevent progression, and treatment of hypoxia and right heart failure are added when these complications occur. In the meantime, because small pulmonary arterioles in CTEPH have the same histological abnormality as those in pulmonary arterial hypertension (PAH), which has been called "small vessel disease," the pulmonary vasodilators used in PAH have started to be administered to patients with inoperable CTEPH with peripheral lesions. Retrospective studies showed effectiveness of these vasodilators in improving the prognosis of CTEPH, and riociguat, a newly developed soluble guanylate cyclase (sGC) stimulator, demonstrated significant clinical benefit in 6-min walk distance (6MWD) and pulmonary hemodynamics. However, the effectiveness of vasodilators in patients with operable CTEPH is not known.

Keywords Chronic thromboembolic pulmonary hypertension (CTEPH) • Anticoagulant • Small vessel disease • Riociguat • Pulmonary vasodilator

14.1 Preface: History of Chronic Thromboembolic Pulmonary Hypertension (CTEPH) Treatment

I first experienced a patient with CTEPH in 1983 when I was a second-year intern in medicine. The patient was a middle-aged man with chief complaint of dyspnea on exertion who was referred from another university hospital because the hospital in which I was trained and worked was a referral center for pulmonary hypertension. The patient was diagnosed as idiopathic pulmonary arterial hypertension and

T. Satoh (✉)
Division of Cardiology, Kyorin University School of Medicine,
6-20-2 Shinkawa, Mitaka 181-8611, Tokyo, Japan
e-mail: tsatoh@ks.kyorin-u.ac.jp

© Springer Science+Business Media Singapore 2017
Y. Fukumoto (ed.), *Diagnosis and Treatment of Pulmonary Hypertension*,
DOI 10.1007/978-981-287-840-3_14

had been treated for this entity. Being in NYHA functional class IV when he was admitted, he died about a month later. Postmortem examination was performed, and I still remember the pathologist swiftly making the diagnosis in the pathology theater, stating that there were lots of new and old thrombi in the patient's pulmonary arteries, leading to PH and death. The clinical diagnosis had been incorrect; however, there was no effective treatment even if the patient had been diagnosed correctly.

I started PH practice in 1994 at the National Cardiovascular Center in Japan, the first center specialized in PH in Japan, at which pulmonary endarterectomy (PEA) was about to be introduced. Several surgeons and internists had visited San Diego and learned and brought back the skills for this new surgery. Over several years, the technique progressed to the present advanced and stable procedure. This course of change in treatment signifies that surgical treatment preceded medical treatment, other than anticoagulants to prevent further thrombi, oxygen inhalation in hypoxic patients, and heart failure treatment such as diuretics, cardiac stimulants, and other general medical measures. Since those development, pulmonary vasodilators, originally used in pulmonary arterial hypertension (PAH) (type 1 PH), have been almost routinely used in patients with CTEPH in Japan.

14.2   Types of Medical Therapy in CTEPH

14.2.1   Anticoagulants

Anticoagulants inhibit thrombus formation in the pulmonary arteries and deep veins, which are possible sources of thrombi in chronic, organized pulmonary emboli [1]. There has been no randomized prospective study to prove the effectiveness of anticoagulants for CTEPH [2]. However, many guidelines state that anticoagulants are absolutely indicated in the treatment of CTEPH [3].

14.2.1.1   Types of Anticoagulants

Because of no prospective randomized study of the effectiveness of anticoagulants for CTEPH, studies on anticoagulants used for maintenance treatment for patients with acute pulmonary embolism may be applied to those with CTEPH. Coumadin has been used for this purpose, *but* there has been no report on the usefulness of new direct oral anticoagulants (DOAC) in this phase of chronic anticoagulation after the acute phase [4]. According to a recently published meta-analysis comparing the overall usefulness among the present anticoagulants, aspirin, Coumadin, and new drug, DOAC, DOAC gave more benefit than control, and the latter two drugs yielded more benefit than the first drug [5].

14.2.2   Oxygen, Treatment for Right Heart Failure, and Other Medical Treatment

There has been no prospective study showing the benefit of oxygen administration, treatment for right heart failure, and other supportive treatment for PH. These treatments are considered obviously necessary when indicated in Western guidelines, suggesting that inhaled ambulatory oxygen should be given when SpO_2 is less than 90–95 %, and loop diuretics, tolvaptan, and cardiotonics are indicated in cases of right heart failure.

14.2.3   Pulmonary Vasodilators

14.2.3.1   Types of Vasodilators

Pulmonay vasodilators have been applied to patients with PAH after they were validated as effective in randomized controlled trials (RCT) in those patients. These drugs are described in detail elsewhere. They are classified into three groups according to their pharmacological mechanism of action: prostaglandin I_2, nitric oxide (NO)-related compounds, and endothelin receptor antagonists. Among these vasodilators, only riociguat (a guanylate cyclase stimulator) demonstrated significant efficacy in patients with CTEPH in RCT.

14.2.3.2   Mechanism of Action of Vasodilators in CTEPH

Because pulmonary arterial lesions, which are histopathologically similar to those in PAH, are also recognized in CTEPH [6], it has been thought that secondary changes in small pulmonary arterioles, thickened vascular medial smooth muscle and proliferated vascular intima, etc., also occur in CTEPH, the so-called small vessel disease.

14.2.3.3   Positioning of Vasodilator Therapy in Chronic Thromboembolic Pulmonary Hypertension (CTEPH) Practice from Guidelines

According to the present guidelines prevailing in Western countries, medical therapy in CTEPH is contemplated when it is impossible to perform surgical treatment (PEA) (Fig. 14.1) [7], which means that surgery always antecedes drug therapy and that the outcome of medical treatment in patients with CTEPH has not been well evaluated. Because reimbursement by medical insurance for drugs in general is more affordable in Japan, medical therapy for patients with CTEPH is readily applied before surgical treatment.

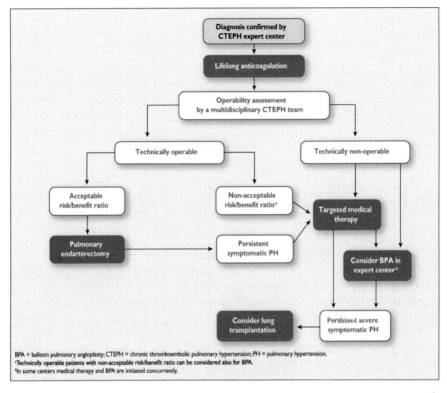

Fig. 14.1 Present treatment guidelines for chronic pulmonary thromboembolic pulmonary hypertension (CTEPH) from 2015 ESC/ERS Guidelines for the diagnosis and treatment of pulmonary hypertension [7]
Medical treatment is chosen when patients are diagnosed as inoperable.

14.2.3.4 Efficacy of Vasodilators in Patients with Inoperable CTEPH

In 2013, one of the most recent retrospective studies on the prognosis of CTEPH using drug therapy was reported in Japan [8]. Ninety-five patients were enrolled from 1986 to 2010, including a majority of patients with peripheral lesions excluded from thromboendarterectomy with mean pulmonary arterial pressure (mPAP) of 43 mmHg. The patients were divided into two groups, one with modern PAH drug therapy including sildenafil and/or bosentan and the other without such therapy. The 5-year survival of the former group was 89 % and that of the latter was 60 %. Inoperable CTEPH patients with drug therapy had a significantly better outcome than those without. The 5-year survival in inoperable CTEPH patients with vasodilatory drugs was comparable to that of those with operable CTEPH [9]. According to other studies on medical therapy for CTEPH, Suntharalingam et al. reported in 2007 that 3-year survival was 53 % in 35 CTEPH patients with distal lesions receiving medical therapy [10]. Condliffe et al. reported in 2008 that 3-year survival was 76 % in 148 patients with distal lesions, with average mPAP of 49 mmHg, 90 % of whom were receiving contemporary pulmonary vasodilators [11]. Without administration of vasodilators or PEA, the famous report concerning the natural history of CTEPH patients by Riedel demonstrated that 5-year survival was 10 % when mPAP exceeded 50 mmHg [12].

14.2.3.5   RCTs of Vasodilators in CTEPH

Prior to riociguat, of which clinical effectiveness in RCT was proved in 2013, there had been no vasodilatory drugs that attained the targets in studies for CTEPH [13]. Before riociguat, bosentan improved the hemodynamics in patients with CTEPH but not 6-minute walk distance (6MWD) resulting in regarded as ineffective, because the drug did not fulfill the primary target of the study (BENEFiT study) [14]. These results mean that vasodilators used for PAH can at least ameliorate the hemodynamics in CTEPH patients. Bosentan is an endothelin receptor blocker and has been used for patients with PAH since 2005 in Japan. A prospective study to investigate its usefulness in patients with inoperable CTEPH was conducted in Western countries, and the results were published in 2008 [14]. One hundred fifty-seven patients were enrolled. Pulmonary vascular resistance (PVR) and cardiac index (CI) were statistically significantly improved compared to placebo, but 6MWD was not. PVR was decreased from baseline by 24.1 % (95 % confidence interval [CI], 31.5 % to 16.0 %; $p = 0.0001$), cardiac index was increased by 0.3 L/min/m^2 (95 % CI, 0.14 to 0.46 L/min/m^2; $p = 0.0007$), and mean change in 6-min walk distance was improved by 2.2 m (95 % CI, 22.5 to 26.8 m; $p = 0.5449$) (Table 14.1).

Table 14.1   Mean treatment effect in patients with or without previous PEA in PVR ($n = 137$[a])

	Placebo ($n = 71$)		Bosentan ($n = 66$)		
	Baseline (dyn·s·cm^{-5})	Change (dyn·s·cm^{-5})	Baseline (dyn·s·cm^{-5})	Change (dyn·s·cm^{-5})	Treatment effect[b] (%)
PEA[c]	700 (561 to 839)	+81 (−21 to 183)	735 (596 to 874)	−193 (−278 to −108)	−34.0 (−45.6 to −20.0)
No PEA[d]	826 (729 to 923)	+7 (−59 to 73)	795 (696 to 894)	−127 (−206 to −48)	−19.5 (−28.7 to −9.1)
Overall	787 (708 to 866)	+30 (−25 to 85)	778 (698 to 857)	−146 (−207 to −85)	−24.1 (−31.5 to −16.0)

Values are mean (95 % confidence interval)
PEA pulmonary endarterectomy, *PVR* pulmonary vascular resistance
[a]Excluding patients considered operable post-randomization by the Operability Evaluation Committee and those with missing baseline or post-baseline assessments
[b]Shown as percentage of baseline
[c]41 patients (22 in placebo group, 19 in bosentan group)
[d]96 patients (49 in placebo group, 47 in bosentan group)

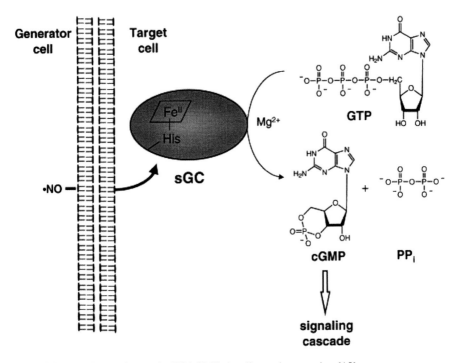

Fig. 14.2 Guanylate cyclase and c NO/cGMP signaling pathway review [15]
cGMP, an arterial dilator, is produced from GTP aided by coenzyme guanylate cyclase, which is
stimulated by NO (nitric oxide)

Riociguat

Riociguat is a direct soluble guanylate cyclase (sGC) stimulant. sGC is an enzyme
that intervenes in the reaction of production of cyclic guanosine monophosphate
(cGMP) from guanosine triphosphate (GTP). Nitric oxide (NO) stimulates sGC and
induces vasodilatation through the pathway mentioned above (Fig. 14.2) [15].
cGMP relaxes smooth muscle located in the pulmonary artery medial layer via
activation of protein kinase G. Other NO-pathway-related vasodilators such as
sildenafil and tadalafil inhibit a cGMP destruction enzyme, phosphodiesterase V.

PATENT-1[13] and PATENT-2[16] studies showed the clinical effect of riociguat. In PATENT-1, 443 patients enrolled were divided into a riociguat group with
administration of 2.5 mg tid and placebo group. After 3 months, 6MWD was
improved by 30 m, as well as significant improvements in PVR, NT-proBNP, WHO
functional class, period until exacerbation, and Borg dyspnea score in exercise test
(Fig. 14.3). Serious adverse events (AE) were syncope, hemoptysis, and pulmonary
hemorrhage. Syncope was experienced by 1 % in the riociguat group and 4 % in
placebo, indicating that it was attributable to PH worsening. Hemoptysis and

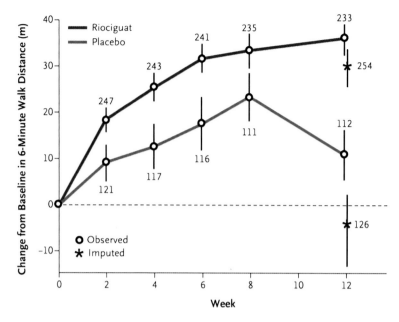

Fig. 14.3 Improvement in 6-minute walk distance from baseline in CTEPH by riociguat [13] Mean (±SE) change from baseline in 6-minute walk distance after 16 weeks' treatment with riociguat is shown compared to placebo. The mean difference in distance at 16 weeks was 46 m (95 % CI, 25 to 67; *P* < 0.001)

pulmonary hemorrhage occurred in seven patients in the riociguat group and none in placebo. In open-label PATENT-2, 396 patients with CTEPH received riociguat, and 6MWD after 1 year was improved by 51 m on average and NYHA functional class by 33 %. Serious AEs were hemoptysis and pulmonary hemorrhage in eight patients in the riociguat group. The causal relationship of riociguat to hemoptysis and pulmonary hemorrhage was not determined; however, a warning regarding hemoptysis and pulmonary hemorrhage with riociguat was made. These two studies confirmed the efficacy of riociguat in inoperable CTEPH in Japan in 2015, as well as in Western countries.

14.2.3.6 Future Direction of Pulmonary Vasodilators

It is not still known how pulmonary vasodilators are effective in patients with operable CTEPH. Considering the progress of newly developed vasodilators, an application of vasodilators to even operable CTEPH patients should be considered. Nevertheless, complete replacement of PEA or pulmonary angioplasty with drug therapy is impossible in the current situation.

References

1. Piazza G, Goldhaber SZ. Chronic thromboembolic pulmonary hypertension. N Engl J Med. 2011;364:351–60.
2. Hoeper MM. Pharmacological therapy for patients with chronic thromboembolic pulmonary hypertension. Eur Respir Rev. 2015;136:272–82.
3. Galiè N, Hoeper MM, Humbert M, Torbicki A, Vachiery J-A, Barbera JA, Beghetti M, Corris P, Gaine S, Gibbs JS, Gomez-Sanchez MA, Jondeau G, Klepetko W, Opitz C, Peacock A, Rubin L, Zellweger M, Simonneau G, Task Force for Diagnosis and Treatment of Pulmonary Hypertension of European Society of Cardiology (ESC), European Respiratory Society (ERS), International Society of Heart and Lung Transplantation (ISHLT). Guidelines for the diagnosis and treatment of pulmonary hypertension. Eur Respir J. 2009;34:1219–63.
4. Limbrey R, Howard L. Developments in the management and treatment of pulmonary embolism. Eur Respir Rev. 2015;24(137):484–97.
5. Marik PE, Cavallazi R. Extended anticoagulant and aspirin treatment for the secondary prevention of thromboembolic disease: a systematic review and meta-analysis. PLoS One. 2015;10(11).
6. Yi ES, Kim H, Ahn H, Strother J, Morris T, Masliah E, Hansen LA, Park K, Friedman PJ. Distribution of obstructive intimal lesions and their cellular phenotypes in chronic pulmonary hypertension. A morphometric and immunohistochemical study. Am J Respir Crit Care Med. 2000;162:1577–86.
7. Galie N, Humbert M, JL V, Gibbs S, Lang I, Torbicki A, Simonneau G, Peacock A, Vonk Noordegraaf A, Beghetti M, Ghofrani A, MA GS, Hansmann G, Klepetko W, Lancellotti P, Matucci M, McDonagh T, LA P, PT T, Zompatori M, Hoeper M. Chronic thromboembolic pulmonary hypertension (group 4) 2015 ESC/ERS guidelines for the diagnosis and treatment of pulmonary hypertension: The Joint Task Force for the Diagnosis and Treatment of Pulmonary Hypertension of the European Society of Cardiology (ESC) and the European Respiratory Society (ERS): endorsed by: Association for European Paediatric and Congenital Cardiology (AEPC), International Society for Heart and Lung Transplantation (ISHLT). Eur Respir J. 2015;46(4):942–5.
8. Nishimura R, Tanabe N, Sugiura T, Shigeta A, Jujo T, Sekine A, Sakao S, Kasahara Y, Tatsumi K. Improved survival in medically treated chronic thromboembolic pulmonary hypertension. Circ J. 2013;77(8):2110–7.
9. Freed DH, Thomson BM, Berman M, et al. Survival after pulmonary thromboendarterectomy: effect of residual pulmonary hypertension. J Thorac Cardiovasc Surg. 2011;141:383–7.
10. Suntharalingam J, Machado RD, Sharples LD, et al. Demographic features, BMPR2 status and outcomes in distal chronic thromboembolic pulmonary hypertension. Thorax. 2007;62:617–22.
11. Condliffe R, Kiely DG, Gibbs JS, et al. Improved outcomes in medically and surgically treated chronic thromboembolic pulmonary hypertension. Am J Respir Crit Care Med. 2008;177:1122–7.
12. Riedel M, Stanek V, Widimsky J, Prerovsky I. Longterm follow-up of patients with pulmonary thromboembolism. Late prognosis and evolution of hemodynamic and respiratory data. Chest. 1982;81(2):151–8.
13. Ghofrani HA, D'Armini AM, Grimminger F, Hoeper MM, Jansa P, Kim NH, Mayer E, Simonneau G, Wilkins MR, Fritsch A, Neuser D, Weimann G, Wang C. Riociguat for the treatment of chronic thromboembolic pulmonary hypertension. N Engl J Med. 2013;369:319–29.
14. Jaïs X, D'Armini AM, Jansa P, et al. Bosentan for treatment of inoperable chronic thromboembolic pulmonary hypertension: BENEFiT (Bosentan Effects in iNopErable Forms of chronIc Thromboembolic pulmonary hypertension), a randomized, placebo-controlled trial. J Am Coll Cardiol. 2008;52:2127–34.
15. Denninger JW, Marletta MA. Guanylate cyclase and the c NO/cGMP signaling pathway review. Biochim Biophys Acta. 1999;1411:334–50.
16. Rubin LJ, Galiè N, Grimminger F, Grünig E, Humbert M, Jing ZC, Keogh A, Langleben D, Fritsch A, Menezes F, Davie N, Ghofrani HA. Riociguat for the treatment of pulmonary arterial hypertension: a long-term extension study (PATENT-2). Eur Respir J. 2015;45(5):1303–13.

Chapter 15
Balloon Pulmonary Angioplasty

Hiromi Matsubara and Aiko Ogawa

Abstract Balloon pulmonary angioplasty (BPA) is a promising treatment option for patients with chronic thromboembolic pulmonary hypertension who are considered ineligible for surgical treatment. Since 2012, the effect of balloon pulmonary angioplasty has been reported mainly in Japan, but currently, it is attracting the attention of many pulmonary hypertension specialists worldwide. Since balloon pulmonary angioplasty has not yet been established as an alternative treatment for these patients, we briefly explain its history, indication, fundamental techniques, complications and prevention methods, and treatment effects. Additionally, we address the limitations and future perspective of balloon pulmonary angioplasty in this chapter.

Keywords Angioplasty • Inoperable chronic thromboembolic pulmonary hypertension • Pulmonary injury

15.1 Introduction

Chronic thromboembolic pulmonary hypertension (CTEPH) is classified as group 4 pulmonary hypertension, according to the clinical classification of pulmonary hypertension [1]. The main cause of this disorder is angiographically visible stenoses or obstructions of the pulmonary arteries due to organized thrombus formation. When an organized thrombus becomes a part of the vascular structures, thrombolytic therapy or anticoagulation is no longer effective for treating CTEPH. The surgical

H. Matsubara (✉)
Department of Cardiology, National Hospital Organization Okayama Medical Center, Okayama, Japan

Department of Clinical Science, National Hospital Organization Okayama Medical Center, Okayama, Japan
e-mail: matsubara.hiromi@gmail.com

A. Ogawa
Department of Clinical Science, National Hospital Organization Okayama Medical Center, Okayama, Japan

© Springer Science+Business Media Singapore 2017
Y. Fukumoto (ed.), *Diagnosis and Treatment of Pulmonary Hypertension*,
DOI 10.1007/978-981-287-840-3_15

removal of organized thrombi (i.e., pulmonary endarterectomy [PEA]) can resolve the stenoses or obstructions of the pulmonary arteries, and thus cure CTEPH [2]. However, some patients cannot be treated by PEA because of surgically inaccessible lesions or comorbidities [3, 4]. Although patients who are ineligible for PEA have been treated with pulmonary hypertension-specific vasodilators, none of these drugs can sufficiently decrease pulmonary arterial pressure [5–7]. Thus, alternative treatment for these patients is needed.

Balloon pulmonary angioplasty (BPA) was first used to treat CTEPH in 1988 [8]. In 2001, the results of BPA in 18 cases of inoperable CTEPH were reported [9]; however, the procedure was not yet widely used, because its effect was inferior to PEA, and it was associated with a high in hospital mortality rate. Recently, a few research groups, including ours, have reported results of various refinements to the BPA technique [10–12]. The efficacy and safety of BPA have been dramatically improved compared to those reported by Feinstein and colleagues in 2001. Now BPA would be a promising treatment option for patients with CTEPH who are ineligible for PEA.

15.2   Indications and Contraindications of BPA

Although some facilities have initiated a BPA program and reported favorable outcomes [13–16], BPA is not yet an established treatment for CTEPH [1]. It is still uncertain whether patients' characteristics such as age, sex, and the duration of the disease affect the results of BPA. Currently, the standard treatment for CTEPH is PEA [1, 17]. Therefore, patients with CTEPH who are ineligible for PEA would be candidates for BPA. Even patients with residual pulmonary hypertension after PEA would be candidates for BPA [18].

The use of contrast medium is essential for performing BPA; thus, it is difficult to perform BPA in patients with an iodine allergy. The benefits of performing BPA in light of these aforementioned risks must be considered in cases with renal dysfunction, even though there was a reported case of improvement of renal function after BPA [19]. Patients with complete obstruction (i.e., a pouching defect) in one of the pulmonary artery trunks may not be candidates for BPA, because recanalization of thick organized thrombi without resection is almost impossible in such cases.

15.3   Technique of BPA

Anticoagulants, which are commonly used in patients with CTEPH, can be replaced with heparin, but they may be continued during BPA. Also, pulmonary hypertension-targeted drugs can be continued if the drugs have been already prescribed before BPA. However, it can be expected that those drugs will only achieve minor reductions in the mean pulmonary arterial pressure [5–7, 11]. Thus, the additional use of pulmonary hypertension-targeted drugs immediately before BPA should be avoided to save time and money.

The BPA procedure is approached either through the right internal jugular vein or the right femoral vein. For inexperienced operators, the internal jugular vein approach is recommended, because manipulation of the guiding catheter is easier. For those with sufficient experience, the femoral vein approach is recommended, because one operator can manipulate both the guiding catheter and the guidewire via the guiding catheter with little difficulty. After inserting a 6–7 French long introducer sheath through the vein into the pulmonary artery, 500–2500 units of heparin are administered to reach an activated clotting time of around 200 s, and an additional 500–1000 units of heparin are administered hourly. A 6–7 French guiding catheter (e.g., a multipurpose type, Judkins right type, or Amplatz left type) is advanced into the segmental pulmonary artery. After performing selective pulmonary angiography (Fig. 15.1a), a 0.014-in. guidewire is used to cross the lesion. Then a balloon catheter of an appropriate diameter (1.5–10 mm) is selected to dilate the lesion (Fig. 15.1b). The balloon size is determined according to findings on various diagnostic images, including selective pulmonary angiography [12, 20], intravascular ultrasound [11, 16], and optical coherence tomography [21, 22]. Each imaging technique has advantages and disadvantages; therefore, it is difficult to determine which technique is the best. Whichever imaging technique is used, it is important to select a smaller-sized balloon to prevent overdilatation of the lesion, especially during initial treatment of the lesion [23]. Since lesions usually exist in almost all segments, the treatment of all lesions in one procedure is impossible. The number and distribution of targets for treatment should be decided according to the operator's experience and the patients' condition. In previous reports, the target area for one procedure was reported to be 2–4 segments in the unilateral lung [10–13]. To obtain sufficient reduction of the pulmonary arterial pressure, the procedure had to be repeated 4–8 times.

Special care after the BPA procedure would be unnecessary if no complications occurred during the procedure. However, if a BPA-related pulmonary injury occurs, appropriate devices such as artificial ventilation via intubation or extracorporeal membrane oxygenation should be used to maintain the patient's oxygenation [11]. In cases with evident pulmonary bleeding (e.g., when the extravasation of contrast medium is observed during pulmonary angiography or when massive hemoptysis occurs after dilatation of the lesion), achieving hemostasis with these treatments is challenging. Stopping the bleeding with intravascular treatments may be required [11, 24]. In cases that experience pulmonary hemorrhage during or after the procedure, pulmonary edema may occur ≥24 h after the BPA procedure. In such cases, methylprednisolone administration may be needed.

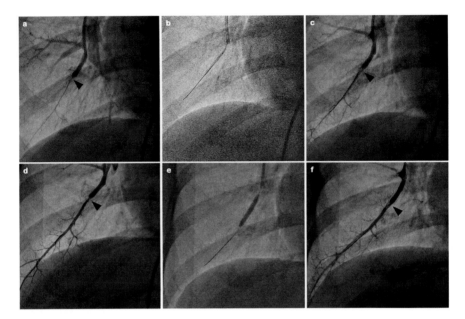

Fig. 15.1 Representative fluoroscopic images before, during, and immediately after balloon pulmonary angioplasty for chronic thromboembolic pulmonary hypertension

The target was the lateral branch of the right basal artery (A9). The *upper panels* (**a–c**) are images from the initial treatment of the lesion. The *lower panels* (**d–f**) are images from the second treatment of the lesion (i.e., the third procedure, 1 month after the initial treatment). Before the initial procedure, the patient's mean pulmonary arterial pressure was 40 mmHg, and it decreased to 33 mmHg after treating 14 segments during two procedures with a 2-mm diameter balloon catheter. To complete the patient's treatment, four procedures were required. After the fourth procedure, the patient's mean pulmonary arterial pressure decreased to 24 mmHg

(a) Subtotal occlusion (*arrowhead*) was observed at the mid-part of the segmental artery

(b) The lesion was dilated with a 2-mm diameter balloon catheter

(c) Flow distal to the lesion was restored, although stenosis (*arrowhead*) remained

(d) The lesion (*arrowhead*) and the vessel distal to the lesion were spontaneously expanded without additional dilatation

(e) The lesion was dilated again with a 3.5-mm diameter balloon catheter

(f) The lesion (*arrowhead*) was optimally dilated

15.4 Complications after BPA and Prevention Methods

Pulmonary injury after the procedure is a unique and major complication of BPA. It is characterized by a newly developed chest radiographic opacity that corresponds to the treated segment and the worsening of oxygen saturation (Fig. 15.2) [9, 11–13]. The incidence of BPA-related pulmonary injury was reported to be 9.6–51.9 % [9, 11–13]. Thus, BPA is an invasive treatment for CTEPH, although the percutaneous approach of BPA seems minimally invasive. Previously, it was believed that reperfusion itself was the cause of BPA-related pulmonary injury; therefore, it was considered to be unavoidable. To minimize the occurrence or severity of pulmonary

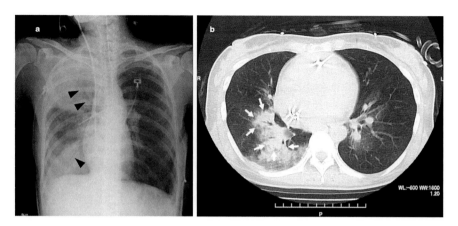

Fig. 15.2 Representative chest radiography and computed tomography images of the pulmonary injury after the initial balloon pulmonary angioplasty procedure
Treated segments included the apical branch of the right upper lobe (A1), anterior branch of the right basal artery (A8), and posterior branch of the right basal artery (A10)
(a) Chest radiography image obtained about 4 h after the procedure. Radiographic opacities were observed that corresponded to the treated segments. It appeared to be pulmonary edema, because an air bronchogram (*arrowheads*) was observed within the radiographic opacity
(b) Computed tomography image obtained immediately after the procedure. A high-density area (*arrows*) was observed only around A8 and A10, indicating the local hemorrhage around the treated site

injury after BPA, the number of treated segments in a procedure was restricted to 2–4 segments in previous reports [10–13]. However, the incidence of pulmonary injury after BPA was not decreased by limiting the number of treated segments [9, 11]. Conversely, the incidence of pulmonary injury after BPA was reported to decrease with the operator's experience [11]. This indicates that the main cause of pulmonary injury after BPA is a technical issue. Unlike systemic or coronary arteries, the vessel wall of the pulmonary artery is very thin. In patients with CTEPH, the vessel wall proximal to the lesion may be remodeled by being exposed to a high pulmonary arterial pressure and covered by mural organized thrombi. In contrast, the vessel wall distal to the lesion would maintain its original fragility because of the absence of a high internal pressure. Mechanical minor injury of the vessel wall caused by the tip of the wire and an abrupt increase in internal pressure due to dilatation of the lesion may result in a hemorrhage distal to the treated segment. Inserting the guidewire too deep and injecting contrast medium too strongly may be a cause of pulmonary injury after BPA. Both of these situations can be avoided by improving the operator's experience.

Another cause of pulmonary injury after BPA may be overdilatation of the lesion. Organized thrombi in patients with CTEPH mainly consists of collagen fibers. It is hardly compressed by balloon dilatation. According to the pathological findings of post-BPA lesions, balloon dilatation seems to increase the lumen cross-sectional area of the lesion by detaching the organized thrombus partially from the vessel wall and stretching the thin vessel wall [23]. Although dilatation using a larger balloon seems to decrease residual stenosis at the lesion site, it also increases local dissection of the pulmonary artery at the treated lesion site, which may result in an oozing hemorrhage from the lesion. Dilatation using a smaller balloon would decrease the risks of an oozing hemorrhage at the treated site, and it would protect the fragile vessel wall distal to the lesion from an abrupt increase in perfusion pressure [25]. Currently, the most reasonable way to prevent pulmonary injury after BPA is by restricting the balloon size, not the number of target segments [26]. Of course, stenosis remains immediately after dilatation when using a smaller balloon compared to the vessel diameter at the lesion site (Fig. 15.1c). However, the lumen at the treated lesion site and the vessel distal to the lesion spontaneously expand over time [11], probably because the thin vessel wall caused by detachment of the organized thrombi may be progressively stretched by a high pulmonary arterial pressure (Fig. 15.1d). Additional dilatation using an optimal-sized balloon can be performed 1–3 months after the initial treatment without the risk of vascular injury, if it is necessary (Fig. 15.1e, f).

15.5   Effect of BPA

The effect of BPA depends on the degree of restoration of lung perfusion. It has already been reported that the number of treated segments is directory correlated with the decrease in pulmonary arterial pressure [11]. In 2001, Feinstein et al. reported that with an average of six dilations during 2.7 BPA procedures, the mean pulmonary arterial pressure of their patient group decreased by 9.3 mmHg [9]. In 2012, we reported that with an average of 12 dilations during four BPA procedures, the mean pulmonary arterial pressure of the patient group decreased by 21.4 mmHg [11]. The effect of BPA in reducing pulmonary arterial pressure was approximately doubled by doubling the target segments. The degree of residual stenosis at the target lesion would also influence the effect of BPA. To maintain the treatment effect of the procedure using a smaller balloon, it may be necessary to increase the number of target segments treated in one procedure.

The number of target segments and procedures should be determined according to the treatment goal at each facility. Currently at our facility, the treatment goal of BPA for patients with CTEPH is to cure the disorder (i.e., achieve a mean pulmonary arterial pressure <25 mmHg and stopping home oxygen therapy) (Fig. 15.3). We need to treat more lesions than we used to, in order to achieve this goal. The effectiveness of BPA is expected to be maintained in the long term, because restenosis of the treated lesion after BPA is uncommon [11]. From November 2004 to December 2015, 1700 BPA procedures were performed at our hospital on 294 patients with CTEPH who were deemed ineligible for PEA. Among them, 252 patients completed BPA and 197 returned for a follow-up (range 0.2–6 years, average 1.8 years after the final BPA procedure) right heart catheter examination. Table 15.1 shows changes in the hemodynamics and 6-minute walking distances before and

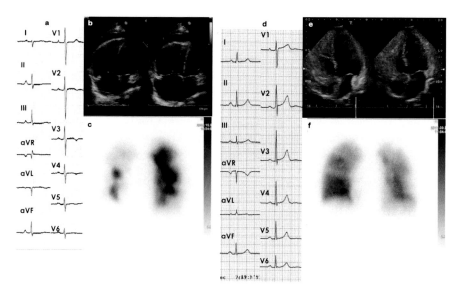

Fig. 15.3 Representative electrocardiograms, echocardiograms, and lung perfusion scintigrams before (**a–c**) and 6 months after (**d–f**) the final balloon pulmonary angioplasty (BPA) procedure in the same patient shown in Fig. 15.2

To complete the patient's treatment, 15 segments were needed to be treated in six procedures. The patient's mean pulmonary arterial pressure decreased from 63 to 23 mmHg

(a) Electrocardiogram before BPA indicating a right axial deviation and marked right ventricular hypertrophy

(b) Echocardiogram before BPA showing marked dilatation of the right atrium and ventricle

(c) Lung perfusion scintigram before BPA indicating multiple perfusion defects in bilateral lungs

(d) The right axial deviation and right ventricular hypertrophy on electrocardiogram disappeared after BPA

(e) The size of the right atrium and ventricle normalized after BPA

(f) Perfusion of bilateral lungs was remarkably improved after BPA

Table 15.1 The latest outcomes of balloon pulmonary angioplasty at Okayama Medical Center

	Before BPA (n = 294)	After BPA (n = 252)	Follow-up (n = 197)
6MWD (m)	264 ± 138	380 ± 95*	409 ± 111*
Systolic PAP (mmHg)	73.9 ± 21.2	39.6 ± 10.1*	34.5 ± 8.5*
Mean PAP (mmHg)	42.6 ± 12.0	23.3 ± 5.4*	20.5 ± 4.9*
RAP (mmHg)	7.3 ± 4.5	3.2 ± 2.5*	3.7± 3.0*
CI (L/min/m²)	2.7 ± 0.8	3.0 ± 0.8*	2.6 ± 0.6
PVR (dyne·sec·cm⁻⁵)	727 ± 373	321 ± 130*	274 ± 109*

BPA, balloon pulmonary angioplasty; *follow-up*, 1.8 ± 1.3 years (range, 0.2–6.0 years) after the final BPA; *6MWD*, 6-minute walking distance; *PAP*, pulmonary artery pressure; *RAP*, right atrial pressure; *CI*, cardiac index; *PVR*, pulmonary vascular resistance; * $p < 0.05$ vs. before BPA

The patient numbers before BPA include seven cases of inhospital death (inhospital mortality rate, 2.4 %)

after BPA and at the follow-up right heart catheter examination. Patients' hemodynamics and exercise capacity were significantly improved after BPA. The improvement was maintained at the time of follow-up. Similarly, recent studies have shown evidence of an improvement in hemodynamics and exercise capacity [11–13, 27]. The 2-year survival rate after BPA treatment has been reported to be 100 % [10]. The 1-, 3-, and 5-year survival rates at our hospital are 97 %, 95 %, and 92 %, respectively. Thus, the long-term prognosis of patients with CTEPH treated with BPA seems to be comparable to the prognosis of those who have undergone PEA. All these effects of BPA are superior to those of medicinal treatment.

15.6   Limitations of BPA

As previously mentioned, there is a learning curve for reducing pulmonary injury after BPA [11]. In our experience, the effect of BPA is also influenced by the operator's proficiency. Arteries in the middle or lingular lobes are difficult for inexperienced operators to treat. When these four segments are left untreated, patients' hemodynamic improvement will be insufficient. Accordingly, the safety and efficacy of BPA depend on the operator's experience and skill. This is the most difficult problem with BPA, which is similar to PEA. Since CTEPH is a rare disease, it would be necessary to accumulate enough patients at BPA centers so that operators can experience a sufficient number of BPA procedures. Currently, devices (e.g., guiding catheters, guidewires, and balloon catheters) for coronary or peripheral arteries are diverted for BPA [11–13]. Of course, the anatomy of the pulmonary arteries is totally different from those of the coronary or peripheral arteries. Therefore, the development of BPA-specific devices is necessary to standardize the BPA procedure. Although the recently reported effects of BPA are superior to those of medicinal treatment, a prospective randomized control trial is necessary to confirm the superiority of BPA over medicinal treatment. The cost-effectiveness of the BPA procedures also needs clarification.

15.7   Conclusions

BPA would be an alternative treatment for patients with CTEPH who are ineligible for PEA. We believe that in the near future, BPA will be a standard treatment for patients, although further progress in the field of clinical research is needed.

References

1. Galie N, Humbert M, Vachiery JL, Gibbs S, Lang I, Torbicki A et al. 2015 ESC/ERS Guidelines for the diagnosis and treatment of pulmonary hypertension: The Joint Task Force for the Diagnosis and Treatment of Pulmonary Hypertension of the European Society of Cardiology (ESC) and the European Respiratory Society (ERS): Endorsed by: Association for European Paediatric and Congenital Cardiology (AEPC), International Society for Heart and Lung Transplantation (ISHLT). Eur Heart J. 2016;37(1):67–119. doi:10.1093/eurheartj/ehv317.
2. Madani MM, Auger WR, Pretorius V, Sakakibara N, Kerr KM, Kim NH et al. Pulmonary endarterectomy: recent changes in a single institution's experience of more than 2,700 patients. Ann Thorac Surg. 2012;94(1):97–103; discussion doi:10.1016/j.athoracsur.2012.04.004.
3. Pepke-Zaba J, Delcroix M, Lang I, Mayer E, Jansa P, Ambroz D et al. Chronic thromboembolic pulmonary hypertension (CTEPH): results from an international prospective registry. Circulation. 2011;124(18):1973–81. doi:10.1161/CIRCULATIONAHA.110.015008.
4. Hurdman J, Condliffe R, Elliot CA, Davies C, Hill C, Wild JM et al. ASPIRE registry: assessing the spectrum of pulmonary hypertension identified at a referral centre. Eur Respir J. 2012;39(4):945–55. doi:10.1183/09031936.00078411.
5. Reichenberger F, Voswinckel R, Enke B, Rutsch M, El Fechtali E, Schmehl T et al. Long-term treatment with sildenafil in chronic thromboembolic pulmonary hypertension. Eur Respir J. 2007;30(5):922–7. doi:10.1183/09031936.00039007.
6. Jais X, D'Armini AM, Jansa P, Torbicki A, Delcroix M, Ghofrani HA et al. Bosentan for treatment of inoperable chronic thromboembolic pulmonary hypertension: BENEFiT (Bosentan Effects in iNopErable Forms of chronIc Thromboembolic pulmonary hypertension), a randomized, placebo-controlled trial. J Am Coll Cardiol. 2008;52(25):2127–34. doi:10.1016/j.jacc.2008.08.059.
7. Ghofrani HA, D'Armini AM, Grimminger F, Hoeper MM, Jansa P, Kim NH et al. Riociguat for the treatment of chronic thromboembolic pulmonary hypertension. N Engl J Med. 2013;369(4):319–29. doi:10.1056/NEJMoa1209657.
8. Voorburg JA, Cats VM, Buis B, Bruschke AV. Balloon angioplasty in the treatment of pulmonary hypertension caused by pulmonary embolism. Chest. 1988;94(6):1249–53.
9. Feinstein JA, Goldhaber SZ, Lock JE, Ferndandes SM, Landzberg MJ. Balloon pulmonary angioplasty for treatment of chronic thromboembolic pulmonary hypertension. Circulation. 2001;103(1):10–3.
10. Sugimura K, Fukumoto Y, Satoh K, Nochioka K, Miura Y, Aoki T et al. Percutaneous transluminal pulmonary angioplasty markedly improves pulmonary hemodynamics and long-term prognosis in patients with chronic thromboembolic pulmonary hypertension. Circ J. 2012;76(2):485–8. doi:JST.JSTAGE/circj/CJ-11-1217 [pii].
11. Mizoguchi H, Ogawa A, Munemasa M, Mikouchi H, Ito H, Matsubara H. Refined balloon pulmonary angioplasty for inoperable patients with chronic thromboembolic pulmonary hypertension. Circ Cardiovasc Interv. 2012;5(6):748–55. doi:10.1161/CIRCINTERVENTIONS.112.971077.
12. Kataoka M, Inami T, Hayashida K, Shimura N, Ishiguro H, Abe T et al. Percutaneous transluminal pulmonary angioplasty for the treatment of chronic thromboembolic pulmonary hypertension. Circ Cardiovasc Interv. 2012;5(6):756–62. doi:10.1161/CIRCINTERVENTIONS.112.971390.
13. Andreassen AK, Ragnarsson A, Gude E, Geiran O, Andersen R. Balloon pulmonary angioplasty in patients with inoperable chronic thromboembolic pulmonary hypertension. Heart. 2013;99(19):1415–20. doi:10.1136/heartjnl-2012-303549.
14. Bouvaist H, Thony F, Jondot M, Camara B, Jais X, Pison C. Balloon pulmonary angioplasty in a patient with chronic thromboembolic pulmonary hypertension. Eur Respir Rev. 2014;23(133):393–5. doi:10.1183/09059180.00000514.

15. Darocha S, Kurzyna M, Pietura R, Torbicki A. Balloon pulmonary angioplasty for inoperable chronic thromboembolic pulmonary hypertension. Kardiol Pol. 2013;71(12):1331. doi:10.5603/KP.2013.0343.

16. Kopec G, Waligora M, Stepniewski J, Zmudka K, Podolec P, Matsubara H. In vivo characterization of changes in composition of organized thrombus in patient with chronic thromboembolic pulmonary hypertension treated with balloon pulmonary angioplasty. Int J Cardiol. 2015;186:279–81. doi:10.1016/j.ijcard.2015.03.203.

17. Kim NH, Delcroix M, Jenkins DP, Channick R, Dartevelle P, Jansa P et al. Chronic thromboembolic pulmonary hypertension. J Am Coll Cardiol. 2013;62(25 Suppl):D92–9. doi:10.1016/j.jacc.2013.10.024.

18. Japanese Circulation Society Joint Working Group. Statement for balloon pulmonary angioplasty for chronic thromboembolic pulmonary hypertension (JCS 2014). http://www.j-circ.or.jp/guideline/pdf/JCS2014_ito_d.pdf

19. Kimura M, Kataoka M, Kawakami T, Inohara T, Takei M, Fukuda K. Balloon pulmonary angioplasty using contrast agents improves impaired renal function in patients with chronic thromboembolic pulmonary hypertension. Int J Cardiol. 2015;188:41–2. doi:10.1016/j.ijcard.2015.04.030.

20. Inami T, Kataoka M, Shimura N, Ishiguro H, Yanagisawa R, Taguchi H et al. Pulmonary edema predictive scoring index (PEPSI), a new index to predict risk of reperfusion pulmonary edema and improvement of hemodynamics in percutaneous transluminal pulmonary angioplasty. JACC Cardiovasc Interv. 2013;6(7):725–36. doi:10.1016/j.jcin.2013.03.009.

21. Tatebe S, Fukumoto Y, Sugimura K, Miura Y, Nochioka K, Aoki T et al. Optical coherence tomography is superior to intravascular ultrasound for diagnosis of distal-type chronic thromboembolic pulmonary hypertension. Circ J. 2013;77(4):1081–3.

22. Sugimura K, Fukumoto Y, Miura Y, Nochioka K, Miura M, Tatebe S et al. Three-dimensional-optical coherence tomography imaging of chronic thromboembolic pulmonary hypertension. Eur Heart J. 2013;34(28):2121. doi:10.1093/eurheartj/eht203.

23. Kitani M, Ogawa A, Sarashina T, Yamadori I, Matsubara H. Histological changes of pulmonary arteries treated by balloon pulmonary angioplasty in a patient with chronic thromboembolic pulmonary hypertension. Circ Cardiovasc Interv. 2014;7(6):857–9. doi:10.1161/CIRCINTERVENTIONS.114.001533.

24. Ejiri K, Ogawa A, Matsubara H. Bail-out technique for pulmonary artery rupture with a covered stent in balloon pulmonary angioplasty for chronic thromboembolic pulmonary hypertension. JACC Cardiovasc Interv. 2015;8(5):752–3. doi:10.1016/j.jcin.2014.11.024.

25. Inami T, Kataoka M, Shimura N, Ishiguro H, Yanagisawa R, Fukuda K et al. Pressure-wire-guided percutaneous transluminal pulmonary angioplasty: a breakthrough in catheter-interventional therapy for chronic thromboembolic pulmonary hypertension. JACC Cardiovasc Interv. 2014;7(11):1297–306. doi:10.1016/j.jcin.2014.06.010.

26. Ogawa A, Matsubara H. Balloon pulmonary angioplasty: a treatment option for inoperable patients with chronic thromboembolic pulmonary hypertension. Front Cardiovasc Med. 2015;2:4. doi:10.3389/fcvm.2015.00004.

27. Taniguchi Y, Miyagawa K, Nakayama K, Kinutani H, Shinke T, Okada K et al. Balloon pulmonary angioplasty: an additional treatment option to improve the prognosis of patients with chronic thromboembolic pulmonary hypertension. EuroIntervention. 2014;10(4):518–25. doi:10.4244/EIJV10I4A89.

Chapter 16
Pulmonary Endarterectomy for Chronic Thromboembolic Pulmonary Hypertension

Hitoshi Ogino

Abstract For chronic thromboembolic pulmonary hypertension (CTEPH), well-established and standardized pulmonary endarterectomy (PEA) is still the first-line therapy with the favorable early and late outcome, particularly, for the proximal lesions of CTEPH. Reperfusion lung injury and residual pulmonary hypertension (PH) remain problematic as the complications related to adverse outcome. However, with the recent advancement of PEA including the adequate patients' selection, the perioperative management, and the technical refinement with accumulation of experiences, the early outcome has been improved with the significant hemodynamic improvement and the lower mortality rates of 5–10 % in general and of less than 5 % in experienced centers. The late outcome is also promising with the low rates of recurrence of CTEPH. On the other hand, an alternative procedure of balloon pulmonary angioplasty (BPA) has been emerging as a less-invasive treatment mainly for difficult patients with inaccessible distal CTEPH lesions and for patients with residual PH after PEA. In these situations, it has been more important to choose the most adequate procedure for each patient and to do, if necessary, the combination therapies of PEA and BPA associated with medical treatments.

Keywords Chronic thromboembolic pulmonary hypertension • Pulmonary endarterectomy

16.1 Introduction

For chronic thromboembolic pulmonary hypertension (CTEPH), pulmonary thrombo-endarterectomy was first performed at the University of California, San Diego (UCSD), in 1970 [1], which was followed by the current techniques of pulmonary endarterectomy (PEA) with deep hypothermic circulatory arrest (DHCA)

H. Ogino, MD, PhD (✉)
Department of Cardiovascular Surgery, Tokyo Medical University,
6-7-1 Nishishinjuku, Shinjuku-ku, Tokyo 160-0023, Japan
e-mail: hogino@tokyo-med.ac.jp

© Springer Science+Business Media Singapore 2017
Y. Fukumoto (ed.), *Diagnosis and Treatment of Pulmonary Hypertension*,
DOI 10.1007/978-981-287-840-3_16

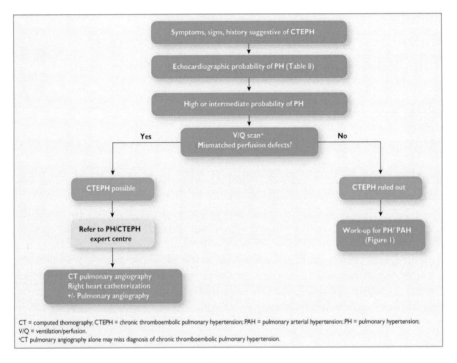

CT = computed thomography; CTEPH = chronic thromboembolic pulmonary hypertension; PAH = pulmonary arterial hypertension; PH = pulmonary hypertension;
V/Q = ventilation/perfusion.
*CT pulmonary angiography alone may miss diagnosis of chronic thromboembolic pulmonary hypertension.

Fig. 16.1 ESC/FRS diagnostic guideline of CTEPH

through a median sternotomy [2, 3]. Since then, this well-established and sophisticated procedure of PEA has already been performed there for over 3200 cases up to 2015 [4–6]. The recently published outcome of 500 patients was more favorable with only 2.2 % of the hospital mortality [6]. In Japan, Nakajima et al. at the National Cardiovascular (Research) Center (NCVC), Osaka, firstly reported on the similar type of surgery, mainly without cardiopulmonary bypass (CPB), through a lateral thoracotomy in 1986 [7]. In the 1990s, the UCSD original method of PEA with CPB and DHCA was introduced at NCVC and Chiba University [8–10]. According to the annual reports of the Japanese Association for Thoracic Surgery, PEA has been carried out for approximately 50 cases per year with favorable outcome of 6.5 % (n= 4/65) in-hospital mortality in 2013 [11].

The two major international guidelines of AHA/ACCF [12] in 2011 and ESC/ ERS in 2015 [13] and the Japanese one in 2012 [14] on PH recommended PEA as the first-line treatment for CTEPH (Figs. 16.1 and 16.2). However, in Japan, less-invasive balloon pulmonary angioplasty (BPA) was revived and has aggressively been attempted as the standard treatment, predominantly for inoperable or high-risk patients having inaccessible distal CTEPH lesions, on which the Japanese guideline has already recommended in 2012 [14]. In addition, medical treatment with the use of riociguat also has provided some beneficial effects to any types of CTEPH since the release. In these recent settings, the indication of each treatment has become more controversial.

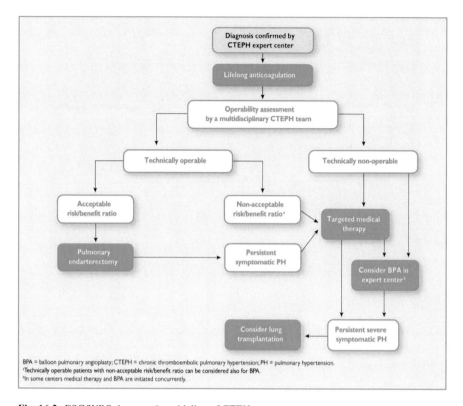

Fig. 16.2 ESC/WRS therapeutic guideline of CTEH

In this chapter, regarding PEA for CTEPH, the current indications, the surgical techniques with perioperative management, the early and long-term outcomes, and the risk factors for mortality and poor hemodynamic improvement after PEA would be described.

16.2   Diagnosis Including Assessment of Operability and Indication of PEA

CTEPH is diagnosed by cardiac echo, enhanced computed tomographic scans (CT scans), pulmonary ventilation/perfusion (V/Q) scintigraphy, right heart catheterization, and pulmonary angiography (PAG) [15, 16]. Predominantly according to the findings of the last two examinations, an adequate therapy is determined as follows: (1) mean pulmonary artery pressure (mPAP) >30 mmHg and pulmonary vascular resistance (PVR) >300 dyne/sec/cm^{-5}, (2) WHO functional class (NYHA classification) III or IV, (3) surgically accessible proximal lesions in the main-lobar or segmental pulmonary artery (PA), and (4) absence of severe comorbidities [4]. In

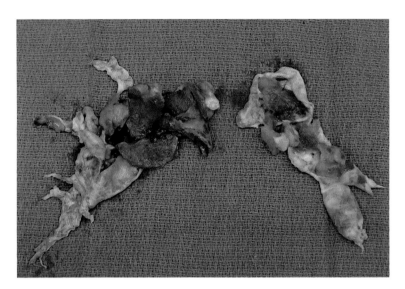

Fig. 16.3 Proximal type

addition, it is more important to assess the operability of each patient based on the institutional and surgeons' experiences as well as the various patient's imaging and hemodynamic data [15–17]. Unfortunately, in Japan, the number of PEA is much smaller and its experienced centers are also limited [11]. Without experienced PEA surgeons, it should be difficult for cardiologists and pulmonologists to independently evaluate the operability, particularly, at less-experienced hospitals. This situation seems to be one reason for recent predominant prevalence of BPA rather than PEA.

In making decision of treatment such as PEA, BPA, and medical treatment, the location of PA disease is one of the most important determinants, which is measured with findings of enhanced CT scans, PAG, and pulmonary V/Q scintigraphy [15–17]. Based on the predominant locations of PA lesions, CTEPH is morphologically classified into two categories such as the proximal and the distal types (Figs. 16.3 and 16.4). Similarly, according to the findings of PEA specimens, CTEPH is classified into four categories: type 1 (incidence at UCSD <25 %), fresh thrombus in the main-lobar pulmonary arteries; type 2 (<40 %), intimal thickening and fibrosis proximal to the segmental arteries; type 3 (<30 %), disease within distal segmental arteries only; and type 4 (<5 %), distal arteriolar vasculopathy without visible thromboembolic disease [18]. Type 1 or 2 lesion, that is, the easily accessible proximal type, should obviously be indicated for PEA. On the other hand, in cases with the distal lesions of the type 3 or 4, PEA is too difficult to resect PA lesions precisely with remarkable reduction of PH. In terms of the location of CTEPH lesion, there seems to be some differences between the Western countries and Japan [16–20]. In the author's experience, the proximal diseases were found in 58 % and the distal

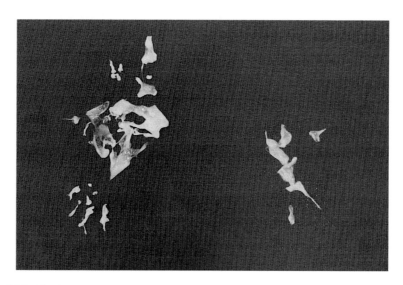

Fig. 16.4 Distal type

ones in 42 % [20]. In contrary, the proximal lesions were considerably predominant with the prevalence of type 1 in 37.4 %, type 2 in 49.0 %, type 3 in 12.0 %, and type 4 in 1.6 % in the UCSD cohort [18]. One article from USCD dealing with the recent PEA series between 2006 and 2010 stated the increased incidence of type 3 lesions from 13.1 to 21.4 % through their more aggressive approach to difficult distal PA lesions with the favorable outcome [6]. However, the incidence of the distal PA lesion was still lower than that of Japanese patients, which is presumably due to racial differences in blood coagulation [16–20]. In CTEPH, vascular obstruction is caused by two mechanisms as follows: direct occlusion of the vessel lumen and inducing secondary endothelial changes of cellular hyperplasia, webbing, and incomplete clot remodeling. The incidence of CTEPH caused by the first mechanism seems to be lower in Japanese patients. Actually, the number of Japanese patients having the past history of significant acute pulmonary embolism is much smaller, compared with Western patients: 37.2 % vs. 74.8 % [16]. As a result, a considerable number of difficult cases having distal PA diseases are involved in the Japanese CTEPH or PEA series. This setting is obviously another reason for widely spreading of BPA [21–23]. Furthermore, in the international registry, over one third of patients having CTEPH were also assessed as inoperable for high risks or difficulties [19], some of whom should be good candidates for BPA. Consequently, with whether PEA or BPA, our own therapeutic strategy needs to be established for better entire outcome of treatment for CTEPH in Japan.

Another considerable determinant for making decision of treatment is degree of PH. Preoperative PVR measured with cardiac output is considered a more important predictor of the postoperative outcome after PEA than an absolute value of mPAP. Previous reports demonstrated PVR > 1100 dyne $\cdot$ sec $\cdot$ cm^{-5} and mPAP >

50 mmHg as risk factors for mortality [24]. However, due to evolving PEA with the accumulation of experience and the advances of PEA techniques and perioperative management, the upper limit of mPAP and PVR for safe PEA was not determined in the guideline [12–14]. In particular, proximal and easily accessible PA lesions would allow us to perform PEA successfully, even with severer PH such as mPAP > 60 mmHg and PVR > 2000 dyne/sec/cm $^{-5}$, because remarkable PH reduction after PEA is expected [25]. However, in the author's practice, there have been four interesting exceptional cases with the proximal PA lesions associated with extremely high PVR > 2000 dyne/sec/cm^{-5}. Despite of technically successful PEA, three of them died from unexpected residual PH and pulmonary bleeding. Only one patient managed to survive the PEA but required BPA eventually for residual PH. All of them had the longer duration of illness of CTEPH over 15 years, and two of them were at bed rest with support of dobutamine and prostaglandin I_2 before surgery. Presumably, they had already developed "small arteriopathy" during such a long-term period of illness and pulmonary infarction with some collateral circulation, which adversely affected on the postoperative courses after PEA [26].

There have been no clear criteria of right ventricular function for PEA. The right ventricle is severely dilated, which causes secondary tricuspid regurgitation (TR). The right ventricular function also deteriorates due to long-standing severe PH. However, with successful PEA, the overload of the right ventricle would decrease, resulting in significant size reduction and improvement of wall motion of the right ventricle [27–29]. Subsequently, the TR grade would reduce naturally after successful PEA and tricuspid valve repair would not be required in most.

Some of patients are in emergency settings with rapidly deteriorated heart and respiratory failure due to "acute on chronic" status of recurrent pulmonary embolism. The outcome of PEA is relatively poorer on such an emergency basis [30]. It is more profitable to initially improve respiratory and hemodynamic conditions with adequate medical treatment. After the conditions are stabilized enough, PEA should be attempted. If impossible, prompt PEA would be the only alternative. Concerning other patient factors, PEA with prolonged CPB and DHCA is too invasive particularly for the elderly. Advanced age is one independent predictor for poor outcome of PEA [20, 31]. Regarding the other conditions such as reoperation [32], PEA for pediatric cases [33], and PEA accompanied with cardiac surgical procedures for coexisting cardiac lesions [34], PEA can be successfully performed with favorable outcome.

As described above, the assessment for operability is based on the experience and skill of the surgeons and the institution with sufficient system for preoperative imaging and diagnosis, decision-making, surgery, and perioperative care [35]. For more favorable outcome of CTEPH treatment, the centralization of institutions dealing with both PEA and BPA would be necessary to perform multidisciplinary therapies by a CTEPH team of each center.

16.3   PEA Procedures

At anesthesia, a twin-lumen endotracheal tube is routinely intubated in preparation for potential risk of serious respiratory tract hemorrhage. In addition with a central venous catheter, a Swan-Ganz catheter is inserted to monitor PA pressure and cardiac output consistently during the perioperative care. At surgery [4–6], the bilateral PA lesions are approached through a median sternotomy. CPB is established with ascending aortic cannulation and bicaval venous drainage. PA venting from the main PA and left ventricular/atrial venting through the right upper pulmonary vein are carried out. The patient is cooled down to 16–18 °C with surface head cooling with ice bags. Initially, the right atrium is opened to recognize the presence of atrial septal defect or patent foramen ovale. If any, they are closed. The right PA is approached between the ascending aorta and the superior vena cava (SVC). It is incised longitudinally and the correct plane for PEA is found in the media of the posterior surface. The ascending aorta is clamped and cardiac arrest is achieved with cardioplegia. PEA is performed down to the segmental and sub-segmental branches using special suction dissectors [4]. Establishment of the correct plane is most crucial because an excessively deep plane is associated with a risk of pulmonary artery perforation and massive airway bleeding, whereas a too superficial plane would result in poor PEA causing residual PH. PEA is carried out using a cycle of 15 min of DHCA followed by 10 min of systemic reperfusion. After PEA, the right PA is closed with double-layered fine stitches. PEA of the left PA is followed with the similar technique. PEA of the left lower lobe is however technically difficult. After PEA, rewarming is commenced and the left PA and the right atrium are closed. The ascending aorta is de-clamped. After the gradual rewarming taking over 1 h, the patient is weaned from CPB carefully, because the hemodynamics is unstable in most as a result of residual PH arising from the adverse effect of hypothermia, CPB, and reperfusion lung injury.

For patients having difficulty in CPB weaning due to hypotension, hypoxia, and/or pulmonary bleeding, percutaneous cardiopulmonary support or extracorporeal membrane oxygenation (ECMO) is indicated using a femoro-femoral circuit or the same unit of CPB [20, 35–37]. The latter, so-called central ECMO, is more preferable for relief of the heart and lung, although the sternal closure is delayed. Intra-aortic balloon pumping (IABP) is also routinely used to produce a pulsatile arterial flow for beneficial organ perfusion. The weaning from it is tried after improvement of hemodynamics and oxygenation is obtained. Another argues regarding DHCA have emerged. Some articles reported on temporary or cognitive neurological dysfunction due to either deep hypothermia or circulatory arrest [38]. The safety and impact of moderate hypothermia with balloon occlusion of the bronchial arteries in the descending thoracic aorta was addressed, which did not any remarkable advantages. One randomized control trial was done between DHCA alone and HCA with selective cerebral perfusion [39]. There were no significant shortcomings of the current brain protection with DHCA alone on the neurological function. The current PEA is consequently still carried out with DHCA alone.

16.4 Perioperative Care

Although the guidelines did not recommend, postoperative outcome seems to be favorably affected by preoperative use of medical therapy including prostacyclin analogs, endothelin receptor antagonists, or phosphodiesterase-5 inhibitors to improve hemodynamic parameters before surgery [40, 41]. However, this has not been rigorously assessed in randomized, controlled trials. The author has already employed this strategy with administration of PGI_2 in the past or currently riociguat before surgery to stabilize the conditions, in particular, for high-risk patients having distal PA lesions and high PVR [41]. After PEA, significant residual PH occurs at the incidences of 10–20 % mainly due to the inaccessible distal PA pathology and/or of secondary small-vessel arteriopathy [42]. Another mechanism is inevitable reperfusion pulmonary injury of the PEA parts of the lung. Adequate mechanical ventilation with high PEEP of 10 cmH_2O [43] and fluid restriction with diuretics are of great importance. If possible, nitric oxide is also used to reduce PH and to improve gas exchange [44, 45]. For serious complication of pulmonary bleeding, ECMO, particularly without use of anticoagulation, is indicated to reduce hemorrhage by decreasing the pulmonary circulation. Postoperatively, anticoagulation therapy involved intravenous heparin for the first week followed by oral warfarin therapy with the target INR around 2.0–3.0 for Japanese patients. Normally, postoperative cardiac catheterization and PAG are carried out before discharge to determine the impact of PEA.

16.5 Outcome

In terms of early outcome, the hospital mortality rates reportedly ranged from 2.2 to 23.0 % [46]. Due to the establishment of PEA indications and the improvement of surgical techniques and perioperative management, the early outcome of PEA has been improved, even though higher-risk patients having distal PA disease and/or high PVR are increasingly accepted for surgery with the accumulation of experiences. In the recent series of 500 patients at UCSD, the hospital mortality rate was only 2.2 % [6]. Even at the other institutions, the mortality rates have achieved between 5 and 10 %. According to the annual summary of the Japanese Association for Thoracic Surgery in 2013, the mortality rate was 6.5 % [11].

Regarding risk factors for mortality, location of PA disease and preoperative hemodynamics are important predictors of the postoperative outcome. At the beginning of this procedure around the 1990s, preoperative mPAP >50 mmHg and PVR >1100 dyne/sec/cm^{-5} were predictors for hospital mortality [24]. In the 2000s, the risk factors were advanced age, high right atrial pressure, poor NYHA class, many lesions in PA branches [31], and preoperative blood gas with low-oxygen partial pressure [47]. In the UCSD report on the location of PA lesion, the mortality rates were type 1 = 1.3 %, type 2 = 2.5 %, type 3 = 13.2 %, and type 4 = 14.3 %, respectively, which means higher mortality and morbidity rates in cases with distal PA lesions of type 3/4 [18]. In another UCSD report, postoperative PVR > 500 dyne/sec/cm^{-5} was an independent predictor for adverse outcome [5]. In the author's practice, the multivariate analysis dealing with 88 patients demonstrated high age > 60 years old as an independent predictor for mortality [20].

In assuming PVR > 500 dyne/sec/cm^{-5} immediately after PEA as residual PH, its incidence was reportedly from 10.1 to 16.0 % [46]. Given more strict criteria of PVR > 400 dyne/sec/cm^{-5}, 33.7 % developed residual PH [47]. In the author's experience of 130 patients at NCVC between 1995 and 2008, the incidence of residual PH (mPAP > 30 mmHg) was 17.7 % [20]. Advanced age, high right atrial pressure, and female gender were independent predictors for persistent PH in the multivariate analysis [31].

With regard to the long-term results, in the recent report from UCSD, the survival rates were reported to be 82 % at 5 years and 75 % at 10 years [6]. The author first reported that the survival rate was 90.7 % at 3 years and 86.4 % at 5 years [19]. Ishida et al. also reported the favorable outcome with survival rate of 84.0 % at 5 years and 82.0 % at 10 years [48]. In terms of the event-free rate in the long-term, in the author's experience, it was 97.1 % at 3 years and 93.5 % at 5 years [20]. In another report, it was 78.0 % at 5 years and 70.0 % at 10 years [48]. Concerning the recurrences of CTEPH after successful PEA, Mayer et al. first reported some hemo-dynamic deterioration in three patients (4.6 %) [49]. In the author's experience, three patients (2.5 %) developed recurrence of PH. Two of them had been suffered from residual PH due to unsuccessful PEA for the distal PA lesions. Ishida et al. demonstrated postoperative mPAP >34 mmHg leading to some deterioration of NHYA class and late death [48].

16.6   Conclusions

Although PEA is invasive and depending on the high level of surgical expertise and the appropriate patients' selection, it is favorably associated with the significant improvements in hemodynamics and exercise capacity and with the lower early and late mortality rates. Consequently, PEA is still the first-line therapy for CTEPH, particularly for the proximal PA lesions. Multidisciplinary therapies including PEA, BPA, and medical treatment by a CTEPH team would be required for more favorable outcome.

References

1. Moser KM, Daily PO, Peterson K, Dembitsky W, Vapnek JM, Shure D, et al. Thromboendarterectomy for chronic, major-vessel thromboembolic pulmonary hypertension. Immediate and long-term results in 42 patients. Ann Intern Med. 1987;107(4):560–5.

2. Daily PO, Johnston GG, Simmons CJ, Moser KM. Surgical management of chronic pulmonary embolism: surgical treatment and late results. J Thorac Cardiovasc Surg. 1980;79(4):523–31.

3. Daily PO, Dembitsky WP, Iversen S. Technique of pulmonary thrombo- endarterectomy for chronic pulmonary embolism. J Card Surg. 1989;4:10–24.

4. Jamieson SW, Auger WR, Fedullo PF, Channick RN, Kriett JM, Moser KM, et al. Experience and results with 150 pulmonary thromboendarterectomy operations over a 29-month period. J Thorac Cardiovasc Surg. 1993;106(1):116–26.

5. Jamieson SW, Kapelanski DP, Sakakibara N, Manecke GR, Thistlethwaite PA, Kerr KM, et al. Pulmonary endarterectomy: experience and lessons learned in 1,500 cases. Ann Thorac Surg. 2003;76(5):1457–62.

6. Madani MM, Auger WR, Pretorius V, Sakakibara N, Kerr KM, Jamieson SW, et al. Pulmonary endarterectomy: recent changes in a single institution's experience of more than 2,700 patients. Ann Thorac Surg. 2012;94(1):97–103.

7. Nakajima N, Kawazoe K, Ando M, Uemura S, Fujita T. An experience in the surgical treatment of chronic pulmonary embolism. Nihon Kyobu Geka Gakkai Zasshi. 1986;34(4):524–31.

8. Ando M, Takamoto S, Okita Y, Matsukawa R, Nakanishi N, Kyotani S, et al. Surgery for chronic pulmonary thromoboembolism accompanied by thrombophilia in eight patients. Ann Thorac Surg. 1998;66:1919–24.

9. Ando M, Okita Y, Tagusari O, Kitamura S, Nakanishi N, Kyotani S. Surgical treatment for chronic thromboembolic pulmonary hypertension under profound hypothermia and circulatory arrest in 24 patients. J Card Surg. 1999;14:377–85.

10. Masuda M, Nakajima N. Our experience of surgical treatment for chronic pulmonary thromboembolism. Ann Thorac Cardiovasc Surg. 2001;7:261–5.

11. Committee for Scientific Affairs. Thoracic and cardiovascular surgery in Japan during 2013: annual report by the Japanese Association for Thoracic Surgery. Gen Thorac Cardiovasc Surg. 2015;63(12):670–701.

12. Jaff MR, McMurtry MS, Archer SL, Cushman M, Goldenberg N, Goldhaber SZ, et al; American Heart Association Council on Cardiopulmonary, Critical Care, Perioperative and Resuscitation; American Heart Association Council on Peripheral Vascular Disease; American Heart Association Council on Arteriosclerosis, Thrombosis and Vascular Biology. Management of massive and submassive pulmonary embolism, iliofemoral deep vein thrombosis, and chronic thromboembolic pulmonary hypertension: a scientific statement from the American Heart Association. Circulation. 2011;123(16):1788–1830.

13. Galiè N, Humbert M, Vachiery JL, Gibbs S, Lang I, Torbicki A, et al. 2015 ESC/ERS Guidelines for the diagnosis and treatment of pulmonary hypertension: The Joint Task Force for the Diagnosis and Treatment of Pulmonary Hypertension of the European Society of Cardiology (ESC) and the European Respiratory Society (ERS): Endorsed by: Association for European Paediatric and Congenital Cardiology (AEPC), International Society for Heart and Lung Transplantation (ISHLT). Eur Heart J. 2016;37(1):67–119.

14. Nakanishi N, Ando M, Ueda H, Ogino H, Saji T, Shiomi T, et al. Guideline for treatment of pulmonary hypertension (Japanese); 2012. p. 50–6.

15. Kim NH, Delcroix M, Jenkins DP, et al. Chronic thromboembolic pulmonary hypertension. J Am Coll Cardiol. 2014;2(25 Suppl):D92–9.

16. Lang IM, Madani M. Update on chronic thromboembolic pulmonary hypertension. Circulation. 2014;130(6):508–18.

17. Jenkins D. Pulmonary endarterectomy: the potentially curative treatment for patients with chronic thromboembolic pulmonary hypertension. Eur Respir Rev. 2015;24(136):263–71.

18. Thistlethwaite PA, Mo M, Madani MM, Blanchard D, Kapelanski DP, Jamieson SW, et al. Operative classification of thromboembolic disease determines outcome after pulmonary endarterectomy. J Thorac Cardiovasc Surg. 2002;124(6):1203–11.

19. Mayer E, Jenkins D, Lindner J, D'Armini A, Kloek J, Meyns B, et al. Surgical management and outcome of patients with chronic thromboembolic pulmonary hypertension: results from an international prospective registry. J Thorac Cardiovasc Surg. 2011;141(3):702–10.

20. Ogino H, Ando M, Matsuda H, Minatoya K, Sasaki H, Nakanishi N, et al. Japanese single-center experience of surgery for chronic thromboembolic pulmonary hypertension. Ann Thorac Surg. 2006;82(2):630–6.

21. Feinstein JA, Goldhaber SZ, Lock JE, Ferndandes SM, Landzberg MJ. Balloon pulmonary angioplasty for treatment of chronic thromboembolic pulmonary hypertension. Circulation. 2001;103(1):10–3.

22. Mizoguchi H, Ogawa A, Munemasa M, Mikouchi H, Ito H, Matsubara H. Refined balloon pulmonary angioplasty for inoperable patients with chronic thromboembolic pulmonary hypertension. Circ Cardiovasc Interv. 2012;5(6):748–55.

23. Kataoka M, Inami T, Hayashida K, Fukuda K, Yoshino H, Satoh T, et al. Percutaneous transluminal pulmonary angioplasty for the treatment of chronic thromboembolic pulmonary hypertension. Circ Cardiovasc Interv. 2012;5(6):756–62.

24. Hartz RS, Byrne JG, Levitsky S, Park J, Rich S. Predictors of mortality in pulmonary thromboendarterectomy. Ann Thorac Surg. 1996;62:1255–9.

25. Thistlethwaite PA, Kemp A, Du L, Madani MM, Jamieson SW. Outcomes of pulmonary endarterectomy for treatment of extreme thromboembolic pulmonary hypertension. J Thorac Cardiovasc Surg. 2006;131(2):307–13.

26. Galiè N, Kim NH. Pulmonary microvascular disease in chronic thrombo- embolic pulmonary hypertension. Proc Am Thorac Soc. 2006;3(7):571–6.

27. Reesink HJ, Marcus JT, Tulevski II, Jamieson S, Kloek JJ, Vonk Noordegraaf A, et al. Reverse right ventricular remodeling after pulmonary endarterectomy in patients with chronic thromboembolic pulmonary hypertension: utility of magnetic resonance imaging to demonstrate restoration of the right ventricle. J Thorac Cardiovasc Surg. 2007;133:58–64.

28. Menzel T, Kramm T, Wagner S, Mohr-Kahaly S, Mayer E, Meyer J, et al. Improvement of tricuspid regurgitation after pulmonary thromboendarterectomy. Ann Thorac Surg. 2002;73:756–61.

29. Thistlethwaite PA, Jamieson SW. Tricuspid valvular disease in the patient with chronic pulmonary thromboembolic disease. Curr Opin Cardiol. 2003;18:111–6.

30. Kitamura T, Morota T, Takamoto S. Emergent pulmonary thromboendarterectomy with percutaneous cardiopulmonary support system for chronic thromboembolic pulmonary hypertension. Eur J Cardiothorac Surg. 2003;24(4):656–8.

31. Tscholl D, Langer F, Wendler O, Wilkens H, Georg T, Schäfers HJ. Pulmonary thromboendarterectomy--risk factors for early survival and hemodynamic improvement. Eur J Cardiothorac Surg. 2001;19(6):771–6.

32. Mo M, Kapelanski DP, Mitruka SN, Auger WR, Fedullo PF, Jamieson SW, et al. Reoperative pulmonary thrombo-endarterectomy. Ann Thorac Surg. 1999;68(5):1770–6.

33. Madani MM, Wittine LM, Auger WR, Fedullo PF, Kerr KM, Jamieson SW, et al. Chronic thromboembolic pulmonary hypertension in pediatric patients. J Thorac Cardiovasc Surg. 2011;141(3):624–30.

34. Thistlethwaite PA, Auger WR, Madani MM, Pradhan S, Kapelanski DP, Jamieson SW. Pulmonary thrombo- endarterectomy combined with other cardiac operations: indications, surgical approach, and outcome. Ann Thorac Surg. 2001;72(1):13–7.

35. Jenkins DP, Madani M, Mayer E, Kerr K, Kim K, Klepetko W, et al. Surgical treatment of CTEPH. ERJ Express. 2012;8

36. Thistlethwaite PA, Madani MM, Kemp AD, Hartley M, Auger WR, Jamieson SW. Venovenous extracorporeal life support after pulmonary endarterectomy: indications, techniques, and outcomes. Ann Thorac Surg. 2006;82:2139–45.

37. Berman M, Tsui S, Vuylsteke A, Snell A, Colah S, Latimer R, et al. Successful extracorporeal membrane oxygenation support after pulmonary thrombo-endarterectomy. Ann Thorac Surg. 2008;86(4):1261–7.

38. Macchiarini P, Kamiya H, Hagl C, Winterhalter M, Barbera J, Haverich A, et al. Pulmonary endarterectomy for chronic thromboembolic pulmonary hypertension: is deep hypothermia required? Eur J Cardiothorac Surg. 2006;30(2):237–41.

39. Vuylsteke A, Sharples L, Charman G, Kneeshaw J, Tsui S, Dunning J, et al. Circulatory arrest versus cerebral perfusion during pulmonary endarterectomy surgery (PEACOG): a randomised controlled trial. Lancet. 2011;378(9800):1379–87.

40. Jensen KW, Kerr KM, Fedullo PF, Kim NH, Test VJ, Ben-Yehuda O, et al. Pulmonary hypertensive medical therapy in chronic thromboembolic pulmonary hypertension before pulmonary thromboendarterectomy. Circulation. 2009;120:1248–54.

41. Nagaya N, Ando M, Ogino H, Sakamaki F, Kyotani S, Nakanishi N, et al. Prostacyclin therapy before pulmonary thromboendarterectomy in patients with chronic thromboembolic pulmonary hypertension. Chest. 2003;123(2):338–43.

42. Freed DH, Thomson BM, Berman M, Tsui SS, Dunning J, Sheares KK, et al. Survival after pulmonary thromboendarterectomy: effect of residual pulmonary hypertension. J Thorac Cardiovasc Surg. 2011;141(2):383–7.

43. Takeuchi M, Imanaka H, Tachibana K, Ogino H, Ando M, Nishimura M. Recruitment maneuver and high positive end-expiratory pressure improve hypoxemia in patients after pulmonary thromboendarterectomy for chronic pulmonary thromboembolism. Crit Care Med. 2005;33(9):2010–4.

44. Haydar A, Malhere T, Mauriat P, Journois D, Pouard P, Denis N, et al. Inhaled nitric oxide for postoperative pulmonary hypertension in patients with congenital heart defects. Lancet. 1992;340(8834–8835):1545.

45. Imanaka H, Miyano H, Takeuchi M, Kumon K, Ando M. Effects of nitric oxide inhalation after pulmonary thromboendarterectomy for chronic pulmonary thromboembolism. Chest. 2000;118(1):39–46.

46. Ogino H. Recent advances of pulmonary endarterectomy for chronic thromboembolic pulmonary hypertension including Japanese experiences. Gen Thorac Cardiovasc Surg. 2014;62(1):9–18.

47. Kunihara T, Gerdts J, Groesdonk H, Sata F, Langer F, Schäfers HJ, et al. Predictors of postoperative outcome after pulmonary endarterectomy from a 14-year experience with 279 patients. Eur J Cardiothorac Surg. 2011;40(1):154–61.

48. Ishida K, Masuda M, Nakajima N. Long-term outcome after pulmonary endarterectomy for chronic thromboembolic pulmonary hypertension. J Thorac Cardiovasc Surg. 2012;144(2):321–6.

49. Mayer E, Dahm M, Hake U, Schmid FX, Pitton M, Kupferwasser I, et al. Mid-term results of pulmonary thromboendarterectomy for chronic thromboembolic pulmonary hypertension. Ann Thorac Surg. 1996;61(6):1788–92.

Part V
Right Ventricular Function

Chapter 17
Right Ventricular Function

Kaoru Dohi, Norikazu Yamada, and Masaaki Ito

Abstract The right ventricle (RV) is highly sensitive to increments of pressure overload. Both acute and chronic excessive pressure overloads lead to right ventricular (RV) maladaptation and subsequent RV failure, which is the main cause of death in patients with pulmonary hypertension (PH). RV function is strongly associated with the exercise capacity of patients and their survival in PH independently of pulmonary arterial pressure. Invasive right heart catheterization including the pressure–volume loop method allows for definition of PH, assessment of pulmonary hemodynamics, RV contractility, and RV-arterial coupling. Noninvasively, echocardiography is widely used for not only screening for PH but also for assessment of the cardiac structure and function in daily clinical practice, and two-dimensional and three-dimensional echocardiography provide comprehensive and quantitative assessments of RV myocardial dynamics. Cardiac magnetic resonance imaging is also increasingly used as a standard tool in the evaluation of RV structure and function. We offer a clinical perspective on RV structure and function and review established and novel methods for measuring RV function in the present section.

Keywords Right ventricular function • Pressure–volume loop • Echocardiography

17.1 Introduction

In normal physiological conditions, the amount of blood ejected by the right ventricle (RV) is equal to that ejected by the left ventricle (LV). However, the structural and functional characteristics of the RV are quite different from those of the LV. The RV has a thin wall with high diastolic compliance to adapt to rapid changes in volume load and discharges blood into a very compliant pulmonary circulation. Conversely, right ventricular (RV) pump function is impaired to a much greater extent in comparison with that of the LV by comparable increases in pressure load. Both acute

K. Dohi (✉) • N. Yamada • M. Ito
Department of Cardiology and Nephrology, Mie University Graduate School of Medicine,
2-174 Edobashi, Tsu 514-8507, Japan
e-mail: dohik@clin.medic.mie-u.ac.jp

© Springer Science+Business Media Singapore 2017   217
Y. Fukumoto (ed.), *Diagnosis and Treatment of Pulmonary Hypertension*,
DOI 10.1007/978-981-287-840-3_17

and chronic excessive pressure overloads lead to RV maladaptation and subsequent RV failure, which is the main cause of death in patients with various types of pulmonary hypertension (PH) including acute pulmonary thromboembolism (APTE) and pulmonary arterial hypertension (PAH). The clinical importance of RV function for the exercise capacity of patients and their survival has been confirmed in PH, and several indices of RV dysfunction and/or signs of RV failure have been identified as significant predictors of mortality. Right heart catheterization (RHC) is the "gold standard" measurement technique in the evaluation of hemodynamic status and is essential for the diagnosis of PH. Pressure–volume loops using a conductance catheter allow for definition of not only RV contractility but also RV-arterial coupling, which indicates the mechanical efficiency of the cardiovascular system and the interaction between cardiac performance and vascular function. Echocardiography is widely used not only in screening for PH but also for the assessment of RV structure and function in daily clinical practice. Longitudinal shortening is the major contributor to overall RV performance, and measures of longitudinal RV function such as tissue Doppler-derived annular systolic velocity wave (S') and tricuspid annular plane systolic excursion (TAPSE) are widely used in the clinical setting. Two-dimensional (2D) speckle-tracking echocardiography (STE) allows rapid and accurate analysis of RV longitudinal systolic mechanics, and global RV longitudinal strain provides prognostic value in patients with PH. Three-dimensional (3D) echocardiography allows for measuring RV volume and EF irrespective of its shape. The new development of 3D-STE provides comprehensive and quantitative assessment of RV myocardial dynamics including the area change of segmental and global endocardial surface that integrates longitudinal and circumferential deformations. Cardiac magnetic resonance imaging (MRI) is also increasingly used as a standard tool in the evaluation of RV structure, function, and tissue characterization. The present chapter reviews the normal RV structural and functional characteristics and then focuses on the pathophysiology, evaluation, and diagnosis of RV dysfunction secondary to PH.

17.2   Anatomy of Right Ventricle

The RV is the most anteriorly situated cardiac chamber and lies immediately behind the sternum in the normal heart. In contrast to the ellipsoidal shape of the LV, the shape of the RV is complex and appears triangular when viewed from the frontal aspect and crescent shaped when viewed in cross section [1, 2] (Fig. 17.1). Anatomically, the RV is divided into three components: (1) the inlet, (2) the trabeculated apical myocardium, and (3) the infundibulum (also known as conus arteriosus) [1, 2]. The inlet consists of the tricuspid valve, chordae tendineae, and papillary muscles. The infundibulum corresponds to the smooth myocardial outflow region. Additionally, the RV can also be divided into anterior, lateral, and inferior walls, as well as basal, mid, and apical sections [1]. The ventricles are composed of multiple layers that form a three-dimensional network of fibers. The RV wall is mainly

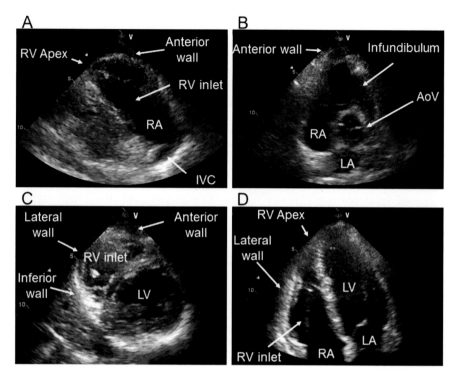

Fig. 17.1 Examples of echocardiography views focusing on the right ventricle.
(**a**) Parasternal right ventricular (RV) three-chamber view, (**b**) parasternal short-axis view at the RV outflow level, (**c**) parasternal short-axis view at the mid ventricular level, (**d**) apical four-chamber view. *AoV* aortic valve, *IVC* inferior vena cava, *LV* left ventricle, *LA* left atrium, *RA* right atrium

composed of superficial and deep muscle layers. The superficial fibers of the RV are arranged circumferentially with the continuity between the both ventricles with the RV being wrapped around the LV, which represents the anatomic basis of free ventricular wall traction caused by LV contraction [1, 2]. The deep muscle fibers are longitudinally aligned from base to apex and contribute to longitudinal shortening of the RV endocardium.

17.3   Mechanical Aspects of Ventricular Contraction

The primary function of the RV is to receive systemic venous blood and to pump it into the pulmonary arteries. The RV contracts by three separate mechanisms: (1) inward movement of the free wall, which produces a bellows effect, (2) contraction of the longitudinal fibers, which shortens the long axis and draws the tricuspid annulus toward the apex, and (3) traction on the free wall at the points of attachment secondary to LV contraction [3]. Shortening of the RV is greater longitudinally than radially, and rotational movements do not contribute significantly to RV contraction. Because of the higher surface-to-volume ratio of the RV, the thin free wall can adequately eject the required stroke volume with a small inward motion. RV contraction is sequential, starting with contraction of the inlet and trabeculated myocardium and ending with the contraction of the infundibulum (approximately 25–50 msec apart). Contraction of the infundibulum is of longer duration than that of the inflow region [1, 4].

In a normal heart, the RV promptly and adequately adapts to dynamic changes in systemic venous return, and an increase in RV volume load leads to an increase in ejection volume according to the Frank–Starling law within physiological limits. The RV is normally connected to a low impedance and highly distensible pulmonary vascular system, and right-sided pressures are significantly lower than comparable left-sided pressures [1, 5]. The RV is vulnerable to any acute rise in wall stress because of its thin-walled and crescent-shaped structure, designed to function as a flow generator accommodating the entire systemic venous return to the heart [1, 6], and a brisk increase in RV pressure load such as massive APTE induces acute dilatation and rapid pump failure of the RV [7, 8]. In contrast, a gradual increase in pressure load to a certain extent allows for RV adaptation to maintain stroke volume or cardiac output (CO) by increasing its wall thickness and contractility. However, when exposed to excessive pressure load even in the chronic form, the RV myocardium has difficulty in normalizing ventricular wall stress (force per unit cross-sectional area) in the process of reactive myocyte hypertrophy, which results in RV dilatation, myocardial ischemia, mechanical dyssynchrony, functional tricuspid regurgitation, and subsequent RV pump failure with high filling pressure. Therefore, in some patients with severe and progressive RV failure, pulmonary artery pressure (PAP) generated by the RV may decrease as a consequence of reduced RV contractility.

RV pressure overload affects LV function not only by limiting the LV preload but also by abnormal pressure interaction via the interventricular septum and the pericardium, known as ventricular interdependence. An inverted transseptal pressure gradient between the LV and RV leads to a leftward displacement and paradoxical motion of the interventricular septum, resulting in impaired LV systolic and diastolic function. Recent clinical observation revealed that the LV myocardial performance index (MPI), described in later sections, is significantly correlated with RV MPI in both acute and chronic RV pressure overload, indicating that LV myocardial performance is regulated by ventricular interdependence [9].

17.4 Hemodynamic Evaluation

Right heart catheterization (RHC) is considered the "gold standard" measurement technique for the evaluation of hemodynamic status and is accepted as essential for the confirmation of PH [1, 10]. RV pressure tracings show an early-peaking and a rapidly declining pressure (Fig. 17.2) in contrast to the rounded contour of LV pressure tracing. RV isovolumic contraction time (ICT) is shorter because the RV systolic

Fig. 17.2 Simultaneously recorded ECG, RV analog signal of pressure development (dP/dt), phasic pulmonary artery flow, pulmonary artery pressure (PAP), and RV pressure (RVP) in a human subject. *ICT* isovolumic contraction time, *ET* ejection time, *HOI* hangout interval (Reproduced from Dell'Italia and Walsh [11] copyright © 1988, with permission from Elsevier)

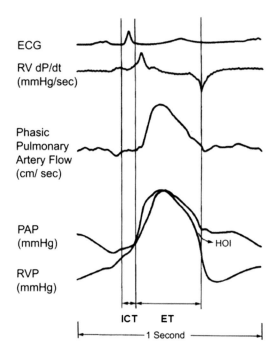

pressure rapidly exceeds the low pulmonary artery diastolic pressure. A careful observation of the hemodynamic tracings and flow dynamics also reveals that end-systolic flow may continue in the presence of a negative ventricular–arterial pressure gradient [1, 4, 11]. This interval, which is referred to as the hangout interval, is most likely explained by the momentum of blood (inertia force) through the outflow. In the highly compliant (low-resistance, high-capacitance) pulmonary vascular bed in healthy individuals, the hangout interval may vary from 30 to 120 msec, contributing significantly to the duration of RV ejection [12]. In the presence of excessive pressure overload, RV ICT becomes longer due to elevated pulmonary artery diastolic pressure, and the RV ejection becomes shorter with the shorter hangout time.

During the course of chronic and progressive PH, rises in pulmonary vascular resistance lead to parallel elevation of PAP until RV CO is maintained. However, the deterioration of RV pump function in the late stages of PH causes a paradoxical decrease in PAP despite steady rises in pulmonary vascular resistance. Finally, RV pump failure in end-stage PH leads to elevated right atrial pressure (Fig. 17.3). Indeed, RHC-derived right atrial pressure, cardiac index, and mixed venous oxygen saturation are the most robust indicators of RV dysfunction and poor prognosis, whereas mean PAP provides little prognostic information [2].

Pressure–volume loops using a conductance catheter depict instantaneous pressure–volume curves under different loading conditions. Suga et al. first showed that the LV end-systolic pressure–volume relationship can be approximated by a linear relationship during inferior vena caval occlusion and that the slope of this relationship represents the end-systolic elastance (Ees), which provides an index of myocardial contractility [13]. Arterial elastance (Ea) is the expression of the total afterload

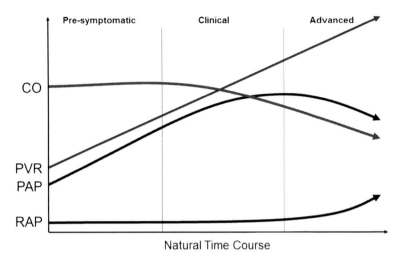

Fig. 17.3 Time course of hemodynamic changes in progressive pulmonary hypertension. *CO* cardiac output, *PVR* pulmonary vascular resistance, *PAP* pulmonary arterial pressure, *RAP* right atrial pressure

imposed on the ventricle and represents the complex association of different arterial properties including vascular wall stiffness, compliance, and outflow resistance [14]. Ventriculo-arterial coupling can be defined as the Ea/Ees ratio and represents the mechanical efficiency of the cardiovascular system and the interaction between ventricular performance and vascular function [14]. Interestingly, many studies have shown that a time-varying elastance model can also be applied to the RV (Fig. 17.4) despite it having markedly different ventricular geometry and hemodynamics to those of the LV [15, 16]. As LV Ees is preserved or even higher despite impaired diastolic relaxation and ventriculo-arterial coupling in patients with arterial hypertension, RV Ees is commonly increased but RV diastolic relaxation is prolonged, and ventriculo-arterial coupling is impaired from the early stages of PH until decompensated RV failure occurs. McCabe et al. performed conductance catheterization in ten patients with chronic thromboembolic pulmonary hypertension (CTEPH), seven with chronic thromboembolic disease without pulmonary hypertension (CTED), and seven controls [17] and revealed that control and CTED groups had lower Ea and Ees compared with the CTEPH group (Ea: 0.30 ± 0.10 vs. 0.52 ± 0.24 vs. 1.92 ± 0.70 mmHg/ml, respectively, $P < 0.001$, and Ees: 0.44 ± 0.20 vs. 0.59 ± 0.15 vs. 1.13 ± 0.43 mmHg/ml, $P < 0.01$) with more efficient ventriculo-arterial coupling (Ees/Ea: 1.46 ± 0.30 vs. 1.27 ± 0.36 vs. 0.60 ± 0.18, respectively, $P < 0.001$). It is well recognized that changes in contractile performance alter Ees, but Ees is also influenced by the chamber geometry and by factors that alter myocardial stiffness. Chronic increase in RV afterload can be associated with tandem increase in both systolic and diastolic RV stiffness. Taken together with the findings of impaired systolic myocardial shortening despite increased Ees in patients with PH, the processes that contribute to diastolic stiffening in PH also influence systolic

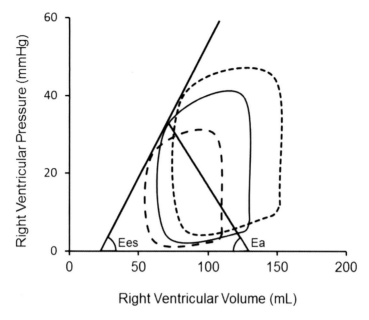

Fig. 17.4 Pressure–volume relation, illustrating the concepts of ventricular elastance (Ees) and arterial elastance (Ea)

stiffness. The clinical utility of this method in the RV functional assessment in PH warrants further investigation mainly because of the nonlinearity and variability in slope values as well as their afterload dependency [18]. Notably, the conductance catheter technique does not take account of volume changes in the longitudinal direction in the assessment of the pressure–volume relationship, which may limit the precise assessment of global ventricular function.

17.5   The Role of the RV Function in Pulmonary Hypertension

RV failure is the main cause of death in patients with PH, and the ability of the RV to adapt to the progressive increase in afterload associated with changes in the pulmonary vasculature is the main determinant of a patient's functional capacity and survival [4, 19]. Excessive RV dilatation secondary to PH also leads to functional tricuspid regurgitation, caused by annular dilatation and chordal traction, which in turn results in RV volume overload, and thus further progressive annular dilation and right ventricle remodeling [19]. Importantly, the relationship between the degree of afterload and RV function is not so strong. Indeed, although endothelin–receptor antagonists, nitric oxide, phosphodiesterase type 5 inhibitors, and prosta-cyclin derivatives have improved the mobility and mortality of PAH, current

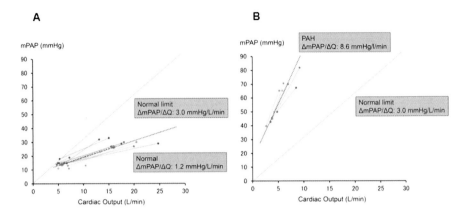

Fig. 17.5 Pulmonary artery pressure-flow relationships. (**a**) In 11 normal studies and (**b**) in five pulmonary arterial hypertension (PAH) studies (Reproduced from Kusunose and Yamada [28] copyright © 2015, with permission from Springer). *ΔmPAP/ΔQ* the slope of the mean pulmonary artery pressure and cardiac output

therapies for right heart failure are still suboptimal [20–25]. In addition, recent clinical observation demonstrated that the RV ejection fraction (RVEF) can deteriorate despite a reduction in pulmonary vascular resistance after PAH-targeted therapy [26]. It is well recognized that right heart failure in PH is accompanied by extensive RV structural and extracellular matrix remodeling, but there is still no ideal therapy that reverses the progression of RV remodeling independent of the RV afterload-reducing effect.

Exercise intolerance and dyspnea upon exertion are the predominant symptoms of patients with PH because of steep mean pressure/flow relationships (Fig. 17.5), and the ability of the RV to increase the CO during exercise is an important determinant of exercise capacity and predicts prognosis in patients with PH [27, 28]. Therefore, measures of RV functional reserve during exercise contain much more important prognostic information than resting variables. Blumberg et al. studied 36 consecutive patients (21 females, 54±15 years) with PAH (n =21) and inoperable CTEPH (n = 15). All patients underwent RHC at rest and during exercise, and cardiopulmonary exercise testing. They revealed that exercise cardiac index was correlated with peak oxygen uptake (peakVO$_2$: r =0.59, P < 0.001) and was the only independent predictor of peakVO$_2$ in multivariate stepwise linear regression analyses (P <0.001). They showed that peakVO$_2$ was the strongest predictor of survival (χ^2 = 14.5, P = 0.003). In addition, only exercise cardiac index (χ^2 = 5.6, P = 0.018) and the slope of the pressure/flow relationship (χ^2 = 4.1, P = 0.04) were significant prognostic indicators among hemodynamic variables [27]. At a given similar pressure/flow relationship among patients with severe PH, an individual with higher RV functional reserve can have a great potential to raise PAP during exercise. Indeed, Grunig et al. revealed that a marked increase (>30 mmHg) of estimated systolic PAP during exercise reflects better RV function and is associated with a better long-term outcome than a modest or no increase [29].

17.6   Assessment of RV Function Using Echocardiography

Accurate echocardiographic assessment of the geometry and function of the RV using conventional techniques is difficult because of its complex shape and trabecular structure. The retrosternal position of the RV also limits echocardiographic imaging. Nevertheless, echocardiography is still used predominantly for the assessment of RV function in daily clinical practice, as it is noninvasive, is relatively inexpensive, and has no adverse side effects [30, 31]. Recent improvements in image quality and new technologies such as tissue Doppler, 2D-STE and 3D-STE show great potential for more accurate measurements of RV structure and function.

Recent guidelines for cardiac chamber quantification by echocardiography provide updated reference values for RV dimensions and most parameters of systolic and diastolic function [31]. The normal ranges in echocardiography-derived RV chamber size and functional parameters are shown in Table 17.1. The guidelines recommend that parameters that can be measured include RV and right atrial (RA)

Table 17.1 Normal values for RV chamber size

Parameter	Mean ± SD	Normal range
RV basal diameter (mm)	33 ± 4	25–41
RV mid diameter (mm)	27 ± 4	19–35
RV longitudinal diameter (mm)	71 ± 6	59–83
RVOT PLAX diameter (mm)	25 ± 2.5	20–30
RVOT proximal diameter (mm)	28 ± 3.5	21–35
RVOT distal diameter (mm)	22 ± 2.5	17–27
RV wall thickness (mm)	3 ± 1	1–5
RVOT EDA (cm^2)		
Men	17 ± 3.5	10–24
Women	14 ± 3	8–20
RV EDA indexed to BSA (cm^2/m^2)		
Men	8.8 ± 1.9	5–12.6
Women	8.0 ± 1.75	4.5–11.5
RV ESA (cm^2)		
Men	9 ± 3	3–15
Women	7 ± 2	3–11
RV ESA indexed to BSA (cm^2/m^2)		
Men	4.7 ± 1.35	2.0–7.4
Women	4.0 ± 1.2	1.6–6.4
RV EDV indexed to BSA (mL/m^2)		
Men	61 ± 13	35–87
Women	53 ± 10.5	32–74
RV ESV indexed to BSA (mL/m^2)		
Men	27 ± 8.5	10–44
Women	22 ± 7	8–36

EDA end-diastolic area, *ESA* end-systolic area, *PLAX* parasternal long-axis view, *RVOT* RV outflow tract

size, a measure of RV systolic function, as assessed by at least one or a combination of the following: RV fractional area change (FAC), tricuspid annular plane systolic excursion (TAPSE), DTI-derived tricuspid lateral annular systolic velocity wave (S'), and RV myocardial performance index (MPI). Given the complex geometry of the RV, none of these variables alone is sufficient to describe RV function, and the overall impression of an experienced physician is often more important than single variables [32]. In addition, the magnitude of tricuspid regurgitation and its peak velocity, velocity time integral of RV outflow tract, inferior vena cava diameter and its respiratory variation, and the LV eccentricity index provide important information on the hemodynamics of the right heart as well as ventricular interdependence.

17.6.1 Right Ventricular Fractional Area Change

RV FAC provides an estimate of global RV systolic function. RV chamber areas are best estimated from a RV-focused apical four-chamber view obtained with either lateral or medial transducer orientation (Fig. 17.6 and Table 17.2). RV areas vary

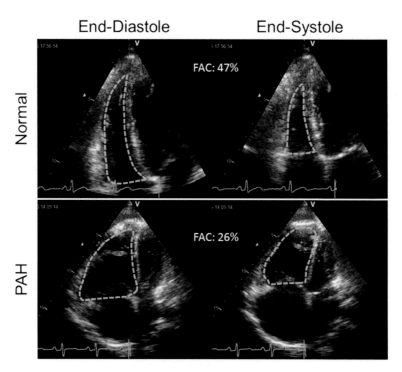

Fig. 17.6 Right ventricular end-diastolic area (RVEDA: *left*) and end-systolic area (RVESA) in a normal subject (*top*) and a patient with pulmonary arterial hypertension (*bottom*). RV fractional area change (RVFAC) is measured by the following formula: (RVEDA–RVESA)/RVEDA

Table 17.2 Normal values for parameters of RV function

Parameter	Mean ± SD	Abnormality threshold
RV fractional area change (%)	49 ± 7	<35
TAPSE (mm)	24 ± 3.5	<17
Pulsed Doppler S wave (cm/sec)	14.1 ± 2.3	<9.5
Pulsed Doppler MPI	0.26 ± 0.085	>0.43
Tissue Doppler MPI	0.38 ± 0.08	>0.54
RV free-wall 2D strain[a](%)	-29 ± 4.5	>−20
RV 3D EF (%)	58 ± 6.5	<45

TAPSE tricuspid annular plane systolic excursion, *RV* right ventricular, *MPI* myocardial performance index, *2D* two dimensional, *3D* three dimensional, *EF* ejection fraction
[a]Limited data; values may vary depending on vendor and software version

widely in the same patient with relatively minor rotations in transducer position, and therefore care should be taken to obtain the image with the largest basal RV diameter without foreshortening. RV FAC < 35 % indicates RV systolic dysfunction [30, 31].

17.6.2   Tricuspid Annular Plane Systolic Excursion

TAPSE is an index of RV longitudinal function, which is measured by M-mode echocardiography with the cursor optimally aligned along the direction of the tricuspid lateral annulus in the apical four-chamber view (Fig. 17.7 and Table 17.2). TAPSE measures displacement of the annular plane toward the transducer. It is easy to measure, reliable, and reproducible and has been shown to correlate well with other measures of global RV systolic function. However, TAPSE is an angle-dependent parameter because of the one-dimensional measurement relative to the transducer position and is influenced by cardiac translation or rotation [31, 33, 34]. While TAPSE values may show minor variations according to age, gender, and physique, the abnormality threshold of TAPSE is <17 mm, which is highly suggestive of RV systolic dysfunction [31].

17.6.3   Tissue Doppler-Derived Tricuspid Lateral Annular Systolic Velocity

The DTI-derived S' wave velocity of tricuspid lateral annulus is another reliable and reproducible index of RV longitudinal function (Fig. 17.8 and Table 17.2). Similar to TAPSE, S' is angle dependent and is influenced by overall heart motion. An S' velocity < 9.5 cm/sec indicates RV systolic dysfunction [31].

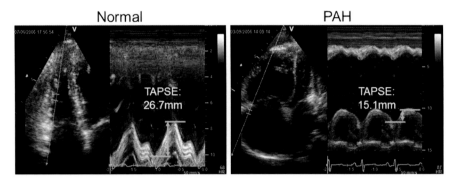

Fig. 17.7 M-mode recording through the lateral tricuspid valve annulus to measure the tricuspid annular plane systolic excursion (TAPSE) in a normal subject (*left*) and a patient with pulmonary arterial hypertension (*right*)

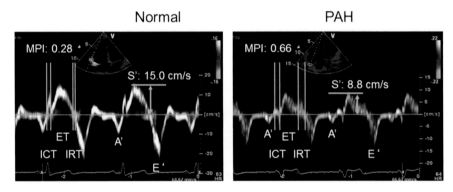

Fig. 17.8 Tissue Doppler image (TDI) of the lateral tricuspid valve annulus in a normal subject (*left*) and a patient with pulmonary arterial hypertension (*right*). S' indicates peak systolic annular motion velocity of the right ventricular free wall. E' and A' indicate peak annular motion velocities at the early diastole and during atrial contraction, respectively. TDI-derived myocardial performance index is measured by the following formula: (ICT+IRT)/ ET. *ICT* isovolumic contraction time, *ET* ejection time, *IRT* isovolumic relaxation time, *MPI* myocardial performance index

17.6.4 Right Ventricular Myocardial Performance Index

RV MPI is a global estimate of both systolic and diastolic function of the RV [30]. It is based on the relationship between ejection and non-ejection work of the RV. The MPI is defined as the ratio of isovolumic time divided by ejection time calculated as MPI = [(IRT + ICT)/ET], where IRT is isovolumic relaxation time and ET is ejection time. These time intervals can be obtained by simultaneous RV inflow and outflow recording. Alternatively, MPI can be calculated by measuring the RV outflow ET (time from the onset to the cessation of flow: Fig. 17.9) and the closure–opening time of the tricuspid valve measured with pulsed Doppler of the tricuspid inflow (time from the end of the transtricuspid A wave to the beginning of the

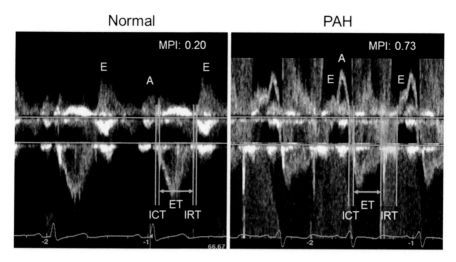

Fig. 17.9 Transtricuspid inflow (*top*) and right ventricular (RV) outflow (*bottom*) signals in a normal subject (*left*) and a patient with pulmonary arterial hypertension (*right*). RV myocardial performance index is measured by the following formula: (ICT+IRT)/ ET. *ICT* isovolumic contraction time, *ET* ejection time, *IRT* isovolumic relaxation time, *MPI* myocardial performance index

transtricuspid E wave: Fig. 17.9). These measurements are taken from different images, and one must therefore attempt to use beats with similar R–R intervals to obtain a more accurate MPI value. RV MPI can also be obtained by the tissue Doppler imaging (TDI) method, and all time intervals are measured from a single beat by recording the velocity of the tricuspid lateral annulus (Fig. 17.8). RV MPI has prognostic value in patients with PH at a single point in time [35], and changes in MPI correlate with changes in clinical status in this patient group [36]. RV MPI > 0.43 by PW Doppler and > 0.54 by TDI indicate RV dysfunction (Table 17.2).

At first, this index was not thought to vary significantly with heart rate and loading conditions. However, recent reports showed that RV MPI increases in response to increased loading conditions in animal models and patients with PH [37, 38]. Ogihara et al. demonstrated that RV MPI was strongly correlated with clinical and pulmonary hemodynamic variables, especially PVR, and the improvement in RV MPI was correlated with the improvement of afterload by PAH-specific therapy [39]. Interestingly, other systolic RV function variables including TAPSE did not significantly change, suggesting that RV MPI is much more sensitive to the response to medical treatment. Therefore, RV MPI can be an index of global RV function that takes into account the status of RV afterload.

17.6.5   RV Strain

RV longitudinal strain (LS) measurement derived from 2D speckle-tracking echocardiography is a relatively novel method for quantifying RV function [40] because longitudinal shortening is the major contributor to overall RV performance (Fig. 17.10).

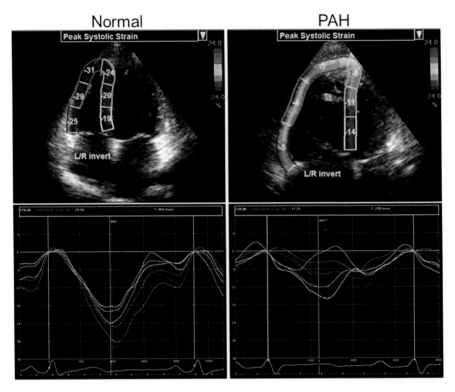

Fig. 17.10 Two-dimensional speckle-tracking strain images for the evaluation of right ventricular (RV) longitudinal deformation (*top*) and corresponding segmental and global time-strain curves. The RV myocardium is automatically divided into six segments (*yellow*, basal septum; *light blue*, mid septum; *green*, apical septum; *magenta*, apical RV free wall; *blue*, mid RV free wall; *red*, basal RV free wall). *White dotted lines* indicate the time-strain curves of global RV myocardium

Pooled data suggest that global longitudinal RV free-wall strain < 20 % in absolute value is likely abnormal. Chia et al. performed RV functional assessment in 142 healthy adult volunteers aged between 20 and 81 years. They revealed that the average of global RVLS was 27.3 ± 3.3 (male: 26.9 ± 3.1 and female: 27.8 ± 3.5) in absolute value, showing a reduction with age [41].

RVLS has been recently reported to have prognostic value in PH. Fine et al. performed prospective echocardiography examinations in 575 patients (mean age, 56±18 years; 63 % women) with known or suspected PH [42]. Eighteen-month survival was 92 %, 88 %, 85 %, and 71 % according to free-wall RV strain quartile (*P*<0.001), with a 1.46 higher risk of death (95 % CI: 1.05–2.12) per 6.7 % decline in RVLS. In addition, free-wall RV strain predicted survival when adjusted for pulmonary pressure, pulmonary vascular resistance, and RA pressure and provided incremental prognostic value over conventional clinical and echocardiographic variables.

17.6.6 Three-Dimensional Echocardiography

RVEF is a powerful predictor of patient survival in PH, and real-time 3D echocardiography allows for measurement of RV volume and EF irrespective of its shape. Recent studies have determined age-, body size-, and sex-specific normal values of RV volumes and EF in a large number of healthy volunteers [43].

The newly developed 3D-STE that features a specialized algorithm for the RV provides comprehensive and quantitative assessment of RV myocardial dynamics including longitudinal strain (LS), circumferential strain (CS), and area change ratio (ACR), determined as the percentage decrease in the size of the endocardial surface area defined by the vectors of longitudinal and circumferential deformations. Atsumi et al. firstly quantified and characterized RV global and regional deformation in an experimental model and confirmed the reliability of this novel 3D-STE system by direct comparison with sonomicrometer measurements [44] (Fig. 17.11). They revealed that pressure overload produced by pulmonary artery banding resulted mainly in changes in the ACR and LS but not in CS in a sheep model, which suggests that longitudinal contraction is more sensitive to pressure overload. A recent

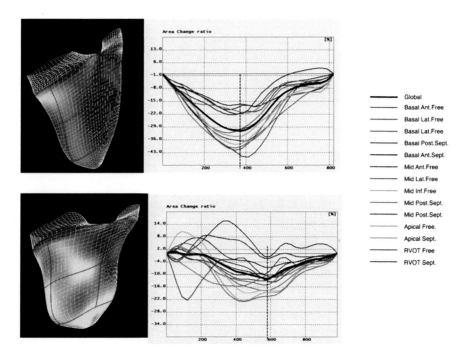

Fig. 17.11 Strain profiles in a representative case. The *top panels* depict baseline global and segmental strain-time curves. The *bottom panels* depict global and segmental strain-time curves during severe pulmonary artery banding. Each vertical broken line shows the surrogate point to measure deformation data corresponding to the maximum deformation point of the global deformation data (Reproduced from Atsumi et al. [44] copyright © 2016, with permission from Elsevier)

clinical study demonstrated that patients with PAH had reduced RV strain with much more dyssynchronous RV deformation pattern compared with controls when assessed by 3D-STE and revealed that ACR correlated best with RVEF and was an independent predictor of death [45]. The clinical applications and prognostic implication of 3D-STE-derived measures warrant further investigation.

17.7 Assessment of RV Volume and Function Using Cardiac Magnetic Resonance

Cardiac magnetic resonance (CMR) imaging is accurate and reproducible in the assessment of RV size, morphology and function, and is the gold standard for the quantitation of RVEF. Short-axis or axial SSFP images and the summation disc method are used for calculations of RV volumes and EF without any geometrical assumption. Normal age and gender-specific values for RV volumes and EF have been published for adult and pediatric populations [46, 47]. Regional RV function can be evaluated qualitatively at rest and during pharmacological stress on SSFP short axis cine loops. It can also be assessed quantitatively by using myocardial tagging or strain-encoding CMR, and both techniques have been shown to be feasible in the RV and correlate well with echocardiographic evaluation [48–50]. However, their application in the RV is technically demanding, due to the thin wall and the need for extensive post processing, which may limit their clinical application [50, 51].

CMR also provides advanced imaging of the RV myocardium including tissue characterization [49]. Late enhancement imaging after gadolinium contrast admin-

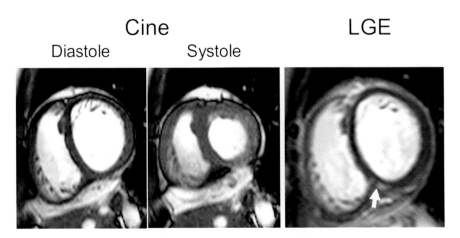

Fig. 17.12 Short-axis cardiac magnetic resonance cine views showing leftward displacement of the interventricular septum (septal bowing) during early diastole (*left*) and late gadolinium enhancement of right ventricular insertion point in a patient with pulmonary arterial hypertension (*right, white arrow*)

istration can be used for tissue characterization of the RV. Recent clinical studies have demonstrated that late gadolinium enhancement (LGE) occurs at the RV insertion point in PAH patients and correlates with CMR-derived RV indices including RVEF and RV stroke volume (Fig. 17.12) [52]. In addition, the presence of LGE in patients with PAH is a marker for more advanced disease and poor prognosis [53].

Velocity-encoded phase contrast imaging is another important CMR tool for RV evaluation. Phase contrast imaging allows quantification of the RV stroke volume, pulmonary and/or tricuspid valve regurgitation, and intracardiac shunts as well as differential lung perfusion [50, 54–56].

References

1. Haddad F, Hunt SA, Rosenthal DN, Murphy DJ. Right ventricular function in cardiovascular disease, part I: anatomy, physiology, aging, and functional assessment of the right ventricle. Circulation. 2008;117:1436–48. doi:10.1161/CIRCULATIONAHA.107.653576.
2. Ho SY, Nihoyannopoulos P. Anatomy, echocardiography, and normal right ventricular dimensions. Heart. 2006;92(Suppl 1):i2–13.
3. Jiang L. Right ventricle. In: Weyman AE, editor. Principle and practice of Echocardiography. Baltimore: Lippincott Williams & Wilkins; 1994. p. 901–21.
4. Dell'Italia LJ. The right ventricle: anatomy, physiology, and clinical importance. Curr Probl Cardiol. 1991;16:653–720.
5. Davidson C, Bonow R. Cardiac catheterization. In: Bonow R, Mann DL, Zipes DP, Libby P, editors. Braunwald's heart disease: a textbook of cardiovascular medicine. 9th ed. Philadelphia: Elsevier; 2011 .Chapter 20
6. Naeije R, Manes A. The right ventricle in pulmonary arterial hypertension. Eur Respir Rev. 2014;23:476–87. doi:10.1183/09059180.00007414.
7. Grifoni S, Olivotto I, Cecchini P, Pieralli F, Camaiti A, Santoro G, et al. Short-term clinical outcome of patients with acute pulmonary embolism, normal blood pressure, and echocardiographic right ventricular dysfunction. Circulation. 2000;101:2817–22.
8. Sugiura E, Dohi K, Onishi K, Takamura T, Tsuji A, Ota S, et al. Reversible right ventricular regional non-uniformity quantified by speckle-tracking strain imaging in patients with acute pulmonary thromboembolism. J Am Soc Echocardiogr. 2009;22:1353–9. doi:10.1016/j. echo.2009.09.005.
9. Ichikawa K, Dohi K, Sugiura E, Sugimoto T, Takamura T, Ogihara Y, et al. Ventricular function and dyssynchrony quantified by speckle-tracking echocardiography in patients with acute and chronic right ventricular pressure overload. J Am Soc Echocardiogr. 2013;26:483–92. doi:10.1016/j.echo.2013.02.010.
10. Galie N, Manes A, Negro L, Palazzini M, Bacchi-Reggiani ML, Branzi A. A meta-analysis of randomized controlled trials in pulmonary arterial hypertension. Eur Heart J. 2009;30:394–403. doi:10.1093/eurheartj/ehp022.
11. Dell'Italia LJ, Walsh RA. Acute determinants of the hangout interval in the pulmonary circulation. Am Heart J. 1988;116(5 Pt 1):1289–97.
12. Felner JM. The second heart sound. In: Walker HK, Hall WD, Hurst JW, editors. Clinical methods: the history, physical, and laboratory examinations. 3rd ed. Boston: Butterworths; 1990 .Chapter 23
13. Suga H, Sagawa K, Shoukas AA. Load independence of the instantaneous pressure-volume ratio of the canine left ventricle and effects of epinephrine and heart rate on the ratio. Circ Res. 1973;32:314–22.

14. Guarracino F, Baldassarri R, Pinsky MR. Ventriculo-arterial decoupling in acutely altered hemodynamic states. Crit Care. 2013;17:213. doi:10.1186/cc12522.
15. Brown KA, Ditchey RV. Human right ventricular end-systolic pressure-volume relation defined by maximal elastance. Circulation. 1988;78:81–91.
16. Dell'Italia LJ, Walsh RA. Application of a time varying elastance model to right ventricular performance in man. Cardiovasc Res. 1988;22:864–74.
17. McCabe C, White PA, Hoole SP, Axell RG, Priest AN, Gopalan D, et al. Right ventricular dysfunction in chronic thromboembolic obstruction of the pulmonary artery: a pressure-volume study using the conductance catheter. J Appl Physiol (1985). 2014;116:355–63. doi:10.1152/japplphysiol.01123.2013.
18. Kass DA, Maughan WL. From 'Emax' to pressure-volume relations: a broader view. Circulation. 1988;77:1203–12.
19. Vonk Noordegraaf A, Galie N. The role of the right ventricle in pulmonary arterial hypertension. Eur Respir Rev. 2011;20:243–53. doi:10.1183/09059180.00006511.
20. Humbert M, Sitbon O, Simonneau G. Treatment of pulmonary arterial hypertension. N Engl J Med. 2004;351:1425–36.
21. Channick RN, Simonneau G, Sitbon O, Robbins IM, Frost A, Tapson VF, et al. Effects of the dual endothelin-receptor antagonist bosentan in patients with pulmonary hypertension: a randomised placebo-controlled study. Lancet. 2001;358:1119–23.
22. Galie N, Ghofrani HA, Torbicki A, Barst RJ, Rubin LJ, Badesch D, et al. Sildenafil citrate therapy for pulmonary arterial hypertension. N Engl J Med. 2005;353:2148–57.
23. Barst RJ, Rubin LJ, McGoon MD, Caldwell EJ, Long WA, Levy PS. Survival in primary pulmonary hypertension with long-term continuous intravenous prostacyclin. Ann Intern Med. 1994;121:409–15.
24. Elias-Al-Mamun M, Satoh K, Tanaka S, Shimizu T, Nergui S, Miyata S, et al. Combination therapy with fasudil and sildenafil ameliorates monocrotaline-induced pulmonary hypertension and survival in rats. Circ J. 2014;78:967–76.
25. Goto I, Dohi K, Ogihara Y, Okamoto R, Yamada N, Mitani Y, et al. Detrimental impact of Vasopressin V2 receptor antagonism in a SU5416/Hypoxia/Normoxia-exposed rat model of pulmonary arterial hypertension. Circ J. 2016;80:989–97. doi:10.1253/circj.CJ-15-1175.
26. van de Veerdonk MC, Kind T, Marcus JT, Mauritz GJ, Heymans MW, Bogaard HJ, et al. Progressive right ventricular dysfunction in patients with pulmonary arterial hypertension responding to therapy. J Am Coll Cardiol. 2011;58:2511–9. doi:10.1016/j.jacc.2011.06.068.
27. Blumberg FC, Arzt M, Lange T, Schroll S, Pfeifer M, Wensel R. Impact of right ventricular reserve on exercise capacity and survival in patients with pulmonary hypertension. Eur J Heart Fail. 2013;15:771–5. doi:10.1093/eurjhf/hft044.
28. Kusunose K, Yamada H. Rest and exercise echocardiography for early detection of pulmonary hypertension. J Echocardiogr. 2016;14:2–12. doi:10.1007/s12574-015-0268-y.
29. Grunig E, Tiede H, Enyimayew EO, Ehlken N, Seyfarth HJ, Bossone E, et al. Assessment and prognostic relevance of right ventricular contractile reserve in patients with severe pulmonary hypertension. Circulation. 2013;128:2005–15. doi:10.1161/CIRCULATIONAHA.113.001573.
30. Rudski LG, Lai WW, Afilalo J, Hua L, Handschumacher MD, Chandrasekaran K, et al. Guidelines for the echocardiographic assessment of the right heart in adults: a report from the American Society of Echocardiography endorsed by the European Association of Echocardiography, a registered branch of the European Society of Cardiology, and the Canadian Society of Echocardiography. J Am Soc Echocardiogr. 2010;23:685–713. quiz 786-8 doi:10.1016/j.echo.2010.05.010.
31. Lang RM, Badano LP, Mor-Avi V, Afilalo J, Armstrong A, Ernande L, et al. Recommendations for cardiac chamber quantification by echocardiography in adults: an update from the American Society of Echocardiography and the European Association of Cardiovascular Imaging. J Am Soc Echocardiogr. 2015;28:1–39.e14. doi:10.1016/j.echo.2014.10.003.
32. Galie N, Humbert M, JL V, Gibbs S, Lang I, Torbicki A, et al. 2015 ESC/ERS Guidelines for the diagnosis and treatment of pulmonary hypertension: The Joint Task Force for the Diagnosis

and Treatment of Pulmonary Hypertension of the European Society of Cardiology (ESC) and the European Respiratory Society (ERS): Endorsed by: Association for European Paediatric and Congenital Cardiology (AEPC), International Society for Heart and Lung Transplantation (ISHLT). Eur Heart J. 2016;37:67–119. doi:10.1093/eurheartj/ehv317.

33. Giusca S, Dambrauskaite V, Scheurwegs C, D'Hooge J, Claus P, Herbots L, et al. Deformation imaging describes right ventricular function better than longitudinal displacement of the tricuspid ring. Heart. 2010;96:281–8. doi:10.1136/hrt.2009.171728.

34. Motoji Y, Tanaka H, Fukuda Y, Sano H, Ryo K, Sawa T, et al. Association of apical longitudinal rotation with right ventricular performance in patients with pulmonary hypertension: insights into overestimation of tricuspid annular plane systolic excursion. Echocardiography. 2016;33:207–15. doi:10.1111/echo.13036.

35. Tei C, Dujardin KS, Hodge DO, Bailey KR, McGoon MD, Tajik AJ, et al. Doppler echocardiographic index for assessment of global right ventricular function. J Am Soc Echocardiogr. 1996;9:838–47.

36. Sebbag I, Rudski LG, Therrien J, Hirsch A, Langleben D. Effect of chronic infusion of epoprostenol on echocardiographic right ventricular myocardial performance index and its relation to clinical outcome in patients with primary pulmonary hypertension. Am J Cardiol. 2001;88:1060–3.

37. Sugiura T, Suzuki S, Hussein MH, Kato T, Togari H. Usefulness of a new Doppler index for assessing both ventricular functions and pulmonary circulation in newborn piglet with hypoxic pulmonary hypertension. Pediatr Res. 2003;53:927–32.

38. Blanchard DG, Malouf PJ, Gurudevan SV, Auger WR, Madani MM, Thistlethwaite P, et al. Utility of right ventricular Tei index in the noninvasive evaluation of chronic thromboembolic pulmonary hypertension before and after pulmonary thromboendarterectomy. JACC Cardiovasc Imaging. 2009;2:143–9. doi:10.1016/j.jcmg.2008.10.012.

39. Ogihara Y, Yamada N, Dohi K, Matsuda A, Tsuji A, Ota S, et al. Utility of right ventricular Tei-index for assessing disease severity and determining response to treatment in patients with pulmonary arterial hypertension. J Cardiol. 2014;63:149–53. doi:10.1016/j.jjcc.2013.07.002.

40. Rajagopal S, Forsha DE, Risum N, Hornik CP, Poms AD, Fortin TA, et al. Comprehensive assessment of right ventricular function in patients with pulmonary hypertension with global longitudinal peak systolic strain derived from multiple right ventricular views. J Am Soc Echocardiogr. 2014;27:657–65.e3. doi:10.1016/j.echo.2014.02.001.

41. Chia EM, Hsieh CH, Boyd A, Pham P, Vidaic J, Leung D, et al. Effects of age and gender on right ventricular systolic and diastolic function using two-dimensional speckle-tracking strain. J Am Soc Echocardiogr. 2014;27:1079–86.e1. doi:10.1016/j.echo.2014.06.007.

42. Fine NM, Chen L, Bastiansen PM, Frantz RP, Pellikka PA, Oh JK, et al. Outcome prediction by quantitative right ventricular function assessment in 575 subjects evaluated for pulmonary hypertension. Circ Cardiovasc Imaging. 2013;6:711–21. doi:10.1161/CIRCIMAGING.113.000640.

43. Maffessanti F, Muraru D, Esposito R, Gripari P, Ermacora D, Santoro C, et al. Age-, body size-, and sex-specific reference values for right ventricular volumes and ejection fraction by three-dimensional echocardiography: a multicenter echocardiographic study in 507 healthy volunteers. Circ Cardiovasc Imaging. 2013;6:700–10. doi:10.1161/CIRCIMAGING.113.000706.

44. Atsumi A, Seo Y, Ishizu T, Nakamura A, Enomoto Y, Harimura Y, et al. Right ventricular deformation analyses using a Three-Dimensional speckle-tracking echocardiographic system specialized for the right ventricle. J Am Soc Echocardiogr. 2016;29:402–11.e2. doi:10.1016/j.echo.2015.12.014.

45. Smith BC, Dobson G, Dawson D, Charalampopoulos A, Grapsa J, Nihoyannopoulos P. Three-dimensional speckle tracking of the right ventricle: toward optimal quantification of right ventricular dysfunction in pulmonary hypertension. J Am Coll Cardiol. 2014;64:41–51. doi:10.1016/j.jacc.2014.01.084.

46. Maceira AM, Prasad SK, Khan M, Pennell DJ. Reference right ventricular systolic and diastolic function normalized to age, gender and body surface area from steady-state free precession cardiovascular magnetic resonance. Eur Heart J. 2006;27:2879–88.

47. Buechel EV, Kaiser T, Jackson C, Schmitz A, Kellenberger CJ. Normal right- and left ventricular volumes and myocardial mass in children measured by steady state free precession cardiovascular magnetic resonance. J Cardiovasc Magn Reson. 2009;11:19. doi:10.1186/1532-429X-11-19.
48. Greil GF, Beerbaum P, Razavi R, Miller O. Imaging the right ventricle: non-invasive imaging. Heart. 2008;94:803–8. doi:10.1136/hrt.2005.079111.
49. Youssef A, el Ibrahim SH, Korosoglou G, Abraham MR, Weiss RG, Osman NF. Strain-encoding cardiovascular magnetic resonance for assessment of right-ventricular regional function. J Cardiovasc Magn Reson. 2008;10:33. doi:10.1186/1532-429X-10-33.
50. Valsangiacomo Buechel ER, Mertens LL. Imaging the right heart: the use of integrated multi-modality imaging. Eur Heart J. 2012;33:949–60. doi:10.1093/eurheartj/ehr490.
51. Menteer J, Weinberg PM, Fogel MA. Quantifying regional right ventricular function in tetralogy of Fallot. J Cardiovasc Magn Reson. 2005;7:753–61.
52. McCann GP, Gan CT, Beek AM, Niessen HW, Vonk Noordegraaf A, van Rossum AC. Extent of MRI delayed enhancement of myocardial mass is related to right ventricular dysfunction in pulmonary artery hypertension. AJR Am J Roentgenol. 2007;188:349–55.
53. Freed BH, Gomberg-Maitland M, Chandra S, Mor-Avi V, Rich S, Archer SL, et al. Late gadolinium enhancement cardiovascular magnetic resonance predicts clinical worsening in patients with pulmonary hypertension. J Cardiovasc Magn Reson. 2012;14:11. doi:10.1186/1532-429X-14-11.
54. Wald RM, Redington AN, Pereira A, Provost YL, Paul NS, Oechslin EN, et al. Refining the assessment of pulmonary regurgitation in adults after tetralogy of Fallot repair: should we be measuring regurgitant fraction or regurgitant volume? Eur Heart J. 2009;30:356–61. doi:10.1093/eurheartj/ehn595.
55. Roman KS, Kellenberger CJ, Farooq S, MacGowan CK, Gilday DL, Yoo SJ. Comparative imaging of differential pulmonary blood flow in patients with congenital heart disease: magnetic resonance imaging versus lung perfusion scintigraphy. Pediatr Radiol. 2005;35:295–301.
56. Beerbaum P, Korperich H, Barth P, Esdorn H, Gieseke J, Meyer H. Noninvasive quantification of left-to-right shunt in pediatric patients: phase-contrast cine magnetic resonance imaging compared with invasive oximetry. Circulation. 2001;103:2476–82.

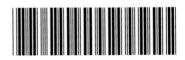